AF846390

The Peripheral Existence and Effects of Corticotropin-releasing Factor Family

Chao Zhu • Rong Wan • Shengnan Li
Editors

The Peripheral Existence and Effects of Corticotropin-releasing Factor Family

Springer

Editors
Chao Zhu
Department of Pharmacology
School of Basic Medical Sciences
Nanjing Medical University
Nanjing, Jiangsu, China

Shengnan Li
Department of Pharmacology
School of Basic Medical Sciences
Nanjing Medical University
Nanjing, Jiangsu, China

Rong Wan
Jiangxi Key Laboratory of Molecular Medicine
The Second Affiliated Hospital of Nanchang University
Nanchang, China

ISBN 978-981-96-5321-8 ISBN 978-981-96-5322-5 (eBook)
https://doi.org/10.1007/978-981-96-5322-5

© The Editor(s) (if applicable) and The Author(s), under exclusive license to Springer Nature Singapore Pte Ltd. 2025

This work is subject to copyright. All rights are solely and exclusively licensed by the Publisher, whether the whole or part of the material is concerned, specifically the rights of translation, reprinting, reuse of illustrations, recitation, broadcasting, reproduction on microfilms or in any other physical way, and transmission or information storage and retrieval, electronic adaptation, computer software, or by similar or dissimilar methodology now known or hereafter developed.
The use of general descriptive names, registered names, trademarks, service marks, etc. in this publication does not imply, even in the absence of a specific statement, that such names are exempt from the relevant protective laws and regulations and therefore free for general use.
The publisher, the authors and the editors are safe to assume that the advice and information in this book are believed to be true and accurate at the date of publication. Neither the publisher nor the authors or the editors give a warranty, expressed or implied, with respect to the material contained herein or for any errors or omissions that may have been made. The publisher remains neutral with regard to jurisdictional claims in published maps and institutional affiliations.

This Springer imprint is published by the registered company Springer Nature Singapore Pte Ltd.
The registered company address is: 152 Beach Road, #21-01/04 Gateway East, Singapore 189721, Singapore

If disposing of this product, please recycle the paper.

Preface

This book is accomplished by the three of us (Dr. Chao Zhu, Dr. Rong Wan, and me myself). My name is Shengnan Li and I am very pleased to write this preface on behalf of all the three authors. It is our honor to have this opportunity to present this book to the readers. Dr. Chao Zhu has been working together with me in Department of Pharmacology, Nanjing Medical University since 2011 and Dr. Rong Wan had 5 years' time with us in the same laboratory during 2018 to 2013 and now is a staff at Nanchang University.

Over the past two decades, our group has carried out the researches on corticotropin-releasing hormone (factor) family peptides (CRF peptides, CRFp) and published 70+ relevant papers, mainly focusing on their peripheral roles in vascular inflammation and tumors, which contributes mostly to the idea that we pick the peripheral roles of CRF peptides as the main subject for this book.

Mammalian CRF-system includes CRF peptides comprising four members, CRH, Urocortin (UCN1), UCN2 and UCN3, CRF receptors (CRFr, CRF_1, and CRF_2), and CRF binding protein (CRF-BP). With the first isolation of brain CRH, a new epoch is made in the research on biological stress. CRH is the main mediator for stress and functions centrally participating in many processes via hypothalamic-pituitary-adrenal (HPA) axis, which is briefly summarized in the first chapter. In recent decades, compiling evidence shows that CRH and UCNs are also widely distributed in peripheral cells/tissues and that they play critical topical roles in digestive system, cardiovascular system, immune/inflammatory system, and cancer development, which has been our work subjects and contributes to the selection of this book's contents and title. The contents of Chaps. 2, 3, 4, 5, 6, 7, and 8 mainly include the features of the CRF peptides (both CRH and UCNs) and the receptors, and their peripheral distributions and functions, in different systems. Moreover, for a comparison among species and wider knowledge of CRF-system, Chap. 9 is added, briefly summarizing the roles of CRF peptides in non-mammals, including vertebrates (fish and frog) and non-vertebrates (insects).

We acknowledge the contribution of more than 30 colleagues and students in our laboratory in Nanjing Medical University over the past 20 years. Many of their published data are cited here. And we are grateful to the publishers, Dr. Yin Chen, making it possible for this book coming into being from the beginning, and Dr. Sudha Ramachandran for the constant liaison for kind reminding.

The aim of this book is to share a basic and relatively complete package (mainly peripheral) about the CRF peptides with the readers, mainly medical students and relevant researchers. Although we tried our utmost to succeed, finding a vast of references and ensuring the correctness of writing and information, negligence may still be inevitable, for which we gratefully welcome criticism. Finally, we hope that the readers, medical students and researchers working in the relevant area, will find their interests in reading.

Nanjing, China — Chao Zhu
Nanchang, China — Rong Wan
Nanjing, China — Shengnan Li
September 30, 2024

Contents

Editors and Contributors

About the Editors

Chao Zhu The author graduated from Nanjing Medical University and got a bachelor's and doctorate in Medicine in 2011 and 2016, respectively. Since then, he has been working as a lecturer/associate professor in the university. During the 8 years' period, he also worked as a research scholar at the University of Arizona (2019–2021) and Indiana University (2024). He has been studying on CRF peptides and cardiovascular pharmacology for 10+ years. His cardiovascular disease research focuses on the protective effect of CRF peptides on multiple vascular functions. He has been continuously funded by natural science foundation of the university, province, and nation since 2017 when he received his first award.

Rong Wan After getting her bachelor's degree in Pharmacy in Nanchang University (Jiangxi Province, China) in 2008, Dr. Rong Wan pursued further study in Nanjing Medical University and got a Doctorate in Medicine in 2013. Thereafter she has been working in Jiangxi Key Laboratory of Molecular Medicine, the Second Affiliated Hospital of Nanchang University. Her research focuses on the area of the underlying mechanisms in cardiovascular diseases, including CRF peptides and proteins post-translational modification.

Shengnan Li The author graduated from Jiangxi Medical College and got a bachelor's degree in Clinical Medicine in 1986, after which she studied in China Medical University (Shenyang, China) and got her Master in Medicine in 1989. Then she worked as a lecture in the Department of Pharmacology, Jiangxi Medical College for 6 years. Thereafter she studied further in the Institute of Pharmacology/Toxicology, Technological University of Dresden, and got her Doctorate in Medicine in 1999, further working as a research fellow in the Institute of Neuroscience, National University of Singapore till 2001. And then she has been working as a professor in Nanjing Medical University ever since. The main research interest is about CRF peptides' roles in cardiovascular functions and tumor development

Contributors

Shengnan Li Department of Pharmacology, School of Basic Medical Sciences, Nanjing Medical University, Nanjing, China

Rong Wan Jiangxi Key Laboratory of Molecular Medicine, The Second Affiliated Hospital of Nanchang University, Nanchang, China

Chao Zhu Department of Pharmacology, School of Basic Medical Sciences, Nanjing Medical University, Nanjing, China

Chapter 1
The Hypothalamic-Pituitary-Adrenal Axis and Its Regulation

Shengnan Li and Chao Zhu

The hypothalamic releasing and inhibitory hormones include five major types, which exert stimulating effects on the pituitary gland, leading to the release of five types of corresponding pituitary hormones, of which thyroid-stimulating hormone and adrenocorticotropin (ACTH) in turn stimulate the hormone secretion from thyroid and adrenal cortex, constituting the often referenced hypothalamic-pituitary-thyroid (HPT) axis and hypothalamic-pituitary-adrenal (HPA) axis, respectively, of which the latter will be mainly focused on in this chapter. The HPA axis is one of the most essential pathways among the central nervous system (CNS)'s influence on the peripheral endocrine functions. The hypothalamic corticotropin-releasing hormone (CRH), together with the arginine vasopressin (AVP), controls the HPA axis' activity. CRH is the main member among corticotropin-releasing hormone (factor) family peptides (CRF peptides, CRFp) existing and functioning in the brain. Since HPA activation, i.e., CRH (+AVP)-ACTH-cortisol promotion, is a main response of stress, hence the central CRH, as a stress mediator, participates in many physiological and pathological processes. In this chapter, the HPA axis constitution and centrally produced CRH and function will be relatively simply summarized since this book will mainly focus on CRH and the other CRFp's peripheral existence/origin and their direct peripheral effects (see the following chapters).

S. Li (✉) · C. Zhu
Department of Pharmacology, School of Basic Medical Sciences,
Nanjing Medical University, Nanjing, Jiangsu, China
e-mail: snli@njmu.edu.cn

© The Author(s), under exclusive license to Springer Nature Singapore Pte Ltd. 2025
C. Zhu et al. (eds.), *The Peripheral Existence and Effects of Corticotropin-releasing Factor Family*, https://doi.org/10.1007/978-981-96-5322-5_1

1 The Hypothalamic-Pituitary-Adrenal Axis (HPA Axis)

1.1 The Hypothalamus and Hypothalamic Releasing/ Inhibitory Hormones

The hypothalamus, which represents less than 1 percent of the brain mass and 2 percent of the brain volume, is a very important part of the CNS, which modulates significant activities of the body [1, 2]. The hypothalamus contains cells secreting neurohormones to act on the pituitary gland, controlling the entire endocrine system and autonomic nervous system, modulating most of the autonomic activities and endocrine functions, the secreted endocrine-controlling neurohormones being the releasing and inhibitory hormones [3–5]. The hypothalamus can be divided into the preoptic, anterior, tuberal, and mammillary regions. Different from the cerebral cortex with the relatively flat laminar structure, the hypothalamus is populated by nuclei, with the anterior region being composed of supraoptic (SON), suprachiasmatic (SCN), and paraventricular (PVN) nuclei [2, 6, 7]. There exist two major neurosecretory cell types in the hypothalamus, the parvocellular neurons (PvCs) in PVN and magnocellular neurons (MgCs) in both PVN and SON. PvCs are the main cells producing the hypothalamic releasing and inhibitory hormones while MgCs mainly produce AVP and oxytocin secreted at the posterior pituitary level [8, 9]. However, colocalization of neuroendocrine substances in both PvCs and MgCs exists [10, 11], e.g., AVP and CRH colocalize in PvCs [10, 12]. The major hypothalamus-produced releasing and inhibitory hormones are summarized as follows [1, 2] (Fig. 1.1).

(a) Thyrotropin-releasing hormone (TRH), the inducer of thyroid-stimulating hormone (TSH) secretion by the anterior pituitary gland.
(b) CRH, the stimulator of ACTH secretion by the anterior pituitary gland.
(c) Growth hormone-releasing hormone (GHRH) and growth hormone inhibitory hormone (GHIH, also called somatostatin), which causes growth hormone (GH) secretion and GH secretion's inhibition, respectively, by the anterior pituitary gland.
(d) Gonadotropin-releasing hormone (GnRH), which induces two gonadotropic hormones' secretion, i.e., luteinizing hormone (LH) and follicle-stimulating hormone (FSH) by the anterior pituitary gland.
(e) Prolactin-inhibitory hormone (PIH), which causes the inhibition of prolactin secretion by the anterior pituitary gland.

Conversely, the induced pituitary gland hormones have a negative feedback effect on the secretion of the hypothalamic releasing/inhibitory hormones [13].

Among the five major hypothalamic releasing and inhibitory hormones, CRH is the main one which will be discussed in this chapter. CRH is a peptide composed of 41 amino acids, first isolated by Vale and colleagues from ovine brain [14]. The cell bodies of the neurons (PvCs) that synthetize CRH are located mainly in PVN of the hypothalamus while the fiber endings of PvCs secret CRH at the eminence in the

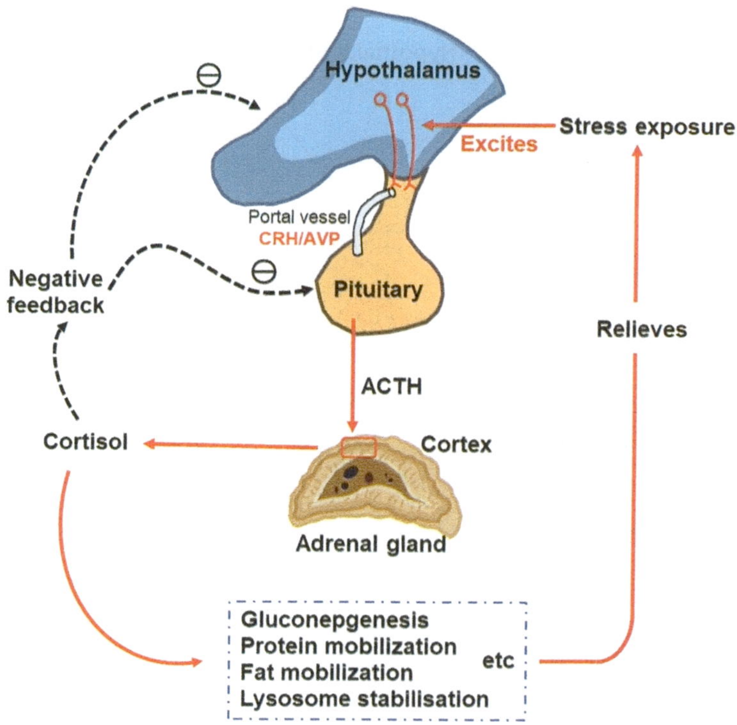

Fig. 1.1 The hypothalamic-pituitary-adrenal axis (CRH/AVP-ACTH-cortisol hormone signaling pathway) in response to stress

pituitary stalk. The secreted CRH is then carried to the anterior pituitary through the long hypophysial portal system [15] (Fig. 1.2, also see Sect. 2). CRH is a major regulator of HPA axis by modulating ACTH release. It is noteworthy that AVP is also a hypothalamic hormone (but not releasing/inhibitory hormone) since it originates from the hypothalamus, although it is normally classified into the posterior pituitary hormones. Both PvCs and MgCs in PVN express AVP, the former projecting to the eminence while the latter to posterior pituitary [11]. In fact, AVP colocalizes with CRH in hypothalamic PvCs and synergistically work with CRH regulating ACTH release [12, 16]. Moreover, hypothalamic MgCs' secretory AVP at the posterior pituitary can also reach the anterior lobe by the vascular link between the two parts (the *short portal system*, Fig. 1.2) [17, 18] and co-act with CRH, stimulating ACTH release from the anterior pituitary and participating in HPA axis regulation. In addition, although there exists evidence that AVP colocalizes with CRH only in PvCs [12], researches also show that CRH may be synthesized in AVP-producing MgCs, and the MgCs-secreted CRH may participate in modulating neurohypophysial (posterior) functions [10, 18] (Fig. 1.3).

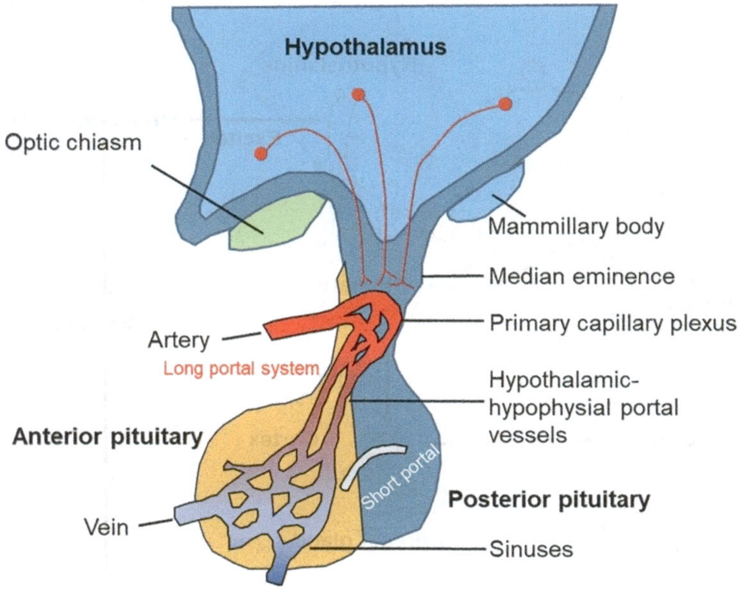

Fig. 1.2 Hypothalamic-hypophysial long portal system and the short portal system between the anterior and posterior pituitary

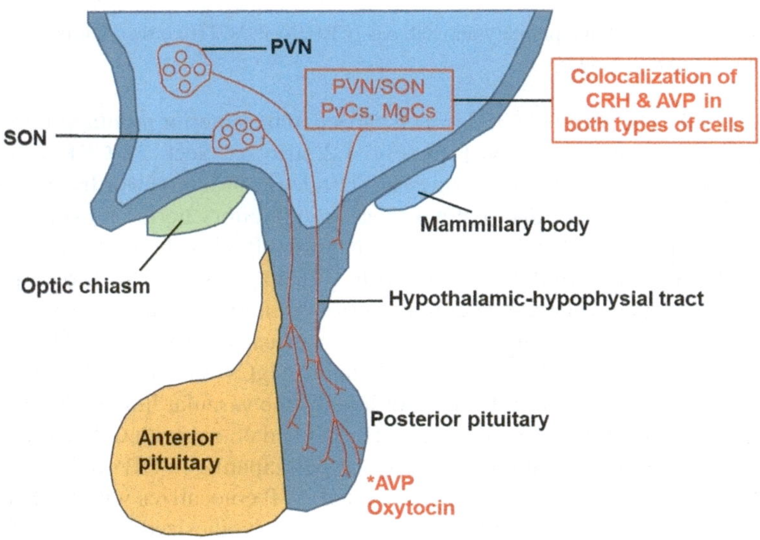

Fig. 1.3 The hypothalamus controlling of the posterior pituitary. (PvCs and MgCs in PVN and SON with colocalization of CRH and AVP; MgCs with fibers terminating at posterior pituitary secreting AVP and oxytocin)

1.2 The Pituitary and the Hormones

The human pituitary gland is a small bean-shaped gland connected to the hypothalamus, which is about 1 centimeter in diameter and 0.5 to 1 gram in weight [1, 19, 20]. The pituitary gland is divisible into two distinct parts: the anterior pituitary (the adenohypophysis) and the posterior pituitary (the neurohypophysis), embryologically originating from different sources—the anterior pituitary from Rathke's pouch, an embryonic invagination of the pharyngeal epithelium, and the posterior pituitary from the evagination of neural tissue from the floor of the third ventricle (outgrowth of the hypothalamus), respectively [21, 22]. The gland has wide functions via secreting hormones regulating essential homeostatic processes ranging from growth to stress [1, 21, 23, 24]. Pathologic conditions, most commonly the benign gland adenoma, affect the pituitary gland and produce endocrinologic and neurologic abnormalities [24, 25].

1.2.1 The Anterior Pituitary and the Hormones

Six major peptide hormones are secreted by the anterior pituitary, i.e., TSH, GH, ACTH, LH&FSH, and prolactin. The anterior pituitary gland contains five different cell types (thyrotropes, lactotropes, corticotropes, somatotropes, and gonadotropes) that synthesize and secrete hormones, with one cell type for each major hormone, e.g., ACTH, which will be focused in this section, is synthesized and secreted by corticotropes [1, 26–29]. Consistently, secretory anterior pituitary cells exhibit cell-type specific electrical activity, differing in the patterns of firing and associated calcium signaling and hormone secretion [30].

As shown in Fig. 1.2, the pituitary gland is connected to the hypothalamus by the pituitary stalk. Hypothalamic releasing/inhibitory hormones (TRH, CRH, GHRH/GHIH, GnRH, PIH) are secreted into the median eminence, an extension of hypothalamus into the pituitary stalk, where the hypothalamic neurons' nerve fibers link between the hypothalamus and the pituitary via the hypophysial portal vessels (*the long portal system*) [31]. The secreted releasing and inhibitory hormones are immediately absorbed into the hypothalamic hypophysial portal system that is first identified in 1933 [32] and carried directly to the sinuses of the anterior pituitary gland, the adenohypophysis, stimulating the adenohypophysis to influence on the secretion of relevant pituitary hormones, TSH, ACTH, GH, LH&FSH, and prolactin, respectively [32–34].

ACTH is an important component of HPA axis. ACTH secretion is mainly controlled by CRH (and AVP, see below), which is secreted into the primary capillary plexus of the hypophysial portal system in the median eminence of the hypothalamus and then carried to the anterior pituitary gland. The secreted ACTH in turn goes into the circulation reaching the adrenal gland and activates adrenocortical cells to secrete steroid hormones (see Sect. 2).

1.2.2 The Posterior Pituitary and the Hormones

Two important peptide hormones are secreted by the posterior pituitary, antidiuretic hormone (also called arginine vasopressin, AVP), and oxytocin (Fig. 1.3).

AVP controls the rate of water excretion into the urine, thus helping to control the concentration of water in the body fluids, insufficiency of which may result in diabetes mellitus [35, 36]. Noticeably, the posterior AVP can also reach the anterior lobe by the short portal system [17] (Fig. 1.2), acting alone [37] or co-acting with CRH regulating HPA axis [38]. Furthermore, AVP colocalizes with CRH in parvocellular neurons and synergistically acts with CRH influencing ACTH secretion, which in a feedback pattern inhibits both CRH and AVP as its down-stream hormone cortisol [10, 12, 13, 16, 39].

1.3 The Adrenal Cortex and Related Hormones

The two adrenal glands lie at the superior poles of the kidneys [40]. The gland, constituted by the adrenal cortex and the adrenal medulla, is one of the most important endocrine organs, producing steroid hormones with a 17-carbon nucleus following a series of hydroxylation reactions [41]. With the adrenal medulla being functionally related to the sympathetic nervous system, the adrenal cortex is mostly influenced by ACTH and angiotensin II, ACTH stimulating the production and secretion of steroid hormones, the HPA-derived end hormone products that are crucial through lifetime, supporting glucose homeostasis, immune response, salt balance, and sexual maturation [1, 42, 43]. Moreover, long-term ACTH stimulation of the adrenal cortex not only results in increased secretory activity but also in hypertrophy and proliferation of the adrenocortical cells [44], which is the reason that chronic excessive ACTH results in Cushing's syndrome [45]. The adult adrenal cortex, which undergoes a series of development processes from a fetal adrenal, is an endocrine structure comprising three concentric zones (layers) specialized to produce specific steroid hormones [46–48]. The adrenal cortex's three layers are the zona glomerulosa, zona fasciculata, and zona reticularis, among which the latter two are where cortisol and gonadal hormone are secreted under the stimulation of ACTH [1, 49]. The layers and their related functions are listed as follows:

(a) The zona glomerulosa lies just underneath the capsule and constitutes about 15 percent of the adrenal cortex. Cells in this layer secrete significant amounts of aldosterone stimulated by angiotensin II [1, 47].
(b) The zona fasciculata possesses about 75 percent of the adrenal cortex and secretes the glucocorticoids cortisol and corticosterone. The secretion by cells in this layer is controlled in large part by HPA axis via ACTH [1, 47, 50].
(c) The zona reticularis is the inner zone of the cortex, which secretes the adrenal androgens dehydroepiandrosterone and androstenedione and small amounts of estrogens and some glucocorticoids as well, also mainly regulated by ACTH [1, 47].

Briefly summarized, the HPA axis is constituted by hypothalamus, pituitary, and adrenal cortex involving relevant hormones' secretion (CRH-ACTH-Cortisol) and their interactions. PvCs of the hypothalamic PVN send out fibers to the median eminence, where the fiber endings secret CRH and AVP, which are absorbed into the portal system and carried to the pituitary gland resulting in the secretion of ACTH from anterior lobe, which in turn stimulates the adrenal cortex to secret cortisol. Also, MgCs from PVN and SON project to the posterior lobe secreting AVP, part of which can access the anterior lobe by short portal circulation and co-work with CRH to stimulate ACTH secretion, also resulting in cortisol secretion from the adrenal cortex. Conversely, both ACTH and cortisol have an inhibitory effect on the release of CRH and AVP in a negative feedback pattern (Fig. 1.1).

2 The Releasing/Secreting Mechanisms of HPA Axis-Derived Hormones-CRH/AVP, ACTH, and Cortisol

The pituitary adenylate cyclase-activating polypeptide (PACAP) and vasoactive intestinal peptide (VIP) are the two important peptides modulating HPA-derived hormones at multi-levels. Both PACAP and VIP exist in nerve fibers and neurons of the hypothalamus, and VIP, but not PACAP, is also synthesized in the pituitary gland. In addition, both peptides are expressed in the adrenal gland and especially in medullary chromaffin cells. PACAP and VIP share the same PACAP/VIP receptors (PVRs), including three subtypes, PAC1, VPAC1, and VPAC2, which belong to G-protein-coupled protein family and share 60% homology [51–53]. The PVRs are associated with adenylate cyclase via cAMP, activating protein kinase A (PKA), which in turn stimulate the mitogen-activated protein kinase (MAPK) pathway. PAC1 is also coupled to phospholipase C, resulting in Ca^{2+} mobilization and protein kinase C activation [53, 54]. PACAP binds with high affinity to all three PVRs, while VIP binds with much higher affinity (1000 fold) to VPAC1 and VPAC2 [53, 55], VIP and PACAP mainly act in a autocrine or paracrine manner in that their blood concentration is very low [56]. PACAP/VIP and PVRs exist in all the components of the HPA axis (hypothalamus, pituitary, and adrenal gland) [57–59].

2.1 CRH/AVP Release Is Controlled by PACAP and VIP

2.1.1 PACAP Regulates CRH/AVP Release

PACAP, a 27- or 38-amino-acid polypeptide, is found to be a master regulator of stress responses modulating hypothalamic CRH/AVP release and hence HPA axis [57, 60, 61]. PACAP deletion from forebrain excitatory neurons impairs CRH elevation in PVN in the hypothalamus [60]. However, intracerebroventricular injection of PACAP elevates CRH levels, which is completely prevented by the concomitant injection of the PACAP antagonist, PACAP(6–38) [61]. PACAP agonizes PVRs and stimulates the production of cAMP via activating adenylate cyclase and hence enhances CRH synthesis. The effect of PACAP on AVP release investigated in conscious rats shows that intracerebroventricular administration of PACAP raises the plasma AVP level dose-dependently, which is not due to blood pressure fall, increase of plasma Na^+, or decrease of plasma volume [62].

2.1.2 VIP Regulates CRH/AVP Release

VIP is 70% homologous to PACAP, binding with very high affinity to VPAC1 and VPAC2, and has a thousand-fold lower affinity for PAC1 compared to PACAP [53, 55]. Therefore, it is understood that VIP also activates adenylate cyclase (though maybe via different receptors), increasing cAMP level and hence stimulates CRH/AVP release [59]. Recently, a critical circuit from VIP-producing neurons in the suprachiasmatic nucleus (SCN) to CRH-producing neurons in PVN is revealed in an in vivo recording, timing the daily release of corticosterone, which also confirms that VIP participates in CRH release [63]. VIP also raises the plasma AVP concentration by intracerebroventricular injection, and the antagonist for VIP receptor, [Lys, Pro, Arg, Tyr]-VIP, inhibits the VIP-induced AVP increase, but not the PACAP-induced AVP increase, suggesting that VIP and PACAP stimulate AVP release via different receptors [62].

2.1.3 Interleukin-6 Participates in CRH Release and HPA Axis

In vivo studies (in mice and rats) demonstrate that the cytokine, interleukin 6 (IL-6), can influence central CRH release and HPA axis activity [64–66]. IL-6 is observed to stimulate CRH release (but not AVP) at the eminence site in the pituitary stalk where PVN neurons' axons end [67]. Furthermore, IL-6 is also involved in PACAP signaling. PACAP functions via IL-6 signal since PACAP or VIP stimulate the production of IL-6 in neurons [68–70]. These observations suggest that PACAP also modulates CRH release via cytokines like IL-6 besides its direct stimulation pathway described above.

In addition, importantly, central CRH levels are modulated by CRF binding protein (CRF-BP), which has a high affinity to CRH [71, 72].

2.2 ACTH Release Is Controlled by CRH/AVP and VIP/PACAP

2.2.1 CRH/AVP Simulate ACTH Release

CRH and AVP released from both PvCs and MgCs can reach the anterior pituitary, stimulating ACTH release [12, 73–75]. In the anterior pituitary, CRH binds to corticotropin-releasing factor family peptides' s type 1 receptor (CRF_1) and AVP to

V1b of the corticotropes [76], resulting in ACTH release [76–78]. The classical mechanism of CRH/AVP's ACTH simulation is mediated by the cAMP/PKA signaling pathway [79]. Binding of CRH to CRF_1 results in adenyl cyclase activation, leading to an increase in intracellular cAMP concentration and PKA activation [79, 80]. Experimental data indicate that CRH-induced ACTH release is suppressed by CRF_1 antagonist, antalarmin [81]. Interestingly, CRH is also reported to directly stimulate adrenocortical cells to release ACTH and cortisol with enhanced cAMP level via CRF_1, which is blocked by antalarmin [82].

2.2.2 VIP/PACAP Stimulate ACTH Release

As precedingly described, both VIP and PACAP, regulate CRH release and hence indirectly enhance pituitary ACTH secretion. Moreover, PACAP can directly stimulate the pituitary corticotropes releasing ACTH [59]. It is reported that mouse AtT-20/D16v corticotrope cells possess PVR2 (VPAC1, VPAC2), which bind PACAP (both 27- and 38-) and VIP with equal affinity, while both PACAP and VIP enhance ACTH release [83]. Moreover, also in mouse corticotrope tumor cells, PACAP and VIP are found to stimulate cAMP generation and ACTH secretion dose and time dependently [84].

2.3 Cortisol Secretion Is Regulated by ACTH, VIP/PACAP, and CRH

2.3.1 ACTH Controls Cortisol Secretion from the Adrenal Cortex

The adult adrenal cortex comprises three zones, zona glomerulosa, zona fasciculata, and zona reticularis (Sect. 1). The adrenal cortex cells have lipid droplets containing cholesteryl esters as precursors for steroidogenesis. ACTH binds to and activates ACTH receptor on the adrenocortical cells, the melanocortin type 2 receptor (MC2R) [85], which is first discovered by Cone and colleagues [86] and later obtained with the functional type [87]. Activation of MC2R by ACTH then stimulates adenyl cyclase inducing the formation of cAMP in the cell cytoplasm [43, 88, 89]. The enhanced cAMP in turn activates PKA, resulting in initial conversion of cholesterol to pregnenolone and then the production of steroid hormones [90, 91]. However, cAMP-independent way of ACTH is also reported in neonatal rats [92], which may be due to the insufficient development of the cortex [3]. Moreover, ACTH, via activation of the cAMP pathway, also regulates adrenal cortical cell proliferation/differentiation, and an alteration in cAMP signaling may be associated with malignancies of the adrenal cortex [93]. In addition, MC2R upregulation in late gestation is essential for the increase in adrenal steroidogenic capacity while MC2R downregulation blocks the ability of ACTH to stimulate early steps in the steroidogenic pathway [94].

2.3.2 PACAP/VIP Influence Cortisol Secretion

Besides the indirect control of cortisol secretion via CRH-ACTH axis, PACAP/VIP directly influence cortisol secretion. PACAP/VIP and PVRs exist in adrenal gland, directly stimulating the secretion of cortisol [95, 96]. In porcine adrenal glands, PACAP can reach about 14 pmol/g tissue. Furthermore, PACAP and VIP are found originated from PACAP immunoreactive nerve fibers among the splanchnic nerves. And exogenous PACAP stimulates cortisol secretion dose-dependently, which is strongly inhibited by the PAC1/VPAC2 receptor antagonist [95]. In human adrenocortical carcinoma (H295) cell line, both VIP and PACAP increase cortisol secretion, coupled with a parallel increase in cAMP accumulation, which is abolished by VPAC1-specific antagonist [96]. In vivo experiments in calf indicate a significant response of adrenal gland to PACAP, since exogenous PACAP causes a dose-related increase in adrenal cortisol output, which is even more obvious in the absence of ACTH [97].

2.3.3 CRH Directly Stimulates the Secretion of Cortisol

Besides its indirect stimulation of cortisol secretion via ACTH, CRH is found to be able to directly stimulate secretion of adrenal cortex [98, 99]. Accumulating evidence suggests that CRH and its related peptides form paracrine regulatory loops in the adrenal cortex, affecting the cortex directly, strengthened by the fact that CRF_1 and CRF_2 as well as CRF-BP are all expressed in adrenal cortical cells [100–102]. In human adrenal cortical cells, CRH binds to CRF_1, causing increases in cortisol production, which can be completely abolished by antalarmin, the CRF_1 antagonist [103]. In microdissected preparations of normal human adrenal glands and in adrenocortical and adrenomedullary tumors, immunoreactive CRF_1 is found primarily within the zona reticularis. Moreover, stimulation of the adrenal tumor cell line NCI-H295R with CRH elicits an increase in dehydroepiandrosterone (DHEA) secretion, which is reproduced in a culture of primary human adrenocortical cells, indicating that CRH directly acts on adrenal DHEA production [104].

Taken together, traditionally, CRH/AVP-ACTH-cortisol cascade is the HPA-derived hormone cascade. However, this cascade is complicatedly modulated at all levels. Firstly, PACAP and VIP are important regulators of HPA axis, involving in regulation of all the HPA-derived hormones including CRH/AVP, ACTH, and cortisol. Therefore, PACAP/VIP may become a therapeutic target for HPA disorder. In fact, a number of synthetic PACAP peptides and a small molecular antagonist have been generated. Also, relevant genetically modified animals are produced for further research [51]. Moreover, CRH/AVP not only stimulate ACTH and hence cortisol secretion, but also directly promote cortisol secretion. In addition, the down-stream hormones have a feedback inhibitory effect on the release of upper ones. Therefore, with all factors considered, central CRH's effect is extremely complicated. Modulated by a pack of things and modulating many down-stream factors, CRH, as an important component of HPA axis, functions in a complex pattern.

3 Functions of Central CRH via HPA Axis

As described above, traditionally, CRH-ACTH-Cortisol cascade is considered as the functional axis of HPA axis. Central effects of CRH are very complicated and involved in many physiological and pathological functions, which will be briefly summarized in this section.

3.1 CRH and Stress

The researcher Selye pioneers the concept of biological stress in 1930s, which culminates in the discovery of CRH signaling pathway later in 1980s [14, 105, 106]. A stress response is elicited by physical or psychological stimuli (stressors) disrupting the body homeostasis [107]. Physiological and behavioral changes in response to stressor exposure constitute the stress response, mediated by a complex interplay, which involves activation of the sympathetic-adreno-medullar (SAM) axis, HPA axis, and immune system [107, 108]. The beneficial role of a stress response is helping the body handle the stressor challenges. However, if the exposure to a stressor is actually or perceived as intense, repetitive (repeated acute stress), or prolonged (chronic stress), the stress response becomes maladaptive and detrimental to the body, resulting in a variety of problems such as depression, anxiety, cognitive impairment, heart disease, etc. [107, 109, 110].

A stress response has two components: a fast response, mediated by the SAM axis, and a slow response, mediated by the HPA axis [107]. The fast response is a sympathomimetic effect due to activation of SAM resulting in increased secretion of norepinephrine and epinephrine, and the slow response of a stress is due to activation of the HPA axis [107]. In terms of HPA axis, stressors cause the release of CRH from the PVN of the hypothalamus at its nerve endings in median eminence, which is carried to the pituitary gland through the portal vessel (Sect. 1, Fig. 1.2). CRH is a selective agonist of CRF_1, which is widely expressed in the brain of mammals and is the key receptor for the stress-induced ACTH release from the anterior pituitary [78, 111]. The CRH level is regulated by CRF binding protein (CRF-BP) in the brain, which has a high affinity for CRH [112, 113]. About half of CRH (40–60%) is found bound with CRF-BP [114], which may serve as a therapeutic target for stress- and cognition-related disorders [115–117]. In exposure to stress, the expression of CRF-BP increases, which is thought to be a negative feedback mechanism to decrease the interaction of CRH with CRF_1 modulating HPA axis [118, 119].

As well recognized, during exposure to stressors, the body shows Selye's general adaptation syndrome [120] through three different stages, i.e., alarm reaction, resistance, and exhaustion stage, with the last two exhibiting the pathological changes of extended stress [121–124]. After the initial shock of the stressful event, the body begins to repair itself by HPA-derived hormones, during which the body remains on alert until the stressful event is no longer a problem, with CRH from PVN playing a defensive role [107, 125]. However, if the stressing disturbances persist for extended periods of time, the body will adapt to cope with higher level of stress, continuing to secrete CRH and other stress hormones and changing the reactiveness of the receptors [107, 126]. If the stressful event stays, dragging the body into the exhaustion stage, symptoms including burnout, fatigue, depression, and anxiety will occur. Furthermore, the immune system will continue to weaken due to the suppressive effects of stress hormones (mainly CRH) on immune cells [107, 127, 128]. Based on the importance of HPA axis in stress responses, interruption on CRH and other stress hormones may be a therapeutical option as important as eliminating stressors for handling the stress-related problems [128].

3.2 *Central CRH's Role in Immune and Inflammation*

The immune/inflammatory response is characterized by enhanced vascular permeability, edema, and leukocytes in extravascular tissues while the immune response balances between pro- and anti-inflammatory actions [129]. The central role of CRH in immune/inflammation is via HPA axis [130]. On the one hand, hypothalamic CRH is recognized to act indirectly as an anti-inflammatory factor, since cortisol, the final product of HPA axis, is known for its anti-inflammatory actions [130]. While on the other hand, central CRH is also reported to have pro-inflammatory actions [130], which may be consistent with the report that glucocorticoids also have a pro-inflammatory effect leading to vascular hyperpermeability under stress [131]. Furthermore, complicated regulation of HPA axis may result in different CRH's effects on immune/inflammation [130]. For instance, the known cytokine IL-6 is a potent stimulator of the HPA axis by modulating CRH and AVP secretion [65, 132, 133]. Peripheral administration of IL-6 causes considerable elevations in plasma ACTH and cortisol [132]. However, in case of severe aseptic inflammation, IL-6 levels are increased while cortisol secretion is deficient [134], suggesting a dysfunction of HPA axis under inflammation stress. Meanwhile, AVP can increase the cortisol level by improving the adrenal response to ACTH [133, 134]. These paradoxical results suggest that different hypothalamic and HPA responses are critical in balancing between the anti- and pro-inflammatory fashion of central CRH. In fact, more and more evidence has been presented for both the anti- and pro-inflammatory effect of central CRH.

3.2.1 The Anti-inflammatory or Non-pro-inflammatory Effect of Central CRH

As described above, central CRH stimulates the release of ACTH, which in turn causes the secretion of cortisol, functioning as an anti-inflammatory factor. A few experiments have shown the direct relationship between central CRH and its indirect anti-inflammatory/or non-pro-inflammatory effects, with some showing CRH's no significant role and others showing its anti-inflammatory role in peripheral inflammation.

For instance, CRH secretion is observed in the hypothalamus to be enhanced during acute colonic inflammation, but the CRH level remains at a high level in the brain after the recovery of colitis [135], suggesting a weak relationship between central CRH effect and colon inflammation. Furthermore, centrally injected CRH does not have an influence on the stress-induced colitis [136] whereas a protective role of brain CRH from stress-induced worsening of colitis is observed [137, 138]. The anti-colon inflammatory effect of central CRH is testified since it is abolished by intracerebroventricular injection of the CRF peptides receptors' antagonist, astressin [138].

3.2.2 The Pro-inflammatory Effects of Central CRH

As a pivotal element in the HPA axis, CRH is reported to exert a pro-inflammatory action responding to stress [5–9]. For example, in a stress-related skin inflammation mouse model, vascular permeability and CRH AND IL-6 levels (IL-6 further stimulates HPA axis increasing central CRH) are increased in association with mast cells [139, 140]. Central CRH is also reported to be related to inflammatory bowel diseases (IBD) involving colon motility enhancement, immune/inflammatory cells, and gut flora via brain-gut-microbes axis under stress [141–144]. And CRH deficiency results in reduced inflammation in a mouse model of colitis [145].

Collectively, the opposite results bring controversies and complexity about the central role of CRH in immune/inflammation. Neuroendocrine and immune system are strictly related in a bidirectional manner [146], as indicated by the shared common signal molecules and receptors [130, 146]. For instance, the presence of and reaction to glucocorticoids, ACTH and CRH have been demonstrated in leukocytes [147–149]. Moreover, CRF_1 has also been detected in mast cells, which are proved to be important targets of CRH in the process of inflammation [150, 151]. On the other hand, specific IL-1 binding sites are found to be widely distributed in the brain influencing CRH release [152–154] while the stress inducible cytokine IL-6 is also a strong HPA activator [65, 155]. Therefore, although hypothalamic CRH is rapidly enzymatically decomposed at the pituitary level or binds to CRF-BP not contributing to its plasma level [156], the role of central CRH in immune/inflammation is extremely complicated, involving both the central responses of HPA axis and peripheral hormones and other factors including immune cells [130, 146]. Moreover, the complexity may also lie in its influence on the balance between Th1 and Th2, i.e., cellular and humoral immunity and in the responsiveness of HPA axis [130, 157]. As well recognized, Fischer and Lewis rats, two highly inbred strains selected for their resistance (Fischer rats) or susceptibility (Lewis rats) to inflammatory disease, are used to study the relationship between HPA axis and inflammatory responses [158–160]. It is observed that an excessive HPA response, e.g., under a state of stress, can increase susceptibility to infectious agents and tumorigenesis but enhance resistance to autoimmune or aseptic inflammatory diseases whereas a defective HPA axis response, e.g., under relative glucocorticoid deficiency, diminishes susceptibility to infections and tumorigenesis but increases susceptibility to autoimmune or aseptic inflammatory diseases [130, 161]. In Lewis rats, hypothalamic CRH neurons respond poorly to stress [162]. Moreover, endogenous glucocorticoid production is found to be disrupted and allergen-induced airway inflammation and lung mechanical dysfunction are enhanced in CRH knock-out mice, suggesting that CRH deficiency could increase asthma severity [163]. In a systemic chronic autoimmune disease (lupus erythematosus) murine model, neuroendocrine alterations are observed to be associated with inflammation, accompanied by altered HPA function and hypothalamic regulation of HPA responses [164]. Furthermore, it is observed that under chronic inflammatory stress, there is an increase in circulating levels of corticosterone and the HPA axis is dominated by AVP instead of CRH [134, 165].

3.3 Central CRH and Depression/Anxiety

As precedingly described, depression is also a result of the later stress adaptation stages [107]. Therefore, it is understandable that HPA axis must be implicated in the pathophysiology of a variety of mood and cognitive disorders. Dysregulation of HPA has been documented as an important factor in depression [166]. Moreover, HPA axis dysfunction is associated with gastrointestinal symptoms in major depression, and patients with depression exhibit HPA axis's hyper-suppression [167]. Although the HPA axis is mostly overactive in depression, an attenuated hormonal response to stress in individuals with a history of multiple suicide attempts (SA) is observed [168, 169]. By the combined dexamethasone suppression/CRH (dex/CRH) test, it is found that patients who are just weary of life show an increased HPA activity, patients with no previous SA show normalization of stress response to the second dex/CRH after acute depression recovery, while patients with multiple previous SA show an increased ACTH response [168, 169].

It is reported that during aging, the activation of CRH neurons is modest compared to the extra activation observed in Alzheimer's disease (AD) and the even stronger increase in major depression [170]. Moreover, CRH neurons in the PVN are hyperactivated in major depressed patients. Also, the number of CRH neurons co-expressing AVP becomes significantly higher, and increased production of AVP in depression occurs both in PVN and SON [171, 172]. The suprachiasmatic nucleus (SCN), i.e., the biological clock of the brain, shows lower AVP production and a smaller circadian amplitude in depression, explaining the sleeping problems in this disorder likely contributing to the strong CRH activation [173–175]. However, no link between AVP and depression is also reported [176]. Moreover, besides the activation of CRH neurons in some depressed patients as described [170, 171], there is evidence for a direct involvement of glucocorticoids, the end HPA axis-derived hormones, in the etiology and symptoms of depression [177].

Interestingly, a synthesized CRF_1-specific peptide agonist, cortagine, is developed and found to be anxiogenic but antidepressive. The pharmacological analysis of cortagine shows that in HEK293 cells transfected with CRF_1, cortagine stimulates the release of cAMP, similarly to CRH. And in behavior experiments, it is observed that intracerebral injection of cortagine enhances anxiety-like behavior. In contrast, cortagine reduces significantly the immobility time in the forced swim test as designed for antidepressive drugs [178]. These results also strongly suggest that CRH-relevant regulation may become a promising approach for depression therapy.

3.4 *Central CRH and Metabolism*

As well known, the CNS plays an important role in the overall metabolic balance although direct hormone action on peripheral tissues mediates the control of nutrient handling [179–181]. HPA axis is well documented to be significant for metabolism maintaining the balance of internal environment of the body through the secretion of related hormones, CRH-ACTH, and glucocorticoids (GCs) [182, 183]. Intracerebral injection of CRH is reported to inhibit gastric secretion, influencing nutrients' absorption [184]. GCs are accepted as being catabolic, liberating energy substrates responding to stress supplying the increased metabolic demand of the body [185]. Abnormality in GC production results in conditions accompanied by metabolism disorder. As well known, endogenous hypercortisolism, Cushing's syndrome, is characterized by excess ACTH or autonomous cortisol release from the adrenal gland, the medical therapy being targeted to the dysregulated HPA axis [186, 187]. On the contrary, in case of Addison's disease, GC deficiency due to the adrenal cortex failure may result in a life-threatening adrenal crisis associated with a pack of things including metabolism disorder [188].

Moreover, the role of HPA axis in glucolipid metabolic disorders has well been reported [189–191]. Hyperactivation of HPA axis is found to be associated with diabetic metabolism disorder, and the stress responsiveness is impaired in diabetes, increasing the metabolic challenge of insulin-induced hypoglycemia [190].

3.5 *Central CRH and Cancers*

Up to date, rare evidence indicates a direct link between the central CRH and the development of cancers. However, the relationship between chronic stress and tumor development has been frequently reported and widely reviewed [192–198]. Therefore, it is reasonable that the central role of CRH in tumor is mainly via the indirect way through HPA axis-mediated stress as a stress mediator.

Clinically, chronic stress is found common among patients with various cancers due to stressors encountered upon diagnosis and during therapy [198–201]. As precedingly described, chronic stress activates the classic neuroendocrine systems, the

HPA axis and the SAM, producing sympathetic hormones and CRH-ACTH-cortisol, excessive of which have been demonstrated to take part in cancer-promoting processes by altering the tumor microenvironment (TME) [193, 196, 202]. For instance, stress hormones can promote colon cancer development through corresponding changes in the body's immune function and inflammatory response [194, 202, 203]. Moreover, stress has significant influence on the gut flora, i.e., the brain-gut-microbiota axis, promoting the composition of pro-inflammatory microbiome and hence resulting in colitis, which is a high risk for colon cancer [204, 205].

4 Summary

As summarized in Fig. 1.4, the HPA axis is regulated at multi-levels and participates in a wide range of functions. The HPA axis-derived corresponding hormones, CRH/AVP-ACTH-Cortisol in sequence, modulated centrally and peripherally by PACAP/VIP (CRH by CRF-BP, too) are life-crucial and exerts much influence on

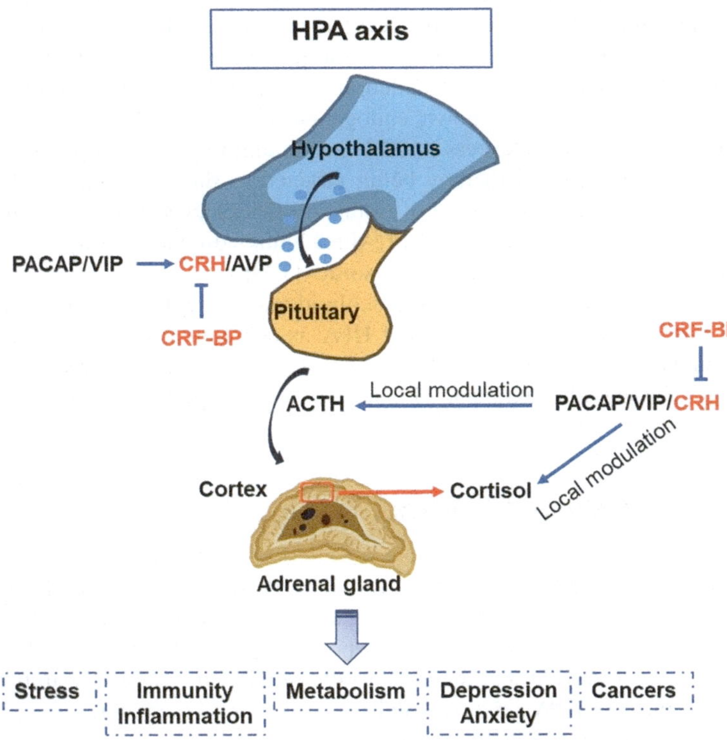

Fig. 1.4 The central and peripheral regulation and functions of HPA axis (and the derived hormones:CRH/AVP-ACTH-Cortisol)

the body including their roles in stress responses, immune activities and inflammation, metabolism, etc. It is noteworthy that central CRH communicates with peripheral cells/systems at many levels via HPA axis. For a relatively long period, the centrally produced and functioning CRH dominates our knowledge linked to HPA axis.

In recent decades, CRH and other CRFp (Urocortins, UCNs) existing and produced peripherally attract wide attention of researchers, which is the focus of the present book and will be discussed in the following chapters.

References

1. Hall JE, Hall ME. Guyton and hall textbook of medical physiology. 14th ed. Elsevier; 2020.
2. Fong H, Zheng J, Kurrasch D. The structural and functional complexity of the integrative hypothalamus. Science. 2023;382(6669):388–94.
3. Clarke IJ. Hypothalamus as an endocrine organ. Compr Physiol. 2015;5(1):217–53.
4. Lechan RM, Toni R. Functional anatomy of the hypothalamus and pituitary. In: Feingold KR, et al., editors. Endotext, vol. 14; 2000. p. 819.
5. Tsigos C, Chrousos GP. Hypothalamic-pituitary-adrenal axis, neuroendocrine factors and stress. J Psychosom Res. 2002;53(4):865–71.
6. Swaab DF, et al. Introduction: the anterior hypothalamus. Handb Clin Neurol. 2021;179:3–5.
7. Loes DJ, et al. MR anatomy and pathology of the hypothalamus. AJR Am J Roentgenol. 1991;156(3):579–85.
8. Hindmarch CCT, Murphy D. The transcriptome and the hypothalamo-neurohypophyseal system. Endocr Dev. 2010;17:1–10.
9. Caldwell HK, et al. Vasopressin: behavioral roles of an "original" neuropeptide. Prog Neurobiol. 2008;84(1):1–24.
10. Sawchenko PE, Imaki T, Vale W. Co-localization of neuroactive substances in the endocrine hypothalamus. Ciba Found Symp. 1992;168:16–30.
11. Kawakami N, et al. Variation of pro-vasopressin processing in parvocellular and magnocellular neurons in the paraventricular nucleus of the hypothalamus: evidence from the vasopressin-related glycopeptide copeptin. J Comp Neurol. 2021;529(7):1372–90.
12. Kawaguchi Y, et al. Knockdown of endoplasmic reticulum chaperone BiP leads to the death of parvocellular AVP/CRH neurons in mice. J Neuroendocrinol. 2023;35(1):e13223.
13. Keller-Wood M. Hypothalamic-pituitary – adrenal axis-feedback control. Compr Physiol. 2015;5(3):1161–82.
14. Vale W, et al. Characterization of a 41-residue ovine hypothalamic peptide that stimulates secretion of corticotropin and beta-endorphin. Science. 1981;213(4514):1394–7.
15. Fink G. 60 years of neuroendocrinology: memoir: Harris' neuroendocrine revolution: of portal vessels and self-priming. J Endocrinol. 2015;226(2):T13–24.
16. Stojiljkovic AS, et al. Influence of arginine vasopressin on the ultradian dynamics of Hypothalamic-Pituitary-Adrenal axis. Front Endocrinol (Lausanne). 2022;13:976323.
17. Gross PM, et al. Topography of short portal vessels in the rat pituitary gland: a scanning electron-microscopic and morphometric study of corrosion cast replicas. Cell Tissue Res. 1993;272(1):79–88.
18. Raff H. Interactions between neurohypophysial hormones and the ACTH-adrenocortical axis. Ann N Y Acad Sci. 1993;689:411–25.
19. Sari S, et al. Measures of pituitary gland and stalk: from neonate to adolescence. J Pediatr Endocrinol Metab. 2014;27(11–12):1071–6.

20. Asa SL. Pituitary histopathology in man: normal and abnormal. In: Feingold KR, et al., editors. Endotext; 2000.
21. Amar AP, Weiss MH. Pituitary anatomy and physiology. Neurosurg Clin N Am. 2003;14(1):11–23. v
22. di Iorgi N, et al. Developmental abnormalities of the posterior pituitary gland. Endocr Dev. 2009;14:83–94.
23. Hodson DJ, Mollard P. Navigating pituitary structure and function – defining a roadmap for hormone secretion. J Neuroendocrinol. 2013;25(7):674–5.
24. Chapman PR, et al. Neuroimaging of the pituitary gland: practical anatomy and pathology. Radiol Clin North Am. 2020;58(6):1115–33.
25. Giraldi E, Allen JW, Ioachimescu AG. Pituitary incidentalomas: best practices and looking ahead. Endocr Pract. 2023;29(1):60–8.
26. Alatzoglou KS, Gregory LC, Dattani MT. Development of the pituitary gland. Compr Physiol. 2020;10(2):389–413.
27. Camilletti MA, et al. From pituitary stem cell differentiation to regenerative medicine. Front Endocrinol (Lausanne). 2020;11:614999.
28. Davis SW, et al. All hormone-producing cell types of the pituitary intermediate and anterior lobes derive from Prop1-expressing progenitors. Endocrinology. 2016;157(4):1385–96.
29. Ooi GT, Tawadros N, Escalona RM. Pituitary cell lines and their endocrine applications. Mol Cell Endocrinol. 2004;228(1–2):1–21.
30. Stojilkovic SS. Pituitary cell type-specific electrical activity, calcium signaling and secretion. Biol Res. 2006;39(3):403–23.
31. Korf HW, Moller M. Arcuate nucleus, median eminence, and hypophysial pars tuberalis. Handb Clin Neurol. 2021;180:227–51.
32. Popa GT, Fielding U. Hypophysio-portal vessels and their colloid accompaniment. J Anat. 1933;67(Pt 2):227–32.
33. Carmel PW, Antunes JL, Ferin M. Collection of blood from the pituitary stalk and portal veins in monkeys, and from the pituitary sinusoidal system of monkey and man. J Neurosurg. 1979;50(1):75–80.
34. Yao Y, et al. Identification of the suprachiasmatic nucleus venous portal system in the mammalian brain. Nat Commun. 2021;12(1):5643.
35. Cuzzo B, Padala SA, Lappin SL. Physiology, vasopressin. StatPearls: Treasure Island (FL) ineligible companies. Disclosure: Sandeep Padala declares no relevant financial relationships with ineligible companies. Disclosure: Sarah Lappin declares no relevant financial relationships with ineligible companies; 2023
36. Hui C et al. Diabetes insipidus. StatPearls. Treasure Island (FL) ineligible companies. Disclosure: Myra Khan declares no relevant financial relationships with ineligible companies. Disclosure: Mahammed Khan Suheb declares no relevant financial relationships with ineligible companies. Disclosure: Jared Radbel declares no relevant financial relationships with ineligible companies; 2023.
37. van de Pavert SA, et al. Effects of vasopressin and elimination of corticotropin-releasing hormone-target cells on pro-opiomelanocortin mRNA levels and adrenocorticotropin secretion in ovine anterior pituitary cells. J Endocrinol. 1997;154(1):139–47.
38. Volpi S, Rabadan-Diehl C, Aguilera G. Vasopressinergic regulation of the hypothalamic pituitary adrenal axis and stress adaptation. Stress. 2004;7(2):75–83.
39. Lee AK, Tse FW, Tse A. Arginine vasopressin potentiates the stimulatory action of CRH on pituitary corticotropes via a protein kinase C-dependent reduction of the background TREK-1 current. Endocrinology. 2015;156(10):3661–72.
40. Slapa RZ, et al. Standards of ultrasound imaging of the adrenal glands. J Ultrason. 2015;15(63):377–87.
41. Rosol TJ, et al. Adrenal gland: structure, function, and mechanisms of toxicity. Toxicol Pathol. 2001;29(1):41–8.

42. Busada JT, Cidlowski JA. Mechanisms of glucocorticoid action during development. Curr Top Dev Biol. 2017;125:147–70.
43. Gallo-Payet N. 60 years Of POMC: adrenal and extra-adrenal functions of ACTH. J Mol Endocrinol. 2016;56(4):T135–56.
44. Menzies RI, et al. Transcription controls growth, cell kinetics and cholesterol supply to sustain ACTH responses. Endocr Connect. 2017;6(7):446–57.
45. Bertagna X. Effects of chronic ACTH excess on human adrenal cortex. Front Endocrinol (Lausanne). 2017;8:43.
46. Abou Nader N, Boyer A. Adrenal cortex development and maintenance: knowledge acquired from mouse models. Endocrinology. 2021;162(12)
47. Xing Y, et al. Development of adrenal cortex zonation. Endocrinol Metab Clin N Am. 2015;44(2):243–74.
48. Freedman BD, et al. Adrenocortical zonation results from lineage conversion of differentiated zona glomerulosa cells. Dev Cell. 2013;26(6):666–73.
49. Pignatti E, et al. Regulation of zonation and homeostasis in the adrenal cortex. Mol Cell Endocrinol. 2017;441:146–55.
50. Hazell G, et al. Dynamics of ACTH-mediated regulation of gene transcription in ATC1 and ATC7 Adrenal Zona fasciculata cell lines. Endocrinology. 2019;160(3):587–604.
51. Shen S, Gehlert DR, Collier DA. PACAP and PAC1 receptor in brain development and behavior. Neuropeptides. 2013;47(6):421–30.
52. Rajbhandari AK, et al. The functional heterogeneity of PACAP: stress, learning, and pathology. Neurobiol Learn Mem. 2023;203:107792.
53. Hirabayashi T, Nakamachi T, Shioda S. Discovery of PACAP and its receptors in the brain. J Headache Pain. 2018;19(1):28.
54. Shioda S, et al. Pleiotropic and retinoprotective functions of PACAP. Anat Sci Int. 2016;91(4):313–24.
55. Lu J, et al. Targeting VIP and PACAP receptor signaling: new insights into designing drugs for the PACAP subfamily of receptors. Int J Mol Sci. 2022;23(15)
56. Conconi MT, Spinazzi R, Nussdorfer GG. Endogenous ligands of PACAP/VIP receptors in the autocrine-paracrine regulation of the adrenal gland. Int Rev Cytol. 2006;249:1–51.
57. Mustafa T. Pituitary adenylate cyclase-activating polypeptide (PACAP): a master regulator in central and peripheral stress responses. Adv Pharmacol. 2013;68:445–57.
58. Pisegna JR, Moody TW, Wank SA. Differential signaling and immediate-early gene activation by four splice variants of the human pituitary adenylate cyclase-activating polypeptide receptor (hPACAP-R). Ann N Y Acad Sci. 1996;805:54–64.
59. Nussdorfer GG, Malendowicz LK. Role of VIP, PACAP, and related peptides in the regulation of the hypothalamo-pituitary-adrenal axis. Peptides. 1998;19(8):1443–67.
60. Jiang SZ, Zhang HY, Eiden LE. PACAP controls endocrine and behavioral stress responses via separate brain circuits. Biol Psychiatry Glob Open Sci. 2023;3(4):673–85.
61. Grinevich V, Fournier A, Pelletier G. Effects of pituitary adenylate cyclase-activating polypeptide (PACAP) on corticotropin-releasing hormone (CRH) gene expression in the rat hypothalamic paraventricular nucleus. Brain Res. 1997;773(1–2):190–6.
62. Murase T, et al. Pituitary adenylate cyclase-activating polypeptide stimulates arginine vasopressin release in conscious rats. Neuroendocrinology. 1993;57(6):1092–6.
63. Jones JR, et al. Circadian neurons in the paraventricular nucleus entrain and sustain daily rhythms in glucocorticoids. Nat Commun. 2021;12(1):5763.
64. Senaris RM, et al. Interleukin-6 regulates the expression of hypothalamic neuropeptides involved in body weight in a gender-dependent way. J Neuroendocrinol. 2011;23(8):675–86.
65. Girotti M, Donegan JJ, Morilak DA. Influence of hypothalamic IL-6/gp130 receptor signaling on the HPA axis response to chronic stress. Psychoneuroendocrinology. 2013;38(7):1158–69.
66. Barkhudaryan N, Dunn AJ. Molecular mechanisms of actions of interleukin-6 on the brain, with special reference to serotonin and the hypothalamo-pituitary-adrenocortical axis. Neurochem Res. 1999;24(9):1169–80.

67. Spinedi E, et al. Cytokines stimulate the CRH but not the vasopressin neuronal system: evidence for a median eminence site of interleukin-6 action. Neuroendocrinology. 1992;56(1):46–53.
68. Ohtaki H, et al. Pituitary adenylate cyclase-activating polypeptide (PACAP) decreases ischemic neuronal cell death in association with IL-6. Proc Natl Acad Sci USA. 2006;103(19):7488–93.
69. Gottschall PE, Tatsuno I, Arimura A. Regulation of interleukin-6 (IL-6) secretion in primary cultured rat astrocytes: synergism of interleukin-1 (IL-1) and pituitary adenylate cyclase activating polypeptide (PACAP). Brain Res. 1994;637(1–2):197–203.
70. Nakamachi T, et al. IL-6 and PACAP receptor expression and localization after global brain ischemia in mice. J Mol Neurosci. 2012;48(3):518–25.
71. Sanson A, et al. CRF binding protein activity in the hypothalamic paraventricular nucleus is essential for stress adaptations and normal maternal behaviour in lactating rats. Neurobiol Stress. 2024;30:100631.
72. Henry BA, Lightman SL, Lowry CA. Distribution of corticotropin-releasing factor binding protein-immunoreactivity in the rat hypothalamus: association with corticotropin-releasing factor-, urocortin 1- and vimentin-immunoreactive fibres. J Neuroendocrinol. 2005;17(3):135–44.
73. Lim CT, Khoo B. Normal physiology of ACTH and GH release in the hypothalamus and anterior pituitary in man. In: Feingold KR, et al., editors. Endotext, vol. 91; 2000. p. 348.
74. Livesey JH, et al. Interactions of CRH, AVP and cortisol in the secretion of ACTH from perifused equine anterior pituitary cells: "permissive" roles for cortisol and CRH. Endocr Res. 2000;26(3):445–63.
75. Matthews SG, Challis JR. CRH and AVP-induced changes in synthesis and release of ACTH from the ovine fetal pituitary in vitro: negative influences of cortisol. Endocrine. 1997;6(3):293–300.
76. Mason D, et al. Acute and chronic regulation of pituitary receptors for vasopressin and corticotropin releasing hormone. Arch Physiol Biochem. 2002;110(1–2):74–89.
77. Aguilera G, et al. Corticotropin releasing hormone receptors: two decades later. Peptides. 2004;25(3):319–29.
78. Papadimitriou A, Priftis KN. Regulation of the hypothalamic-pituitary-adrenal axis. Neuroimmunomodulation. 2009;16(5):265–71.
79. Mo C, et al. Corticotropin-releasing hormone (CRH) stimulates cocaine- and amphetamine-regulated transcript gene (CART1) expression through CRH type 1 receptor (CRHR1) in chicken anterior pituitary. Mol Cell Endocrinol. 2015;417:166–77.
80. Uribe-Marino A, et al. Prefrontal cortex corticotropin-releasing factor receptor 1 conveys acute stress-induced executive dysfunction. Biol Psychiatry. 2016;80(10):743–53.
81. Webster EL, et al. In vivo and in vitro characterization of antalarmin, a nonpeptide corticotropin-releasing hormone (CRH) receptor antagonist: suppression of pituitary ACTH release and peripheral inflammation. Endocrinology. 1996;137(12):5747–50.
82. Valego NK, Rose JC. A specific CRH antagonist attenuates ACTH-stimulated cortisol secretion in ovine adrenocortical cells. Reprod Sci. 2010;17(5):477–86.
83. Braas KM, Brandenburg CA, May V. Pituitary adenylate cyclase-activating polypeptide regulation of AtT-20/D16v corticotrope cell proopiomelanocortin expression and secretion. Endocrinology. 1994;134(1):186–95.
84. Aoki Y, et al. Regulation of the rat proopiomelanocortin gene expression in AtT-20 cells. II: Effects of the pituitary adenylate cyclase-activating polypeptide and vasoactive intestinal polypeptide. Endocrinology. 1997;138(5):1930–4.
85. Fridmanis D, Roga A, Klovins J. ACTH receptor (MC2R) specificity: what do we know about underlying molecular mechanisms? Front Endocrinol (Lausanne). 2017;8:13.
86. Mountjoy KG, et al. The cloning of a family of genes that encode the melanocortin receptors. Science. 1992;257(5074):1248–51.
87. Metherell LA, et al. Mutations in MRAP, encoding a new interacting partner of the ACTH receptor, cause familial glucocorticoid deficiency type 2. Nat Genet. 2005;37(2):166–70.

88. Gallo-Payet N, Payet MD. Mechanism of action of ACTH: beyond cAMP. Microsc Res Tech. 2003;61(3):275–87.
89. Fragoso MC, et al. Genetics of primary macronodular adrenal hyperplasia. Presse Med. 2018;47(7–8 Pt 2):e139–49.
90. Clark BJ. ACTH action on StAR biology. Front Neurosci. 2016;10:547.
91. Rocha KM, et al. Deconstructing the molecular mechanisms of cell cycle control in a mouse adrenocortical cell line: roles of ACTH. Microsc Res Tech. 2003;61(3):268–74.
92. Bodager J, et al. Adrenocortical sensitivity to ACTH in neonatal rats: correlation of corticosterone responses and adrenal cAMP content. Am J Physiol Regul Integr Comp Physiol. 2014;307(3):R347–53.
93. Peri A, et al. Variable expression of the transcription factors cAMP response element-binding protein and inducible cAMP early repressor in the normal adrenal cortex and in adrenocortical adenomas and carcinomas. J Clin Endocrinol Metab. 2001;86(11):5443–9.
94. Su Y, Rose JC. The impact of ACTH receptor knockdown on fetal and adult ovine adrenocortical cell function. Reprod Sci. 2008;15(3):253–62.
95. Tornoe K, et al. PACAP-(1-38) as neurotransmitter in the porcine adrenal glands. Am J Physiol Endocrinol Metab. 2000;279(6):E1413–25.
96. Nicol MR, et al. Vasoactive intestinal peptide (VIP) stimulates cortisol secretion from the H295 human adrenocortical tumour cell line via VPAC1 receptors. J Mol Endocrinol. 2004;32(3):869–77.
97. Edwards AV, Jones CT. Adrenal responses to the peptide PACAP in conscious functionally hypophysectomized calves. Am J Phys. 1994;266(6 Pt 1):E870–6.
98. Fehm HL, et al. Ability of corticotropin releasing hormone to stimulate cortisol secretion independent from pituitary adrenocorticotropin. Life Sci. 1988;42(6):679–86.
99. Smith R, et al. Corticotropin-releasing hormone directly and preferentially stimulates dehydroepiandrosterone sulfate secretion by human fetal adrenal cortical cells. J Clin Endocrinol Metab. 1998;83(8):2916–20.
100. Tsatsanis C, et al. The corticotropin-releasing factor (CRF) family of peptides as local modulators of adrenal function. Cell Mol Life Sci. 2007;64(13):1638–55.
101. Karteris E, et al. Expression and coupling characteristics of the CRH and orexin type 2 receptors in human fetal adrenals. J Clin Endocrinol Metab. 2001;86(9):4512–9.
102. Sirianni R, et al. Corticotropin-releasing hormone (CRH) and urocortin act through type 1 CRH receptors to stimulate dehydroepiandrosterone sulfate production in human fetal adrenal cells. J Clin Endocrinol Metab. 2005;90(9):5393–400.
103. Willenberg HS, et al. Effects of a novel corticotropin-releasing-hormone receptor type I antagonist on human adrenal function. Mol Psychiatry. 2000;5(2):137–41.
104. Willenberg HS, et al. Corticotropin-releasing hormone receptor expression on normal and tumorous human adrenocortical cells. Neuroendocrinology. 2005;82(5–6):274–81.
105. Selye H. A syndrome produced by diverse nocuous agents. J Neuropsychiatry Clin Neurosci. 1936;10(2):230–1.
106. Tache Y, Brunnhuber S. From Hans Selye's discovery of biological stress to the identification of corticotropin-releasing factor signaling pathways: implication in stress-related functional bowel diseases. Ann N Y Acad Sci. 2008;1148:29–41.
107. Chu B et al. Physiology, stress reaction. StatPearls. Treasure Island (FL) ineligible companies. Disclosure: Komal Marwaha declares no relevant financial relationships with ineligible companies. Disclosure: Terrence Sanvictores declares no relevant financial relationships with ineligible companies. Disclosure: Derek Ayers declares no relevant financial relationships with ineligible companies; 2023.
108. Godoy LD, et al. A comprehensive overview on stress neurobiology: basic concepts and clinical implications. Front Behav Neurosci. 2018;12:127.
109. Richardson AE, VanderKaay Tomasulo MM. Stress-induced HPA activation in virtual navigation and spatial attention performance. BMC Neurosci. 2022;23(1):40.

110. Tsuru J, et al. Association of BDNF Val66Met polymorphism with HPA and SAM axis reactivity to psychological and physical stress. Neuropsychiatr Dis Treat. 2014;10:2123–33.
111. Chrousos GP, Zoumakis E. Milestones in CRH research. Curr Mol Pharmacol. 2017;10(4):259–63.
112. Behan DP, et al. Characterization of a sheep brain corticotropin releasing factor binding protein. Brain Res. 1996;709(2):265–74.
113. Turnbull AV, Rivier C. Corticotropin-releasing factor (CRF) and endocrine responses to stress: CRF receptors, binding protein, and related peptides. Proc Soc Exp Biol Med. 1997;215(1):1–10.
114. Ketchesin KD, Stinnett GS, Seasholtz AF. Corticotropin-releasing hormone-binding protein and stress: from invertebrates to humans. Stress. 2017;20(5):449–64.
115. Curley DE, et al. Corticotropin releasing factor binding protein as a novel target to restore brain homeostasis: lessons learned from alcohol use disorder research. Front Behav Neurosci. 2021;15:786855.
116. Behan DP, et al. Displacement of corticotropin releasing factor from its binding protein as a possible treatment for Alzheimer's disease. Nature. 1995;378(6554):284–7.
117. Behan DP, et al. Neurobiology of corticotropin releasing factor (CRF) receptors and CRF-binding protein: implications for the treatment of CNS disorders. Mol Psychiatry. 1996;1(4):265–77.
118. Klampfl SM, et al. Brain CRF-binding protein modulates aspects of maternal behavior under stressful conditions and supports a hypo-anxious state in lactating rats. Horm Behav. 2016;84:136–44.
119. Stinnett GS, Westphal NJ, Seasholtz AF. Pituitary CRH-binding protein and stress in female mice. Physiol Behav. 2015;150:16–23.
120. Selye H. The alarm reaction, the general adaptation syndrome, and the role of stress and of the adaptive hormones in dental medicine. Oral Surg Oral Med Oral Pathol. 1954;7(4):355–67.
121. Ramiro Fde S, et al. Investigation of stress, anxiety and depression in women with fibromyalgia: a comparative study. Rev Bras Reumatol. 2014;54(1):27–32.
122. Alpini D, Cesarani A. Tinnitus as an alarm bell: stress reaction tinnitus model. ORL J Otorhinolaryngol Relat Spec. 2006;68(1):31–6.
123. Szabo S. The post-COVID stress syndrome: from the three-stage stress response of Hans Selye to COVID-19. Inflammopharmacology. 2023;31(6):2799–806.
124. Rochette L, Dogon G, Vergely C. Stress: eight decades after its definition by hans selye: "stress is the spice of life". Brain Sci. 2023;13(2)
125. Daviu N, et al. Paraventricular nucleus CRH neurons encode stress controllability and regulate defensive behavior selection. Nat Neurosci. 2020;23(3):398–410.
126. Grammatopoulos DK, Ourailidou S. CRH receptor signalling: potential roles in pathophysiology. Curr Mol Pharmacol. 2017;10(4):296–310.
127. Friedman EM, Irwin MR. A role for CRH and the sympathetic nervous system in stress-induced immunosuppression. Ann N Y Acad Sci. 1995;771:396–418.
128. Aguilera G. HPA axis responsiveness to stress: implications for healthy aging. Exp Gerontol. 2011;46(2–3):90–5.
129. Jessop DS, Harbuz MS, Lightman SL. CRH in chronic inflammatory stress. Peptides. 2001;22(5):803–7.
130. Nezi M, Mastorakos G, Mouslech Z. Corticotropin releasing hormone and the immune/inflammatory response. In: Feingold KR, et al., editors. Endotext; 2000.
131. Elenkov IJ, et al. Stress, corticotropin-releasing hormone, glucocorticoids, and the immune/inflammatory response: acute and chronic effects. Ann N Y Acad Sci. 1999;876:1–11.
132. Mastorakos G, Chrousos GP, Weber JS. Recombinant interleukin-6 activates the hypothalamic-pituitary-adrenal axis in humans. J Clin Endocrinol Metab. 1993;77(6):1690–4.
133. Mastorakos G, et al. Hypothalamic-pituitary-adrenal axis activation and stimulation of systemic vasopressin secretion by recombinant interleukin-6 in humans: potential implications for the syndrome of inappropriate vasopressin secretion. J Clin Endocrinol Metab. 1994;79(4):934–9.

134. Dimopoulou I, et al. Hypothalamic-pituitary-adrenal axis dysfunction in critically ill patients with traumatic brain injury: incidence, pathophysiology, and relationship to vasopressor dependence and peripheral interleukin-6 levels. Crit Care Med. 2004;32(2):404–8.
135. Greenwood-Van Meerveld B, et al. Long-term expression of corticotropin-releasing factor (CRF) in the paraventricular nucleus of the hypothalamus in response to an acute colonic inflammation. Brain Res. 2006;1071(1):91–6.
136. Gue M, et al. Stress-induced enhancement of colitis in rats: CRF and arginine vasopressin are not involved. Am J Phys. 1997;272(1 Pt 1):G84–91.
137. Million M, Tache Y, Anton P. Susceptibility of Lewis and Fischer rats to stress-induced worsening of TNB-colitis: protective role of brain CRF. Am J Phys. 1999;276(4):G1027–36.
138. Martinez V, et al. Central injection of a new corticotropin-releasing factor (CRF) antagonist, astressin, blocks CRF- and stress-related alterations of gastric and colonic motor function. J Pharmacol Exp Ther. 1997;280(2):754–60.
139. Huang M, et al. Mast cell deficient W/W(v) mice lack stress-induced increase in serum IL-6 levels, as well as in peripheral CRH and vascular permeability, a model of rheumatoid arthritis. Int J Immunopathol Pharmacol. 2002;15(3):249–54.
140. Huang M, et al. Stress-induced interleukin-6 release in mice is mast cell-dependent and more pronounced in Apolipoprotein E knockout mice. Cardiovasc Res. 2003;59(1):241–9.
141. Mawdsley JE, Rampton DS. Psychological stress in IBD: new insights into pathogenic and therapeutic implications. Gut. 2005;54(10):1481–91.
142. Zhao SB, et al. Corticotropin releasing hormone promotes inflammatory bowel disease via inducing intestinal macrophage autophagy. Cell Death Discov. 2021;7(1):377.
143. Gao X, et al. Chronic stress promotes colitis by disturbing the gut microbiota and triggering immune system response. Proc Natl Acad Sci USA. 2018;115(13):E2960–9.
144. Nakade Y, et al. Restraint stress stimulates colonic motility via central corticotropin-releasing factor and peripheral 5-HT3 receptors in conscious rats. Am J Physiol Gastrointest Liver Physiol. 2007;292(4):G1037–44.
145. Gay J, et al. Corticotropin-releasing hormone deficiency is associated with reduced local inflammation in a mouse model of experimental colitis. Endocrinology. 2008;149(7):3403–9.
146. Bamberger CM, Bamberger AM. The peripheral CRH/urocortin system. Ann N Y Acad Sci. 2000;917:290–6.
147. Meyer WJ 3rd, et al. In vivo immunoreactive adrenocorticotropin (ACTH) production by human mononuclear leukocytes from normal and ACTH-deficient individuals. J Clin Endocrinol Metab. 1987;64(1):98–105.
148. Genedani S, et al. Influence of f-MLP, ACTH(1-24) and CRH on in vitro chemotaxis of monocytes from centenarians. Neuroimmunomodulation. 2008;15(4–6):285–9.
149. Tsagarakis S, Grossman A. Corticotropin-releasing hormone: interactions with the immune system. Neuroimmunomodulation. 1994;1(6):329–34.
150. Theoharides TC, et al. Mast cells as targets of corticotropin-releasing factor and related peptides. Trends Pharmacol Sci. 2004;25(11):563–8.
151. Cao J, et al. Human mast cells express corticotropin-releasing hormone (CRH) receptors and CRH leads to selective secretion of vascular endothelial growth factor. J Immunol. 2005;174(12):7665–75.
152. Rivest S, Rivier C. Stress and interleukin-1 beta-induced activation of c-fos, NGFI-B and CRF gene expression in the hypothalamic PVN: comparison between Sprague-Dawley, Fisher-344 and Lewis rats. J Neuroendocrinol. 1994;6(1):101–17.
153. De Souza EB, et al. Corticotropin-releasing factor (CRF) and interleukin-1 (IL-1) receptors in the brain-pituitary-immune axis. Psychopharmacol Bull. 1989;25(3):299–305.
154. Marquette C, et al. Rat interleukin-1 beta binding sites in rat hypothalamus and pituitary gland. Neuroendocrinology. 1995;62(4):362–9.
155. Sweep F, Rijnkels C, Hermus A. Activation of the hypothalamus-pituitary-adrenal axis by cytokines. Acta Endocrinol. 1991;125(Suppl 1):84–91.

156. Schurmeyer TH, et al. Human corticotropin-releasing factor in man: pharmacokinetic properties and dose-response of plasma adrenocorticotropin and cortisol secretion. J Clin Endocrinol Metab. 1984;59(6):1103–8.
157. Abe R, et al. The role of pituitary-adrenal counterregulation of inflammation in cerulein-induced pancreatitis: a comparison between Fischer and Lewis rats. Pancreas. 1996;12(3):280–5.
158. Sternberg EM, et al. Corticotropin releasing hormone related behavioral and neuroendocrine responses to stress in Lewis and Fischer rats. Brain Res. 1992;570(1–2):54–60.
159. Fecho K, Valtschanoff JG. Acute inflammatory and neuropathic pain in Lewis and Fischer rats. J Neuroendocrinol. 2006;18(7):504–13.
160. Frost P, et al. IL-1 receptor type I gene expression in the amygdala of inflammatory susceptible Lewis and inflammatory resistant Fischer rats. J Neuroimmunol. 2001;121(1–2):32–9.
161. Kosten TA, Ambrosio E. HPA axis function and drug addictive behaviors: insights from studies with Lewis and Fischer 344 inbred rats. Psychoneuroendocrinology. 2002;27(1–2):35–69.
162. Chrousos GP. The hypothalamic-pituitary-adrenal axis and immune-mediated inflammation. N Engl J Med. 1995;332(20):1351–62.
163. Silverman ES, et al. Corticotropin-releasing hormone deficiency increases allergen-induced airway inflammation in a mouse model of asthma. J Allergy Clin Immunol. 2004;114(4):747–54.
164. Shanks N, et al. Alterations in hypothalamic-pituitary-adrenal function correlated with the onset of murine SLE in MRL +/+ and lpr/lpr mice. Brain Behav Immun. 1999;13(4):348–60.
165. Berczi I, Quintanar-Stephano A, Kovacs K. Neuroimmune regulation in immunocompetence, acute illness, and healing. Ann N Y Acad Sci. 2009;1153:220–39.
166. Menke A. Is the HPA Axis as target for depression outdated, or is there a new hope? Front Psych. 2019;10:101.
167. Karling P, et al. Hypothalamus-pituitary-adrenal axis hypersuppression is associated with gastrointestinal symptoms in major depression. J Neurogastroenterol Motil. 2016;22(2):292–303.
168. Hennings JM, et al. Recurrent suicide attempts affect normalization of HPA axis dysregulation after recovery from major depression. Front Psych. 2022;13:937582.
169. Hennings JM, et al. Effects of weariness of life, suicide ideations and suicide attempt on HPA axis regulation in depression. Psychoneuroendocrinology. 2021;131:105286.
170. Rana T, et al. Exploring the role of neuropeptides in depression and anxiety. Prog Neuro-Psychopharmacol Biol Psychiatry. 2022;114:110478.
171. Raadsheer FC, et al. Increased numbers of corticotropin-releasing hormone expressing neurons in the hypothalamic paraventricular nucleus of depressed patients. Neuroendocrinology. 1994;60(4):436–44.
172. Meynen G, et al. Increased arginine vasopressin mRNA expression in the human hypothalamus in depression: a preliminary report. Biol Psychiatry. 2006;60(8):892–5.
173. Bao AM, Meynen G, Swaab DF. The stress system in depression and neurodegeneration: focus on the human hypothalamus. Brain Res Rev. 2008;57(2):531–53.
174. Zhou JN, et al. Alterations in arginine vasopressin neurons in the suprachiasmatic nucleus in depression. Arch Gen Psychiatry. 2001;58(7):655–62.
175. Merali Z, et al. Corticotropin-releasing hormone, arginine vasopressin, gastrin-releasing peptide, and neuromedin B alterations in stress-relevant brain regions of suicides and control subjects. Biol Psychiatry. 2006;59(7):594–602.
176. Pitchot W, et al. Vasopressin-neurophysin and DST in major depression: relationship with suicidal behavior. J Psychiatr Res. 2008;42(8):684–8.
177. Swaab DF, Bao AM, Lucassen PJ. The stress system in the human brain in depression and neurodegeneration. Ageing Res Rev. 2005;4(2):141–94.
178. Tezval H, et al. Cortagine, a specific agonist of corticotropin-releasing factor receptor subtype 1, is anxiogenic and antidepressive in the mouse model. Proc Natl Acad Sci USA. 2004;101(25):9468–73.

179. Myers MG Jr, Olson DP. Central nervous system control of metabolism. Nature. 2012;491(7424):357–63.
180. Kullmann S, et al. Central nervous pathways of insulin action in the control of metabolism and food intake. Lancet Diabetes Endocrinol. 2020;8(6):524–34.
181. Farr S, Taher J, Adeli K. Central nervous system regulation of intestinal lipid and lipoprotein metabolism. Curr Opin Lipidol. 2016;27(1):1–7.
182. Kuo T, et al. Regulation of Glucose Homeostasis by Glucocorticoids. Adv Exp Med Biol. 2015;872:99–126.
183. Vegiopoulos A, Herzig S. Glucocorticoids, metabolism and metabolic diseases. Mol Cell Endocrinol. 2007;275(1–2):43–61.
184. Tache Y, et al. Inhibition of gastric acid secretion in rats by intracerebral injection of corticotropin-releasing factor. Science. 1983;222(4626):935–7.
185. Peckett AJ, Wright DC, Riddell MC. The effects of glucocorticoids on adipose tissue lipid metabolism. Metabolism. 2011;60(11):1500–10.
186. Raff H, Carroll T. Cushing's syndrome: from physiological principles to diagnosis and clinical care. J Physiol. 2015;593(3):493–506.
187. Boscaro M, et al. Cushing's syndrome. Lancet. 2001;357(9258):783–91.
188. Barthel A, et al. An update on addison's disease. Exp Clin Endocrinol Diabetes. 2019;127(2–03):165–75.
189. Lin Y, et al. Hypothalamus-pituitary-adrenal Axis in Glucolipid metabolic disorders. Rev Endocr Metab Disord. 2020;21(4):421–9.
190. Chan O, et al. Diabetes and the hypothalamo-pituitary-adrenal (HPA) axis. Minerva Endocrinol. 2003;28(2):87–102.
191. Sharma VK, Singh TG. Chronic stress and diabetes mellitus: interwoven pathologies. Curr Diabetes Rev. 2020;16(6):546–56.
192. Baritaki S, et al. Chronic stress, inflammation, and colon cancer: a CRH system-driven molecular crosstalk. J Clin Med. 2019;8(10)
193. Tian W, et al. Chronic stress: impacts on tumor microenvironment and implications for anticancer treatments. Front Cell Dev Biol. 2021;9:777018.
194. Vignjevic Petrinovic S, et al. Interplay between stress and cancer-A focus on inflammation. Front Physiol. 2023;14:1119095.
195. Dai S, et al. Chronic stress promotes cancer development. Front Oncol. 2020;10:1492.
196. Chen X, et al. Chronic stress-induced immune dysregulation in breast cancer: Implications of psychosocial factors. J Transl Int Med. 2023;11(3):226–33.
197. Cui B, et al. Stress-induced epinephrine enhances lactate dehydrogenase A and promotes breast cancer stem-like cells. J Clin Invest. 2019;129(3):1030–46.
198. Burgess C. Stress and cancer. Cancer Surv. 1987;6(3):403–16.
199. Gil F, et al. First anxiety, afterwards depression: psychological distress in cancer patients at diagnosis and after medical treatment. Stress Health. 2012;28(5):362–7.
200. Chrobak AA, et al. Bipolar spectrum in prostate cancer patients and its role in stress related symptoms. Psychooncology. 2023;32(3):438–45.
201. Atallah M, et al. Psychological symptoms and stress are associated with decrements in attentional function in cancer patients undergoing chemotherapy. Cancer Nurs. 2020;43(5):402–10.
202. Hou N, et al. A novel chronic stress-induced shift in the Th1 to Th2 response promotes colon cancer growth. Biochem Biophys Res Commun. 2013;439(4):471–6.
203. Peters S, et al. Chronic psychosocial stress increases the risk for inflammation-related colon carcinogenesis in male mice. Stress. 2012;15(4):403–15.
204. Tan HE. The microbiota-gut-brain axis in stress and depression. Front Neurosci. 2023;17:1151478.
205. Cryan JF, et al. The microbiota-gut-brain axis. Physiol Rev. 2019;99(4):1877–2013.

Chapter 2
CRF Peptides in the Periphery

Shengnan Li and Chao Zhu

The finding of corticotropin-releasing hormone (CRH) signaling further promotes the study of biological stress since the stress concept pioneering by Selye [1, 2]. After the identification of central CRH signaling pathways by Vale group [3–5], all corticotropin-releasing hormone (factor) family peptides (CRF peptides, CRFp)'s peripheral presence and functions have been widely studied. The discovery of peripheral CRH is interesting and preludes the wide investigations on all CRFp outside the brain. It is found by Hargreaves et al. that pituitary corticotroph secretion of β-endorphin can be either caused by hypothalamic CRH or by a tissue factor from the periphery in response to stressors. Rats' inflamed tissue is observed to release a factor, evoking pituitary secretion of β-endorphin, which is independent of the afferent input with the inability of the hindlimb denervation to block the effect. Also, the subcutaneous perfusates stimulate β-endorphin release in cultured pituitary cells [6]. By analyzing human tissues, it is found that CRH outside the brain is identical to hypothalamic CRH [7]. Afterward, the existence and role of peripheral CRFp have attracted wide attention [8]. Mammalian CRFp include four members, CRH, urocortin (UCN1), UCN2, and UCN3, signaling through two distinct CRF receptors (CRFr) belonging to B1 G protein-coupled receptor (GPCR) types, CRF_1 and/or CRF_2, to modulate a range of peripheral activities [8–12]. This chapter mainly focuses on the structures of CRFp and their overall distributions in important systems including the digestive, cardiovascular, immune/inflammatory, and reproductive system.

S. Li (✉) · C. Zhu
Department of Pharmacology, School of Basic Medical Sciences,
Nanjing Medical University, Nanjing, Jiangsu, China
e-mail: snli@njmu.edu.cn

© The Author(s), under exclusive license to Springer Nature Singapore Pte Ltd. 2025

C. Zhu et al. (eds.), *The Peripheral Existence and Effects of Corticotropin-releasing Factor Family*, https://doi.org/10.1007/978-981-96-5322-5_2

1 Structure of CRF Peptides

The four members of mammalian CRFp have similar peptide chains while they have distinct features [13]. Structure-activity relationship studies support that CRFp show differences in binding affinities, receptor selectivity (for CRF_1 or CRF_2), and nuclear magnetic resonance (NMR) structure [13, 14]. CRFp have common α-helical backbones, with a small kink or a turn-around residues 25–27, resulting in a helix-loop-helix motif. The C-terminal helices are amphipathic, whereas the N-terminal helices have a variety of amphipathicity. Moreover, the C-terminal helices assume a conformation bound to the receptor. And both the C-terminal and N-terminal helices may play a crucial role in ligand-receptor activities, the former interacting along their hydrophobic faces for binding the receptor and the latter being involved in receptor activation. Common and divergent features observed in the 3D structures of CRFp multiple binding models are also proposed, likely explaining their plurality of actions [15, 16].

1.1 The Structure of CRH

1.1.1 The Primary Structure of CRH

CRH is a **41**-amino acid (AA) peptide first purified from sheep hypothalamic extracts, which is observed to have high potency and intrinsic activity for stimulating the secretion of adrenocorticotropin (ACTH)-like and β-endorphin-like peptides in cultured anterior pituitary [3]. Later CRH's wide existence in the periphery is observed [4], which is identical to the hypothalamic CRH in structure and plays significant roles in digestive, cardiovascular, immune and reproductive system, etc. [7].

As shown in Table 2.1, the primary structure of the extracted ovine (sheep) 41-AA residue CRH (oCRH, ACTH- and β-endorphin-releasing molecule) is proposed and determined to be H-Ser-Gln-Glu-Pro-Pro-Ile-Ser-Leu-Asp-Leu-Thr-Phe-His-Leu-Leu-Arg-Glu-Val-Leu-Glu-Met-Thr-Lys-Ala-Asp-Gln-Leu-Ala-Gln-Gln-Ala-His-Ser-Asn-Arg-Lys-Leu-Leu-Asp-Ile-Ala-NH_2 [3], which shows more than 90% homology with the human/ rat CRH (h/rCRH) [3, 17]. Supporting the

Table 2.1 The primary structure of CRH in different species [17]

Species	Amino-acids sequence
Human/ Rat	Ser-Glu-Glu-Pro-Pro-Ile-Ser-Leu-Asp-Leu-Thr-Phe-His-Leu-Leu-Arg-Glu-Val-Leu-Glu-Met-Ala-Arg-Ala-Glu-Gln-Leu-Ala-Gln-Gln-Ala-His-Ser-Asn-Arg-Lys-Leu-Met-Glu-Ile-Ile
Sheep	Ser-Gln-Glu-Pro-Pro-Ile-Ser-Leu-Asp-Leu-Thr-Phe-His-Leu-Leu-Arg-Glu-Val-Leu-Glu-Met-Thr-Arg-Ala-Glu-Gln-Leu-Ala-Gln-Gln-Ala-His-Ser-Asn-Arg-Lys-Leu-Met-Asp-Ile-Ala

Reprinted with permission from Elsevier

analytical proposal, the synthetic replicate of CRH, according to this AA sequence, is observed to be highly potent in stimulating secretion of both ACTH and beta-endorphin-like immunoactivities in vitro [3] and in vivo [18, 19].

The ovine CRH precursor (o-pre-proCRH)' nucleotide sequence of the cloned cDNA reveals the primary structure of it [20]. Then, the primary structure of human CRH precursor (h-pre-proCRH) is analyzed through using a number of computer algorithms to identify the areas of highest predicted antigenicity by Gastro Group [21]. Six areas of high predicted antigenicity are identified in h-pre-proCRH, with two areas corresponding almost exactly to the two putative cleavage sites of the prohormone, and a third one lying within the C-terminal region of the tested product of post-translational processing of the prohormone, i.e., CRH (1–41). Experimental cross-reactivity data indicate that a number of structural factors such as omega loops and peptide conformation are involved in recognition of peptide fragments by antibodies [21]. These results are consistent with the data obtained from studies of antibodies produced in rabbits by immunizing with h-pre-proCRH [22].

The exact AA composition of canine CRH is predicted from the partial sequence of the gene encoding canine CRH by Meloen and colleagues. The CRH gene is amplified from genomic DNA of white blood cells by a polymerase chain reaction (PCR) and subsequently sequenced by using the dideoxy method, resulting in the identical structure to that of human, rat, and equine CRH. Immunological tools confirm the existence of the highest cross-reactivity of a canine hypothalamus extract, known to have a high content of CRH, with antisera directed against h/rCRH [23]. In addition, hamster CRH is also successfully cloned and displays a high sequence similarity to rCRH (unlike hamster UCN1 (see below)) [24], which might be related to the finding that hamsters have a similar distribution of CRH-positive neurons and fibers in hypothalamus to that of rats [25].

1.1.2 The Secondary and 3D Structures of CRH

It is proved that α-helical conformation is important for the recognition and binding of the CRH to CRFr, and stability and content of α-helicity in the structure contribute greatly to its taking effects [26–28], which is supported by the fact that the connection of two existing segregated receptor binding sites at the N and C termini of CRH is essential for its receptor binding and activation, and the connection by an appropriate α-helical linker results in CRH analogs of higher potency [29].

In the laboratory of Darbon and colleagues, the NMR structure of hCRH is determined by proton NMR in a mixed-solvent system of 66% trifluoroethanol (TFE)/34% H_2O at pH 3.8 and 37 °C with complete resonance assignment achieved by using standard two-dimensional methods. The structure of hCRH in this TFE solvent is shown to comprise an extended N-terminal tetrapeptide connected to a well-defined α-helix between residues 6 and 36. It is observed that the first half of the α-helix (residues 6–20) is clearly amphipathic. And the five C-terminal residues are predominantly disordered [30]. Vale and colleagues report that the substitution of His-32 in the oCRH with Ala brings about a four-fold increase in activity [31]. Kim group determine the secondary structure of this Ala-substituted oCRH ([Ala32]oCRH) in the α-helix formation stabilizing TFE solution using circular dichroism (CD) and MR techniques, the results showing that the α-helical structure extends to the C-terminus of oCRH [14]. By further analyzing the C-αH and NH chemical shifts, it is found that oCRH and [Ala32]oCRH have stable α-helical structures in the middle region. However, [Ala32]oCRH displays a more stable α-helical structure than oCRH in the vicinity of the substitution region, which may be the cause of the increased activity of [Ala32]oCRH [14]. Loquet et al. obtain the 3D structure of the microcrystalline model protein CRH derived from solid-state NMR distance restraints for fully labeled protein samples. By proton-mediated rare-spin correlation spectra and carbon-13 spin diffusion experiments, enough short, medium, and long-range structural restraints are provided to get high-resolution structures of the dimeric CRH protein. In addition, because of the ambiguities in resonance assignments induced by the restraints preventing 3D structure determination, an automated iterative assignment algorithm is implemented in a dedicated solid-state NMR version (as shown in Fig. 2.1), permitting to resolve the majority of ambiguities and to calculate a de novo 3D structure [32].

Moreover, the differences between oCRH and hCRH in their conformational properties are also found by CD, spectroscopy, NMR, and dynamic light scattering. oCRH is observed to exist as a monomer in dilute aqueous solution while association at concentrations higher than 10^{-3} mol/L results predominantly in dimers. hCRH exhibits a high tendency of association highly sensitive to the pH value and the tetramers' formation at millimolar concentration is related to a helical content of about 50%. Furthermore, the potentially helical, highly hydrophobic region enlarged by more hydrophobic residues 23 and 25 is proposed to stabilize the hCRH

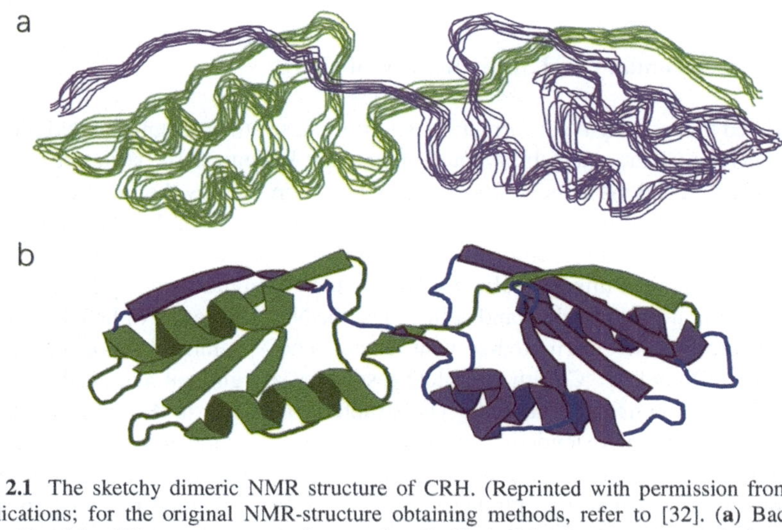

Fig. 2.1 The sketchy dimeric NMR structure of CRH. (Reprinted with permission from ACS Publications; for the original NMR-structure obtaining methods, refer to [32]. (**a**) Backbone ensemble of the 10 lowest energy conformers (bundle-like) of the dimer structure calculated from solid-state NMR data; (**b**) Dimer structure of CRH protein)

associates. In TFE solution, both oCRH and hCRH exist as monomers, oCRH revealing about 72% helicity and hCRH about 85% located in the C-terminal heptapeptide [33]. The higher content in helicity of hCRH may explain, at least to some extent, its higher affinity to the receptors (CRFr), CRH antibodies and CRF-binding protein, and hence different levels of actions compared to oCRH [33–35].

1.1.3 The Synthesized CRH and Analogs

CRH and a series of CRH analogs are successfully synthesized and the synthetic CRH and analogs are active both in vitro and in vivo [36, 37].

The synthetic form of CRH, corticorelin acetate (CrA), is found to exert antiangiogenic effects in vivo, with a very high efficacy either as a single agent or in combination with the antiangiogenic agent, bevacizumab, in three different patient-derived human brain tumor xenografts in athymic mice. Single use of CrA significantly increases the lifespan of mice in the tumor xenograft models while its use in combination with bevacizumab has a better therapeutic outcome [36].

Peptide analogs of CRH can be synthesized by substitution of residues, deletion of the residues, and introduction of lactam rings (or combined ways) in CRH chain (for both CRFr agonists and antagonists, also see Chap. 3), changing the secondary structure while not hindering receptor recognition and binding, such as cyclo(30–33) [Ac-Leu8,DPhe12,Nle21, Glu30,Lys33,Nle38]hCRH(8–41) and cyclo(30–33) [Ac-Pro4,D-Phe2,Nle21,38,Glu30,Lys33]r/hCRH-(4–41) [28, 37–41], and the activity being based on the α-helical conformational structure pattern [4]. Predictive methods and physicochemical measurements indicate that CRH exhibits an internal secondary α-helical conformation spanning about 25 residues and by maximization of α-helix-forming potential through AA substitutions from the native known sequences (r/hCRH and oCRH), much more potent analogs than the parent peptides can be obtained in vitro [4, 39]. On the other hand, replacement of AA residues 12 and 15 by nonprotein AA d-phenylalanine and α-aminoisobutyric acid from r/hCRH, respectively, results in an analog of no activity, since the substitutions seem to perturb the elements of the native 35-residue helix [38]. Moreover, certain N-terminally shortened fragments (by AA residue deletion), such as α-helical CRH (α-helCRH(9–41) or oCRH(8–41), oCRH(9–41) and oCRH(10–41), are found to be competitive CRH inhibitors in vitro and in vivo [4]. Consistently, fragments of hCRH, CRH (6–33) and CRH (9–33), have high affinity for the CRH-modulating molecule (CRF-binding protein), being able to reverse the molecule-inhibited ACTH secretion in vitro [42]. Furthermore, different truncated and conformationally constrained analogs of CRH are synthesized on the basis of the AA sequences of h/rCRH and oCRH and tested for their ability to displace [^{125}I-Tyr0]oCRH or [^{125}I-Tyr0]Sauvagine (Svg) from membrane homogenates of HEK 293 cells stably transfected with cDNA coding for $rCRF_1$, or mouse CRF_2 ($mCRF_2$), resulting in a potent and selective $mCRF_2$ antagonist, [DPhe11, His12] Svg(11–40), named anti-Svg-30 (aSvg30) [43], based on which more aSvg30 analogs are further synthesized with binding ability to CRF_1 or CRF_2 [44].

It is noteworthy that many efforts in CRF system research result in huge amount of data, yet much more work is needed for identifying and marketing diagnostic or therapeutic CRFp and small molecule ligands [45]. CRH binding to its selective receptor (CRF_1) is an important target in drug discovery aiming to develop lead compounds with the potential to treat various disorders [46–48]. Besides the shortened derivatives of CRH such as α-helical-CRH(9–41), several non-peptide CRF_1 antagonists are developed, including CP154526, Antalarmin and NBI27914, which compete with CRH and are frequently used for research or clinical trials [49–51] (see Chap. 3). And more compounds showing promising CRF_1 receptor affinity are developed [52]. For action mechanisms, CRH binding to CRF_1 is associated with adenyl cyclase (AC), leading to cAMP production [53, 54]. Moreover, the mitogen-activated protein kinase extracellular signal-related kinase 1/2 (ERK1/2) is also reported to be implicated in CRH signaling through CRF_1 [55].

1.1.4 CRH Modulation by CRF-Binding Protein

CRH is modulated by a 37-kDa CRF-binding protein (CRF-BP), CRF-BP cDNAs encoding proteins of **322** AA with one putative signal sequence, one N-glycosylation site, and 10 conserved cysteines [42]. CRH binds to CRF-BP, which is a secreted binding protein smaller than CRFr but binds CRH with an equal or greater affinity, blocking CRH-mediated ACTH release in vitro [56]. The binding requirements of CRFr and CRF-BP can be distinguished in that hCRH fragments, such as hCRH (6–33) and hCRH (9–33), have high affinity for CRF-BP but low affinity for CRFr [42, 57]. In human plasma, CRF-BP is reported to bind CRH preventing from its action on the receptor and proposed to prevent inappropriate pituitary-adrenal stimulation in pregnancy [58]. Actually, an inverse correlation between reduced plasma CRF-BP and increased CRH levels in the maternal circulation is observed during pregnancy [59]. And in post-term, maternal plasma CRH levels are significantly lower while CRF-BP significantly higher than in term pregnancies [60].

Vale group isolate, sequence, clone, and characterize the cDNAs of CRF-BP from human liver and rat brain (hCRF-BP, rCRF-BP). Expression of the cDNAs for h/r CRF-BP in COS-7 cells shows that the recombinant CRF-BP binds CRH with the same affinity as the native human protein, inhibiting CRH-induced ACTH release by pituitary cells in vitro [57]. While cloning human and mouse CRF-BP (mCRF-BP), they further find that the protein is mapped to the distal region of chromosome 13 and loci 5q in the mouse and human genomes, respectively. The gene consists of 7 exons and 6 introns, and the mature protein has 10 cysteines and 5 tandem disulfide bridges, the first 3 AA being coded for by an extreme 5′ exon [61]. Moreover, this group also cloned a sheep CRF-BP (oCRF-BP) from sheep brain, with both native o/rCRF-BP and recombinant rCRF-BP being shown to be N-glycosylated. Two native forms of oCRF-BPs (33 and 35 kDa) are purified from sheep brain homogenates, the 35 kDa protein proteolytically cleaved near the N-terminus producing a 33 kDa CRF-BP. Functionally, both of the oCRF-BPs can be specifically cross-linked to ^{125}I-oCRH and ^{125}I-hCRH. In contrast, the recombinant rCRF-BP can only be cross-linked to ^{125}I-hCRH. Furthermore, a 1.7 kb cDNA clone encoding a **324** AA CRF-BP precursor is cloned from a sheep brain lambda gtlO cDNA library, having 85% and 87% AA homology to the r/hCRF-BP, respectively. Interestingly, the recombinant oCRF-BP expressed in CHO cells bind to both hCRH and oCRH, the affinity being approximately 50-fold higher for the former [62]. In addition, CRF-BP existence is found to differentiate in species. In horse plasma, CRH shows no elevation in maternal peripheral serum in late gestation, and there is no evidence for a plasma CRF-BP analogous to that found in human plasma in either peripheral blood from normal or pregnant horses [63].

The pharmaceutical potential of CRF-BP inhibitors has caught much attention [64]. Several regions of CRF-BP expression colocalize with sites of CRH secretion suggesting that CRF-BP may have a profound impact on the biological activity of CRH. Linton et al. first use CRF-BP purified from human plasma to investigate its influence on the physiological activity of CRH. It is observed that the purified CRF-BP reduces ACTH-releasing activity of synthetic hCRH dose-dependently and co-use of hCRH and CRF-BP causes an average 76% reduction in ACTH release. The suppressing effect is indirectly confirmed by that the co-use of oCRH and CRF-BP has no effect since oCRH does not bind to CRF-BP [56]. For investigation on the in vivo role of this modulatory protein, animal models of CRF-BP overexpression or deficiency are developed, which show numerous physiological changes in body responses, parallel with the levels of unbound ("free") CRH and related peptides [65–68]. CRF-BP is strongly conserved throughout evolution (existing in invertebrate and vertebrate species) [69], suggesting the maintenance of a structural conformation in N-terminus necessary for biological activity [70, 71]. While the function of CRF-BP is thought to be primarily inhibitory, some studies indicate that novel functional roles may exist [71]. And as described above, hCRH(6–33) and CRH(9–33) may become useful approaches for CRF-BP relevant states due to their high binding affinity [42]. A more complete understanding of the central and peripheral functions of CRF-BP will help elucidate its potential role in the etiology or treatment of disorders of CRH dysregulation.

1.2 The Structure of Urocortin (UCN1)

1.2.1 The Primary Structure of UCN1

After urotensin I [72], sauvagine [73] and CRH precursor [74, 75] are discovered in fish and amphibians (see Chap. 9), UCN1 is identified in mammalians, which is more closely related to CRH. Human, sheep, rat, and mouse UCN1 possess a **40**-AA sequence [76–79].

Vanghan et al. characterize a mammalian member of CRFp and clone-related cDNAs from a rat midbrain region, which they name urocortin (rat UCN1, rUCN1).

The peptide is related to CRH with 45% sequence identity [76]. A positive clone determined to encode human UCN1 (hUCN1) is obtained from a low stringency hybridization screen of a human genomic library with a probe encoding the mature peptide region of rUCN1. The nucleotide sequence for hUCN1 encodes a 123 AA protein composed of a 79 AA precursor and a putative 40 AA mature peptide. The putative mature 40 AA hUCN1 peptide has 88% identity to rUCN1 at the nucleotide level and 95% identity at the AA level. UCN1 is a potent ligand for both CRF_1 and CRF_2 [77].

The mouse UCN1 (mUCN1) and hUCN1 genes are very similar in structures, having two exons with the entire coding region located in the second exon, as is the case for mouse CRH [78, 80]. Sequence analyses of the mUCN1 and hUCN1 genes also reveal the presence of Mpv17 in the 5′ region upstream of the gene. Functional studies following transient transfection of UCN1 reporter plasmids in PC12 cells show that mUCN1 promoter is controlled by both positive and negative elements, which is important for basal activity as well as responsiveness to forskolin stimulation [78].

In Vale's laboratory, an 18-kb sheep genomic DNA fragment encoding UCN1 is isolated by the hybridization screening of a lambda phage library with a probe generated from rUCN1 cDNA. The sheep clone contains a region that is 83 ~ 84% and 88% homologous to the coding region of rUCN1 and hUCN1, respectively, encoding an ovine UCN1 (oUCN1) identical to the rUCN1 [79]. Competitive binding assays show that the oUCN1 has a high affinity and is the principal ligand for the sheep CRF-BP in ovine brain. Moreover, localization studies by in situ hybridization indicate that the distribution of oUCN1 mRNA in sheep brain is similar to that of rUCN1 in rat brain [79, 81].

Hamster UCN1 mature peptide is found with some difference. Although the deduced hamster CRH AA sequence and cleavage site is identical to that in rat, the UCN1 AA sequence is unique in possessing Asn and Ala in positions 38 and 39, respectively. Moreover, compared to urotensin-1 and sauvagine, the hamster UCN1 C-terminus sequence shows greater similarity in structure to the insect diuretic hormones (DH, see Chap. 9), suggesting either retrogressive mutational changes within the mature peptide or convergent sequence evolution. Regardless of the differences, human and hamster UCN1 are generally equipotent at AC activation resulting in cAMP production, neuronal acidification rate, and CRFr affinities [24]. Moreover, hamster melanoma cells are demonstrated to express UCN1gene, sequencing of which being confirmed identical with the known sequence of the UCN1 gene [82].

The above findings demonstrate that, even across diverse species, UCN1 is highly conserved with respect to its structure and pharmacology, which is different from CRH where significant AA substitutions between the rat/human and sheep peptides may underlie differences in functional regulation [79]. The AA sequences of UCN1 in different species are shown in Table 2.2 [17, 83].

Table 2.2 The primary structure of urocortin (UCN1) [17]

Species	Amino acid sequence
Human	Asp-Asn-Pro-Ser-Leu-Ser-Ile-Asp-Leu-Thr-Phe-His-Leu-Leu-Arg-Thr-Leu-Leu-Glu-Leu-Ala-Arg-Thr-Gln-Ser-Gln-Arg-Glu-Arg-Ala-Glu-Gln-Asn-Arg-Ile-Ile-Phe-Asp-Ser-Val
Mouse/Rat/Sheep	Asp-Asn-Pro-pro-Leu-Ser-Ile-Asp-Leu-Thr-Phe-His-Leu-Leu-Arg-Thr-Leu-Leu-Glu-Leu-Ala-Arg-Thr-Gln-Ser-Gln-Arg-Glu-Arg-Ala-Glu-Gln-Asn-Arg-Ile-Ile-Phe-Asp-Ser-Val

Reprinted with permission from Elsevier

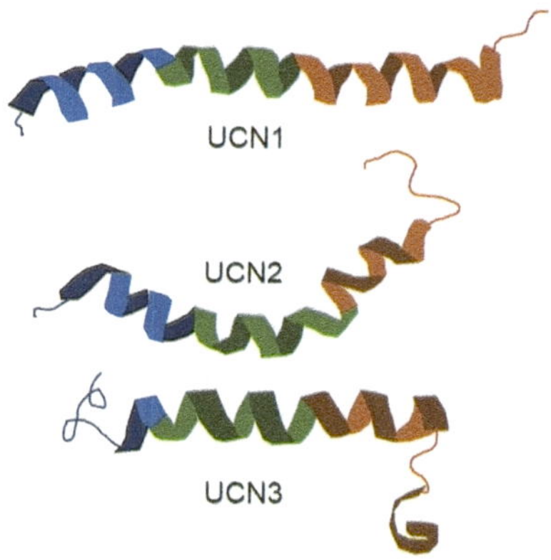

Fig. 2.2 The sketchy NMR structures of UCN1, UCN2 and UCN3 [15, 16] (Reprinted with permission from ACS Publications + open access; methods used for the image obtaining of each peptide are similar to those for determining CRH NMR structures (Fig. 2.1), as depicted in the original article [15], i.e., 20 energy-minimized conformers are like a bundle, and the conformers with the lowest target function are used to represent the NMR structure)

1.2.2 The Secondary and 3D Structures of UCN1

As described above, the α-helical conformation is common among CRFp including UCNs (UCN1, UCN2, and UCN3) and crucial to the binding and activity [15, 26–28]. The α-helical backbones are with a small kink or a turn-around residues 25–27, resulting in a helix-loop-helix motif, with C-terminal helices being of amphipathic nature assuming a conformation bound to CRFr and N-terminal helices differing in the amphipathicity determining activities [15, 84]. The common and divergent features observed in the NMR structures of UCN1, UCN2, and UCN3 in DMSO are as shown in Fig. 2.2 [15, 16].

1.2.3 UCN1 Modulation by CRF-BP

CRF-BP binds UCN1 with high affinity in the same range as for CRH. Co-incubation with CRP-BP prevents the release of ACTH by UCN1. Biologically inactive CRH fragments such as hCRH(9–33), which interfere with the binding ability of CRF-BP to CRH [85], can also restore the UCN1 effect [77, 86].

Functionally, UCN1 has equal affinity for CRF_1 and CRF_2 (both are class B GPCR with Gs) associated with AC activation [13, 77]. It is observed to be potent in inducing intracellular cAMP accumulation in CHO cells stably transfected with CRF_1 and CRF_2 and in stimulating ACTH secretion from rat anterior pituitary cells in vitro [77]. Also, UCN1 can stimulate myometrial mitogen-activated protein kinase MAPK via induction of the Gq/phospholipase C/inositol triphosphates (IP3)/protein kinase C (PKC) pathway, whereas CRH-induced activation of this pathway appears to be insufficient to achieve MAPK activation. The CRF_1 and $CRF_{2\beta}$ are observed to mediate UCN1-induced MAPK activation associated with activation of Gq instead of Gs. UCN1 is 10 times more potent than CRH on Gq activation [87].

1.3 The Structure of UCN2

1.3.1 The Primary Structure

UCN2 is also known as stresscopin-related peptide (SCR), selectively acting on CRF_2 [13, 88].

Like isoforms of UCN1 and UCN3, UCN2 is cloned at the Salk Institute from human and mouse cDNA libraries [89–91]. Searches of the public human genome database identify a region with significant sequence homology to the CRFp. By using homologous primers deduced from the human sequence, a mouse cDNA is isolated from whole brain poly(A)(+) RNA encoding a predicted **38**-AA peptide, structurally related to CRH and UCN1. UCN2 binds selectively to CRF_2, with no appreciable activity on CRF_1. Transcripts encoding UCN2 are expressed in discrete regions of the rodent central nervous system, eliciting activation responses [90]. At the same time, a group of researchers elsewhere identify a similar peptide, which is named stresscopin-related peptide (SCR, homologous with UCN2) [91]. The SCR is found to be discretely expressed in the central nervous system with a pattern distinct from CRH, UCN1, and UCN3 pathways [91].

The structure of UCN2 precursor gene predicts a 38-AA mature peptide [90], although the existence of N-terminally extended peptide of 43 AA in length is also postulated [91]. Since the human and mouse homologues of the precursor are less conserved in the extended N terminus than in the remaining sequence, it seems more likely that UCN2 exists as a 38-AA peptide. Furthermore, the 38- and 43-AA ligands possess similar pharmacological potencies, also supporting the 38 AA version of UCN2 since CRFp rapidly lose agonistic potency upon N-terminal truncation [4, 44]. The AA sequences of UCN2 in different species are as listed in Table 2.3.

Chae et al. clone rat UCN2 (rUCN2) cDNA from rat mid-brain by RT-PCR. The rUCN2 clone contains an open reading frame coding 109 AA which shares 90% and 63% homology with mouse and human homologues, respectively. The

Table 2.3 The primary structures of UCN2 in different species [17]

Species	Amino acid sequences
Human	Ile-Val-Leu-Ser-Leu-Asp-Val-Pro-Ile-Gly-Leu-Leu-Gln-Ile-Leu-Leu-Glu-Gln-Ala-Arg-Ala-Arg-Ala-Ala-Arg-Glu-Gln-Ala-Thr-Thr-N-Ala-Arg-Ile-Leu-Ala-Arg-Val (SRP) His-Pro-Gly-Ser-Arg-Ile-Val-Leu-Ser-Leu-Asp-Val-Pro-Ile-Gly-Leu-Leu-Gln-Ile-Leu-Leu-Glu-Gln-Ala-Arg-Ala-Arg-Ala-Ala-Arg-Glu-Gln-Ala-Thr-Thr-Asn-Ala-Arg-Ile-Leu-Ala-Arg-Val
Mouse	Val-Ile-Leu-Ser-Leu-Asp-Val-Pro-Ile-Gly-Leu-Leu-Arg-Ile-Leu-Leu-Glu-Gln-Ala-Arg-Tyr-Lys-Ala-Ala-Arg-Asn-Gln-Ala-Ala-Thr-Asn-Ala-Gln-Ile-Leu-Ala-His-Val
Rat	Val-Ile-Leu-Ser-Leu-Asp-Val-Pro-Ile-Gly-Leu-Leu-Arg-Ile-Leu-Leu-Glu-Gln-Ala-Arg-Asn-Lys-Ala-Ala-Arg-Asn-Gln-Ala-Ala-Thr-Asn-Ala-Gln-Ile-Leu-Ala-Arg-Val
Sheep	Val-Ile-Leu-Ser-Leu-Asp-Val-Pro-Ile-Gly-Leu-Leu-Arg-Ile-Leu-Leu-Glu-Gln-Ala-Arg-Tyr-Lys-Ala-Ala-Arg-Asp-Gln-Ala-Ala-Thr-Asn-Ala-Gln-Ile-Leu-Ala-His-Val

Reprinted with permission from Elsevier

expression of UCN2 mRNA is mainly distributed in bone marrow, ovary, uterus, hypophysis, adrenal gland, and skin. Rat recombinant UCN2 is expressed in *E. coli* and purified in active form. It is observed that the purified recombinant UCN2 specifically binds to CRF_2 in rat ROS 17/2.8 and GH3 cells by flow-cytometry analysis [92]. Furthermore, Vale group report the identifying of mouse UCN2 (mUCN2) and human UCN2 (hUCN2) by molecular cloning strategies, postulating the primary AA sequence of their mature forms by analogy to closely related members of CRFp. The primary structures are assigned using a combination of Edman degradation sequencing and mass spectrometry. For mUCN2, transduced cells are observed to secrete a 39 AA peptide and the glycosylated prohormone lacking signal peptide. Posttranslational cleavage and C-terminal amidation yield the peptides potent to activate CRF_2, consistent with cleavage of mUCN2 prohormone to a mature form in murine tissue extracts. However, hUCN2 undergoes different posttranslational processes over an 88-AA glycosylated prohormone not amidated at the C-terminus [93].

1.3.2 The Secondary and 3D Structures of UCN2

As precedingly described, the α-helical structure is the backbone of UCN2 [84]. Moreover, like CRH and UCN1 [3, 76], UCN2 possesses biological activity only when it is C-terminally amidated, which might contribute to the amphipathic nature of C-terminal helices [91, 93, 94]. Therefore, compared to the primary structure of UCN2, the secondary structure rather than linear sequence homology most likely determines difference of its biological activity from that of other CRFp [90, 91, 95].

NMR structure of UCN2 in DMSO is as described above in Sect. 1.2.2) [15, 16] (Fig. 2.2).

1.3.3 UCN2 Modification by CRF-BP

UCN2 is also reported to be modulated by CRF-BP. Using chimeric peptides for a structure-affinity relationship study, it is observed that mUCN2 but not mUCN3 has a high affinity for rat CRF-BP [96], indicating UCN2 level may also be impacted by CRF-BP. However, there are not very much additional data adding to this evidence.

1.4 The Structure of UCN3

1.4.1 The Primary Structure

UCN3, also known as stresscopin (SCP), selectively binds to CRF_2 [13].

By searching the public human genome databases, a partial expressed sequence tagged (EST) clone with significant sequence identity to UCN1 is found by Lewis and colleagues. By using primers based on the human EST sequence, a full-length human clone is isolated from genomic DNA encoding a protein including a predicted putative 38-AA peptide (hUCN3) structurally related to other CRFp. Moreover, with a human probe, a mouse ortholog is then cloned from a genomic library (mUCN3). Human and mouse UCN3 share 90% identity [89]. Almost at the same time range, HSU et al. successfully identify human SCP specifically binding to CRF_2. The genes encoding UCN3 are expressed in diverse peripheral tissues and CNS, exerting multiple functions [91]. The AA sequences of UCN3 in different species are as listed in Table 2.4 [17].

1.4.2 The Secondary and 3D Structures of UCN3

UCN3 shares common α-helical backbones of CRFp, both the C-terminal and N-terminal helices playing a crucial part in receptor binding and selectivity [15, 16]. The 3D architecture of CRF_2-peptide-binding site and binding of the α-helical

Table 2.4 The primary structures of UCN3 in different species [17]

Species	Amino acid sequences
Human	Thr-Lys-Phe-Thr-Leu-Ser-Leu-Asp-Val-Pro-Thr-Asn-Ieu-Met-Asn-Leu-Leu-Phe-Asn-Ile-Ala-Lys-Ala-Lys-Asn-Leu-Arg-Ala-Gln-Ala-Ala-Ala-Asn-Ala-His-Leu-Met-Ala-Gln-Ile Thr-Lys-Phe-Thr-Leu-Ser-Leu-Asp-Val-Pro-Thr-Asn-Ile-Met-Asn-Leu-Leu-Phe-Asn-Ile-Ala-Lys-Ala-Lys-Asn-Leu-Arg-Ala-Gln-Ala-Ala-Ala-Asn-Ala-His-Leu-Met-Ala-Gln-Ile (SCP)
Mouse	Thr-Lys-Phe-Thr-Leu-Ser-Leu-Asp-Val-Pro-Thr-Asn-Ile-Met-Asn-Leu-Leu-Phe-Asn-Ile-Asp-Lys-Ala-Lys-Asn-Leu-Arg-Ala-Lys-Ala-Ala-Ala-Asn-Ala-Gln-Leu-Met-Ala-Gln-Ile

Reprinted with permission from Elsevier

UCNs are similar to those of CRF_1-CRH with only a single AA difference in the receptors (CRF_1 Glu104/$CRF_{2\alpha}$ Pro-100) at a site proximate to peptide residue 35 (Arg in CRH/UCN1, Ala in UCN2/3). CRF_1 Glu-104 acts as a selectivity filter preventing UCN2/3 binding because the nonpolar Ala-35 is incompatible with the negatively charged Glu-104 [97]. Moreover, on the basis of secondary structure predictions, it is hypothesized and then confirmed that the AA motifs Pro-Ile-Gly of mUCN2 and Pro-Thr-Asn of mUCN3 decrease α-helicity and thereby impair binding to CRF_1 whereas binding affinity to CRF_2 is not affected, correlated with a decrease in alpha-helicity as indicated by the data of CD spectroscopy [96]. NMR structure of UCN3 is shown as in Fig. 2.2 [15, 16].

1.4.3 UCN3 Modulation by CRF-BP

Rare is reported on UCN3's modulation by CRF-BP. A negative result is presented as described above, i.e., UCN3 has no significant affinity for CRF-BP [96].

2 Peripheral Presence and Functions of CRF Peptides

CRFp are expressed along with CRFr at diverse sites in the periphery, including digestive, cardiovascular, immune/inflammatory, reproductive system, and tumors, playing significant roles in different functions in mammals [13, 98–102]. For instance, it is observed that UCN1 can bind to all three subtypes of CRFr (CRF_1, $CRF_{2\alpha}$, and $CRF_{2\beta}$) in the periphery and plays important roles, as described separately in the relevant systems as follows.

In digestive system, CRFp are widely expressed, in pancreas, liver, gastrointestinal (GI) tract, local immune/inflammatory cells, and enteric nervous system (ENS), participating in digestive functions (insulin secretion, motility, etc.) and some pathological states (colitis, colon cancer, etc.) [103–107]. CRH is shown to occur in endocrine cells of the pancreas, GI tract, and the liver functioning via CRF_1 [108, 109]. UCN1 is also found widely distributed in digestive system [83], including pancreas, liver, upper and lower GI tract, and enteric neurons [110]. Besides UCN3's presence in CNS mediating food intake [111], UCN3 is observed to express in pancreatic beta-cells and in a mouse beta-cell line, MIN6, whose secretion and effects are blocked by a CRF_2 antagonist, astressin2B [112]. Experiments in UCN3-null mice and UCN3-negative beta cells reveal that UCN3 is an excellent mature beta cell marker but not necessary for beta cell maturation [113]. In GI tract, UCN1, 2, and 3 and CRF_2 mRNA are observed to prominently express in various layers of the rat upper gut [114]. Furthermore, transcripts of UCNs and the most common CRF_2 isoform in the periphery, $CRF_{2\beta}$, are detected in all layers in rat colon, including myenteric neurons. Moreover, in a status of inflammation, UCNs/CRF_2 are found in all colonic layers, playing a role in dampening acute inflammatory response [115].

Moreover, CRH and UCNs exist in enteric nervous system exerting their effects on GI tract motility in guinea pig colon [116, 117], suggesting the peripheral CRFp neuron-influencing effects, although exogenous CRH is also observed to stimulate rat colonic secretory-motor function via CNS CRF_1 [118].

CRFp (mainly UCNs) are found to express and play a significant role in cardiovascular system (CVS), acting on CVS itself, and/or via suppressing the renin-angiotensin system (RAS) and influencing the sympathetic nervous system (SNS) [9]. Co-localization of UCN1 and $CRF_{2\beta}$ in the heart and vasculature is shown [100, 119]. UCNs are observed to mainly exert cardiovascular protecting effects such as vasodilation, positive inotropic and lusitropic effects, as well as cardioprotection against ischemia-reperfusion (I/R) injury via CRF_2, supported by the fact that cardiomyocytes isolated from CRF_2-null mice are less resistant to I/R injury [120–122]. UCN1 expression is increased in the ventricles of patients with failing hearts [123] and dysfunctional rat hearts [124], which may account for its complementary role of causing vasodilation and enhancing cardiac functions. Parallelly, in ovine experimental heart failure, UCN1 is found to reduce cardiac preload and afterload increasing cardiac output and inhibit vasopressin, endothelin, and renin-angiotensin-aldosterone axis [123]. UCN2 is also observed to express in heart and show promising therapeutic effects on heart failure as well in mice [125]. Circulating UCN2 is associated with clinical and echocardiographic markers of volume overload and pulmonary hypertension in acute heart failure patients [126]. However, on the other hand, CRH and UCNs may play detrimental roles in cardiovascular activities [127, 128], and in CVS pathologic settings, plasma UCN1 concentrations' elevation may contribute to the pathological processes [129, 130]. With all these effects together, beneficial or harmful, UCNs are recognized as biomarkers of the CVS diseases [121].

In the immune/inflammatory system, CRFp effects are also well documented [8, 131]. CRH, detected in the inflamed area but not in the systemic circulation, is found to promote immune functions in vitro via its receptors [132], suggesting that CRH is produced in peripheral inflammatory sites acting as an autocrine or paracrine inflammatory cytokine [133]. Human mast cells are observed to synthesize and secrete both CRH, UCN1, and CRFr, participating in immune/inflammatory responses via releasing cytokines and other pro-inflammatory mediators [134, 135]. It is reported that CRH modulates the functions of peripheral human leukocytes [136] and monocytic THP-1 cells [137] and participates in IL-6 production modulating immune functions [138]. Furthermore, human lymphocytes show ability to release CRH. However, there is also report that only UCN1 mRNA, but not CRH mRNA, is expressed by unstimulated and stimulated normal human lymphocytes [139]. Furthermore, in the endometrium, locally produced embryonic and endometrial CRH plays a role in both the aseptic inflammatory process of implantation and the anti-rejection process that protects the fetus from the maternal immune system [10].

In the reproductive system, CRFp are highly expressed. Almost all reproductive organs/tissues, such as ovary, endometrium, placenta, myometrium, and prostate and testis, are sources of UCN1 [101, 140–143]. CRH is also reported being produced in placenta, having paracrine effects on mother and fetus. Moreover, CRH is a potent local regulator of myometrial contractility and of prostaglandin release, which to some extent UCN1 mimics. A local CRF-BP modulates the paracrine effects of CRH and UCN1. Plasma CRH and CRF-BP levels change during pregnancy [144]. In addition, it is observed that UCN1, CRH, and CRF_1 and $CRF_{2\alpha}$ are significantly higher in the regressing corpus luteum than in the functioning corpus luteum [143]. In adult male rats, CRH is reported existing in the testes [145, 146], influencing steroidogenic process in the testis Leydig cells (both negative and positive effects are reported) [147–151]. And high level of UCN1 in the male gonads is also shown, while UCN2 and UCN3 mRNA expression is weak [152]. The inhibitory effect of UCN1on testosterone response in rat Leydig cells is reported, too [142].

CRFp are observed to express in different types of tumors contributing to their development, including colon cancer, skin cancer, prostate cancer, endometrial carcinoma, breast cancer, ovarian cancer, thyroid cancer, etc. [102, 153–155]. Moreover, UCN1 is reported to improve osteoporotic bone properties [156], and its effect on skeletal muscle structure in vivo is also observed in osteopenic rats [157], which might have a potential therapeutic role in dealing with postmenopausal osteoporosis and musculoskeletal function decline leading to loss of bone and muscle [158, 159]. UCN2 is also observed to be highly associated with skeletal muscle mass and function [160, 161]. Finally, CRH and UCNs are expressed in the skin [82, 162, 163], and demonstration of the corresponding CRFr in the skin also suggests their para- or autocrine mechanisms of action [164, 165]. Interestingly, mast cells are very often associated with CRFp effects in the skin [166, 167].

3 Summary

This chapter mainly summarizes the structures of CRFp and their overall distribution and functions in the periphery. For primary structures, CRH is a 41-AA peptide, and UCN1 a 40- and UCN2 and UCN3 a 38-AA peptide. The secondary structures of CRFp related to α-helical conformation play a decisive role in their binding to the relevant receptors and subsequent activating effects. Among the CRFp, CRH and UCN1 are significantly modulated by CRF-BP. CRFp are widely distributed in the periphery mainly including the digestive system, cardiovascular system, immune/inflammatory system, reproductive system, and tumors exerting protective or detrimental effects, which is briefly described and will be focused in detail in the following relevant chapters (Chaps. 4, 5, 6, 7, and 8).

References

1. Tache Y, Brunnhuber S. From Hans Selye's discovery of biological stress to the identification of corticotropin-releasing factor signaling pathways: implication in stress-related functional bowel diseases. Ann N Y Acad Sci. 2008;1148:29–41.
2. Selye H. A syndrome produced by diverse nocuous agents. J Neuropsychiatry Clin Neurosci. 1936;10(2):230–1.
3. Vale W, et al. Characterization of a 41-residue ovine hypothalamic peptide that stimulates secretion of corticotropin and beta-endorphin. Science. 1981;213(4514):1394–7.
4. Rivier J, Rivier C, Vale W. Synthetic competitive antagonists of corticotropin-releasing factor: effect on ACTH secretion in the rat. Science. 1984;224(4651):889–91.
5. Bale TL, Vale WW. CRF and CRF receptors: role in stress responsivity and other behaviors. Annu Rev Pharmacol Toxicol. 2004;44:525–57.
6. Hargreaves KM, Costello AH, Joris JL. Release from inflamed tissue of a substance with properties similar to corticotropin-releasing factor. Neuroendocrinology. 1989;49(5):476–82.
7. Suda T, et al. Distribution and characterization of immunoreactive corticotropin-releasing factor in human tissues. J Clin Endocrinol Metab. 1984;59(5):861–6.
8. Bamberger CM, Bamberger AM. The peripheral CRH/urocortin system. Ann N Y Acad Sci. 2000;917:290–6.
9. Walczewska J, et al. The role of urocortins in the cardiovascular system. J Physiol Pharmacol. 2014;65(6):753–66.
10. Ilias I, Mastorakos G. The emerging role of peripheral corticotropin-releasing hormone (CRH). J Endocrinol Investig. 2003;26(4):364–71.
11. Filaretova LP, Morozova OY, Yarushkina NI. Peripheral corticotropin-releasing hormone may protect the gastric musosa against indometacin-induced injury through involvement of glucocorticoids. J Physiol Pharmacol. 2021;72(5)
12. Vuppaladhadiam L, et al. Corticotropin-releasing factor family: a stress hormone-receptor system's emerging role in mediating sex-specific signaling. Cells. 2020;9(4)
13. Perrin MH, Vale WW. Corticotropin releasing factor receptors and their ligand family. Ann N Y Acad Sci. 1999;885:312–28.
14. Ryu KS, et al. Structures of ovine corticotropin-releasing factor and its Ala32 mutant as studied by CD and NMR techniques. J Biochem. 2000;127(4):687–94.
15. Grace CR, et al. Common and divergent structural features of a series of corticotropin releasing factor-related peptides. J Am Chem Soc. 2007;129(51):16102–14.
16. Matsoukas MT, et al. Structural and functional insights into CRF peptides and their receptors. Biology (Basel). 2024;13(2)
17. Fekete EM, Zorrilla EP. Physiology, pharmacology, and therapeutic relevance of urocortins in mammals: ancient CRF paralogs. Front Neuroendocrinol. 2007;28(1):1–27.
18. Jackson RV, et al. Synthetic ovine corticotropin-releasing hormone: simultaneous release of proopiolipomelanocortin peptides in man. J Clin Endocrinol Metab. 1984;58(4):740–3.
19. Rupprecht R, et al. Blunted adrenocorticotropin but normal beta-endorphin release after human corticotropin-releasing hormone administration in depression. J Clin Endocrinol Metab. 1989;69(3):600–3.
20. Furutani Y, et al. Cloning and sequence analysis of cDNA for ovine corticotropin-releasing factor precursor. Nature. 1983;301(5900):537–40.
21. Ringan NS, et al. Prediction of protein antigenic sites in human corticotrophin-releasing hormone precursor. Comp Biochem Physiol B. 1993;104(3):521–9.
22. Castro MG, et al. The use of inclusion bodies, isolated from Escherichia coli expressing corticotrophin-releasing hormone precursor, to raise specific antibodies against the neuropeptide moiety. J Mol Endocrinol. 1990;5(3):221–30.
23. Mol JA, et al. Predicted primary and antigenic structure of canine corticotropin releasing hormone. Neuropeptides. 1994;27(1):7–13.

24. Robinson BM, et al. Cloning and characterization of corticotropin-releasing factor and urocortin in Syrian hamster (Mesocricetus auratus). Peptides. 1999;20(10):1177–85.
25. Delville Y, Stires C, Ferris CF. Distribution of corticotropin-releasing hormone immunoreactivity in golden hamster brain. Brain Res Bull. 1992;29(5):681–4.
26. Miranda A, et al. Conformationally restricted competitive antagonists of human/rat corticotropin-releasing factor. J Med Chem. 1994;37(10):1450–9.
27. Miranda A, et al. Constrained corticotropin-releasing factor antagonists with i-(i + 3) Glu-Lys bridges. J Med Chem. 1997;40(22):3651–8.
28. Gulyas J, et al. Potent, structurally constrained agonists and competitive antagonists of corticotropin-releasing factor. Proc Natl Acad Sci USA. 1995;92(23):10575–9.
29. Beyermann M, et al. A role for a helical connector between two receptor binding sites of a long-chain peptide hormone. J Biol Chem. 2000;275(8):5702–9.
30. Romier C, et al. Solution structure of human corticotropin releasing factor by 1H NMR and distance geometry with restrained molecular dynamics. Protein Eng. 1993;6(2):149–56.
31. Kornreich WD, et al. Alanine series of ovine corticotropin releasing factor (oCRF): a structure-activity relationship study. J Med Chem. 1992;35(10):1870–6.
32. Loquet A, et al. 3D structure determination of the Crh protein from highly ambiguous solid-state NMR restraints. J Am Chem Soc. 2008;130(11):3579–89.
33. Dathe M, et al. Conformational differences of ovine and human corticotropin releasing hormone. A CD, IR, NMR and dynamic light scattering study. Int J Pept Protein Res. 1996;47(5):383–93.
34. Marini M, Rey F, Gomez F. Test with ovine corticotropin-releasing hormone (oCRH): clinical application and reference values in the young adult and the postmenopausal women. Schweiz Med Wochenschr. 1991;121(18):653–9.
35. Smith SR, et al. Peripheral administration of human corticotropin-releasing hormone: a novel method to increase energy expenditure and fat oxidation in man. J Clin Endocrinol Metab. 2001;86(5):1991–8.
36. Gamez I, Ryan RP, Keir ST. Corticorelin acetate, a synthetic corticotropin-releasing factor with preclinical antitumor activity, alone and with bevacizumab, against human brain tumor models. Anticancer Res. 2010;30(12):5037–42.
37. Papazacharias S, et al. Synthesis and biological evaluation of new CRH analogues. Bioinorg Chem Appl. 2010;2010
38. Spyroulias GA, et al. Monitoring the structural consequences of Phe12->D-Phe and Leu15->Aib substitution in human/rat corticotropin releasing hormone. Implications for design of CRH antagonists. Eur J Biochem. 2002;269(24):6009–19.
39. Rivier J, et al. Minimal-size, constrained corticotropin-releasing factor agonists with i-(i+3) Glu-Lys and Lys-Glu bridges. J Med Chem. 1998;41(14):2614–20.
40. Rivier JE, et al. Constrained corticotropin releasing factor antagonists (astressin analogues) with long duration of action in the rat. J Med Chem. 1999;42(16):3175–82.
41. Koerber SC, et al. Constrained corticotropin-releasing factor (CRF) agonists and antagonists with i-(i+3) Glu-Xaa-DXbb-Lys bridges. J Med Chem. 1998;41(25):5002–11.
42. Behan DP, et al. Corticotropin releasing factor (CRF) binding protein: a novel regulator of CRF and related peptides. Front Neuroendocrinol. 1995;16(4):362–82.
43. Ruhmann A, et al. Structural requirements for peptidic antagonists of the corticotropin-releasing factor receptor (CRFR): development of CRFR2beta-selective antisauvagine-30. Proc Natl Acad Sci USA. 1998;95(26):15264–9.
44. Brauns O, et al. Secondary structure of antisauvagine analogues is important for CRF receptor antagonism: development of antagonists with increased potency and receptor selectivity. Peptides. 2002;23(10):1817–27.
45. Rivier JE. Prospective clinical applications of CRF peptide antagonists. Curr Mol Pharmacol. 2017;10(4):264–9.
46. Holsboer F. Prospects for antidepressant drug discovery. Biol Psychol. 2001;57(1–3):47–65.

47. Kojima T, et al. Discovery of 1,2,3,4-tetrahydropyrimido[1,2-a]benzimidazoles as novel class of corticotropin releasing factor 1 receptor antagonists. Bioorg Med Chem. 2018;26(9):2229–50.
48. Shekhar MS, et al. Computational investigation of binding mechanism of substituted pyrazinones targeting corticotropin releasing factor-1 receptor deliberated for anti-depressant drug design. J Biomol Struct Dyn. 2019;37(12):3226–44.
49. Rivier JE, Rivier CL. Corticotropin-releasing factor peptide antagonists: design, characterization and potential clinical relevance. Front Neuroendocrinol. 2014;35(2):161–70.
50. Carr JA, et al. An intrinsic CRF signaling system within the optic tectum. Gen Comp Endocrinol. 2013;188:204–11.
51. Wang XB, et al. Corticotropin-releasing hormone 1 receptor antagonism attenuates chronic unpredictable mild stress-induced depressive-like behaviors in rats. Neuroreport. 2020;31(1):1–8.
52. Kuppast B, et al. Synthesis of substituted pyrimidines as corticotropin releasing factor (CRF) receptor ligands. Eur J Med Chem. 2014;78:1–9.
53. Inda C, et al. Different cAMP sources are critically involved in G protein-coupled receptor CRHR1 signaling. J Cell Biol. 2016;214(2):181–95.
54. Olianas MC, Lampis G, Onali P. Coupling of corticotropin-releasing hormone receptors to adenylyl cyclase in human Y-79 retinoblastoma cells. J Neurochem. 1995;64(1):394–401.
55. Refojo D, et al. Corticotropin-releasing hormone activates ERK1/2 MAPK in specific brain areas. Proc Natl Acad Sci USA. 2005;102(17):6183–8.
56. Linton EA, et al. Corticotropin-releasing hormone (CRH)-binding protein: reduction in the adrenocorticotropin-releasing activity of placental but not hypothalamic CRH. J Clin Endocrinol Metab. 1990;70(6):1574–80.
57. Potter E, et al. Cloning and characterization of the cDNAs for human and rat corticotropin releasing factor-binding proteins. Nature. 1991;349(6308):423–6.
58. Zhao XJ, et al. Corticotropin-releasing hormone-binding protein and its possible role in neuroendocrinological research. Horm Metab Res. 1997;29(8):373–8.
59. Petraglia F, et al. High levels of corticotropin-releasing factor (CRF) are inversely correlated with low levels of maternal CRF-binding protein in pregnant women with pregnancy-induced hypertension. J Clin Endocrinol Metab. 1996;81(2):852–6.
60. Florio P, et al. Maternal plasma corticotropin-releasing factor (CRF) and CRF-binding protein (CRF-BP) levels in post-term pregnancy: effect of prostaglandin administration. Eur J Endocrinol. 2007;157(3):279–84.
61. Behan DP, et al. Cloning and structure of the human corticotrophin releasing factor-binding protein gene (CRHBP). Genomics. 1993;16(1):63–8.
62. Behan DP, et al. Characterization of a sheep brain corticotropin releasing factor binding protein. Brain Res. 1996;709(2):265–74.
63. Ellis MJ, Livesey JH, Donald RA. Horse plasma corticotrophin-releasing hormone (CRH): characterisation and lack of a late gestational rise or a plasma CRH-binding protein. J Endocrinol. 1994;143(3):455–60.
64. Jahn O, et al. Corticotropin-releasing factor binding protein – a ligand trap? Mini Rev Med Chem. 2005;5(10):953–60.
65. Karolyi IJ, et al. Altered anxiety and weight gain in corticotropin-releasing hormone-binding protein-deficient mice. Proc Natl Acad Sci USA. 1999;96(20):11595–600.
66. Lovejoy DA, et al. Ectopic expression of the CRF-binding protein: minor impact on HPA axis regulation but induction of sexually dimorphic weight gain. J Neuroendocrinol. 1998;10(7):483–91.
67. Burrows HL, et al. Excess corticotropin releasing hormone-binding protein in the hypothalamic-pituitary-adrenal axis in transgenic mice. J Clin Invest. 1998;101(7):1439–47.
68. Seasholtz AF, et al. Mouse models of altered CRH-binding protein expression. Peptides. 2001;22(5):743–51.

69. Huising MO, Flik G. The remarkable conservation of corticotropin-releasing hormone (CRH)-binding protein in the honeybee (Apis mellifera) dates the CRH system to a common ancestor of insects and vertebrates. Endocrinology. 2005;146(5):2165–70.
70. Woods RJ, et al. Cleavage of recombinant human corticotropin-releasing factor (CRF)-binding protein produces a 27-kilodalton fragment capable of binding CRF. J Clin Endocrinol Metab. 1999;84(8):2788–94.
71. Westphal NJ, Seasholtz AF. CRH-BP: the regulation and function of a phylogenetically conserved binding protein. Front Biosci. 2006;11:1878–91.
72. Lederis K, et al. Complete amino acid sequence of urotensin I, a hypotensive and corticotropin-releasing neuropeptide from Catostomus. Science. 1982;218(4568):162–5.
73. Montecucchi PC, Henschen A. Amino acid composition and sequence analysis of sauvagine, a new active peptide from the skin of Phyllomedusa sauvagei. Int J Pept Protein Res. 1981;18(2):113–20.
74. Okawara Y, et al. Cloning and sequence analysis of cDNA for corticotropin-releasing factor precursor from the teleost fish Catostomus commersonii. Proc Natl Acad Sci USA. 1988;85(22):8439–43.
75. Stenzel-Poore MP, et al. Characterization of the genomic corticotropin-releasing factor (CRF) gene from Xenopus laevis: two members of the CRF family exist in amphibians. Mol Endocrinol. 1992;6(10):1716–24.
76. Vaughan J, et al. Urocortin, a mammalian neuropeptide related to fish urotensin I and to corticotropin-releasing factor. Nature. 1995;378(6554):287–92.
77. Donaldson CJ, et al. Cloning and characterization of human urocortin. Endocrinology. 1996;137(5):2167–70.
78. Zhao L, et al. The structures of the mouse and human urocortin genes (Ucn and UCN). Genomics. 1998;50(1):23–33.
79. Cepoi D, et al. Ovine genomic urocortin: cloning, pharmacologic characterization, and distribution of central mRNA. Brain Res Mol Brain Res. 1999;68(1–2):109–18.
80. Seasholtz AF, et al. Nucleotide sequence and expression of the mouse corticotropin-releasing hormone gene. Mol Cell Neurosci. 1991;2(3):266–73.
81. Baigent SM, Lowry PJ. Urocortin is the principal ligand for the corticotrophin-releasing factor binding protein in the ovine brain with no evidence for a sauvagine-like peptide. J Mol Endocrinol. 2000;24(1):53–63.
82. Slominski A, et al. The skin produces urocortin. J Clin Endocrinol Metab. 2000;85(2):815–23.
83. Oki Y, Sasano H. Localization and physiological roles of urocortin. Peptides. 2004;25(10):1745–9.
84. Grace CR, et al. Structure of the N-terminal domain of a type B1 G protein-coupled receptor in complex with a peptide ligand. Proc Natl Acad Sci USA. 2007;104(12):4858–63.
85. Sutton SW, et al. Ligand requirements of the human corticotropin-releasing factor-binding protein. Endocrinology. 1995;136(3):1097–102.
86. Donaldson CJ, et al. Cloning and characterization of human urocortin. Endocrinology. 1996;137(9):3896.
87. Grammatopoulos DK, et al. Urocortin, but not corticotropin-releasing hormone (CRH), activates the mitogen-activated protein kinase signal transduction pathway in human pregnant myometrium: an effect mediated via R1alpha and R2beta CRH receptor subtypes and stimulation of Gq-proteins. Mol Endocrinol. 2000;14(12):2076–91.
88. Hauger RL, et al. International Union of Pharmacology. XXXVI. Current status of the nomenclature for receptors for corticotropin-releasing factor and their ligands. Pharmacol Rev. 2003;55(1):21–6.
89. Lewis K, et al. Identification of urocortin III, an additional member of the corticotropin-releasing factor (CRF) family with high affinity for the CRF2 receptor. Proc Natl Acad Sci USA. 2001;98(13):7570–5.

90. Reyes TM, et al. Urocortin II: a member of the corticotropin-releasing factor (CRF) neuropeptide family that is selectively bound by type 2 CRF receptors. Proc Natl Acad Sci USA. 2001;98(5):2843–8.
91. Hsu SY, Hsueh AJ. Human stresscopin and stresscopin-related peptide are selective ligands for the type 2 corticotropin-releasing hormone receptor. Nat Med. 2001;7(5):605–11.
92. Chae JI, et al. cDNA cloning and analysis of tissue-specific gene expression of rat urocortin II. Mol Biol (Mosk). 2009;43(1):91–6.
93. Vaughan JM, et al. Posttranslational processing of human and mouse urocortin 2: characterization and bioactivity of gene products. Endocrinology. 2013;154(4):1553–64.
94. Dautzenberg FM, Hauger RL. The CRF peptide family and their receptors: yet more partners discovered. Trends Pharmacol Sci. 2002;23(2):71–7.
95. Tillinger A, Mravec B. Vagotomy affects lipopolysaccharide-induced changes of Urocortin 2 gene expression in the brain and on the periphery. Neurochem Res. 2021;46(2):159–64.
96. Jahn O, et al. Three-amino acid motifs of urocortin II and III determine their CRF receptor subtype selectivity. Neuropharmacology. 2004;47(2):233–42.
97. Pal K, et al. Structural basis for hormone recognition by the human CRFR2alpha G protein-coupled receptor. J Biol Chem. 2010;285(51):40351–61.
98. Chatoo M, et al. Involvement of corticotropin-releasing factor and receptors in immune cells in irritable bowel syndrome. Front Endocrinol (Lausanne). 2018;9:21.
99. Larauche M, Kiank C, Tache Y. Corticotropin releasing factor signaling in colon and ileum: regulation by stress and pathophysiological implications. J Physiol Pharmacol. 2009;60(Suppl 7):33–46.
100. Huang Y, et al. Urocortin and cardiovascular protection. Acta Pharmacol Sin. 2004;25(3):257–65.
101. Florio P, Vale W, Petraglia F. Urocortins in human reproduction. Peptides. 2004;25(10):1751–7.
102. Kaprara A, et al. The corticotropin releasing factor system in cancer: expression and pathophysiological implications. Cell Mol Life Sci. 2010;67(8):1293–306.
103. Zhang H, et al. Understanding the connection between gut homeostasis and psychological stress. J Nutr. 2023;153(4):924–39.
104. Tache Y, Perdue MH. Role of peripheral CRF signalling pathways in stress-related alterations of gut motility and mucosal function. Neurogastroenterol Motil. 2004;16(Suppl 1):137–42.
105. Perrelli M, et al. Stress and the CRH system, norepinephrine, depression, and type 2 diabetes. Biomedicines. 2024;12(6)
106. Kawahito Y, et al. Corticotropin releasing hormone in colonic mucosa in patients with ulcerative colitis. Gut. 1995;37(4):544–51.
107. Huang X, et al. Corticotropin-releasing factor receptor agonists decrease interstitial cells of Cajal in murine colon. Neurogastroenterol Motil. 2023;35(3):e14499.
108. Petrusz P, et al. Central and peripheral distribution of corticotropin-releasing factor. Fed Proc. 1985;44(1 Pt 2):229–35.
109. Paschos KA, et al. The corticotropin releasing factor system in the liver: expression, actions and possible implications in hepatic physiology and pathology. Hormones (Athens). 2013;12(2):236–45.
110. Yamato S, et al. Urocortin 1: a putative excitatory neurotransmitter in the enteric nervous system. Neurogastroenterol Motil. 2020;32(10):e13842.
111. Li C, et al. Urocortin III-immunoreactive projections in rat brain: partial overlap with sites of type 2 corticotrophin-releasing factor receptor expression. J Neurosci. 2002;22(3):991–1001.
112. Li C, et al. Urocortin III is expressed in pancreatic beta-cells and stimulates insulin and glucagon secretion. Endocrinology. 2003;144(7):3216–24.
113. Huang JL, et al. Genetic deletion of Urocortin 3 does not prevent functional maturation of beta cells. J Endocrinol. 2020;246(1):69–78.
114. Boorse GC, Denver RJ. Widespread tissue distribution and diverse functions of corticotropin-releasing factor and related peptides. Gen Comp Endocrinol. 2006;146(1):9–18.

115. Yuan PQ, et al. Urocortins and CRF receptor type 2 variants in the male rat colon: gene expression and regulation by endotoxin and anti-inflammatory effect. Am J Physiol Gastrointest Liver Physiol. 2016;310(6):G387–98.
116. Liu S, et al. Distribution and chemical coding of corticotropin-releasing factor-immunoreactive neurons in the Guinea pig enteric nervous system. J Comp Neurol. 2006;494(1):63–74.
117. Liu S, et al. Differential actions of urocortins on neurons of the myenteric division of the enteric nervous system in Guinea pig distal colon. Br J Pharmacol. 2010;159(1):222–36.
118. Yuan PQ, et al. Activation of CRF(1) receptors expressed in brainstem autonomic nuclei stimulates colonic enteric neurons and secreto-motor function in male rats. Neurogastroenterol Motil. 2021;33(11):e14189.
119. Wiley KE, Davenport AP. CRF2 receptors are highly expressed in the human cardiovascular system and their cognate ligands urocortins 2 and 3 are potent vasodilators. Br J Pharmacol. 2004;143(4):508–14.
120. Brar BK, et al. Urocortin-II and urocortin-III are cardioprotective against ischemia reperfusion injury: an essential endogenous cardioprotective role for corticotropin releasing factor receptor type 2 in the murine heart. Endocrinology. 2004;145(1):24–35.
121. Kuizon E, et al. Mechanisms of action and clinical implications of cardiac urocortin: a journey from the heart to the systemic circulation, with a stopover in the mitochondria. Int J Cardiol. 2009;137(3):189–94.
122. Hashimoto K, et al. Urocortins and corticotropin releasing factor type 2 receptors in the hypothalamus and the cardiovascular system. Peptides. 2004;25(10):1711–21.
123. Charles CJ, Rademaker MT, Richards AM. Urocortins: putative role in cardiovascular disease. Curr Med Chem Cardiovasc Hematol Agents. 2004;2(1):43–7.
124. Nishikimi T, et al. Urocortin, a member of the corticotropin-releasing factor family, in normal and diseased heart. Am J Physiol Heart Circ Physiol. 2000;279(6):H3031–9.
125. Lai NC, et al. Intravenous AAV8 encoding Urocortin-2 increases function of the failing heart in mice. Hum Gene Ther. 2015;26(6):347–56.
126. Pintalhao M, et al. Urocortin-2 in acute heart failure: role as a marker of volume overload and pulmonary hypertension. Curr Probl Cardiol. 2022;47(4):100860.
127. Zhu C, Li S. The peripheral corticotropin releasing factor family's role in vasculitis. Vasc Pharmacol. 2024;154:107275.
128. Wu Y, et al. Enhanced expression of vascular cell adhesion molecule-1 by corticotrophin-releasing hormone contributes to progression of atherosclerosis in LDL receptor-deficient mice. Atherosclerosis. 2009;203(2):360–70.
129. Wan R, et al. Urocortin increased LPS-induced endothelial permeability by regulating the cadherin-catenin complex via corticotrophin-releasing hormone receptor 2. J Cell Physiol. 2013;228(6):1295–303.
130. Wan R, et al. Sex difference in urocortin production is contributory to the gender disparity in a rat model of vasculitis induced by sodium laurate. Endocrinology. 2013;154(12):4663–74.
131. Karalis K, et al. CRH and the immune system. J Neuroimmunol. 1997;72(2):131–6.
132. Karalis K, et al. Autocrine or paracrine inflammatory actions of corticotropin-releasing hormone in vivo. Science. 1991;254(5030):421–3.
133. Kalantaridou S, et al. Peripheral corticotropin-releasing hormone is produced in the immune and reproductive systems: actions, potential roles and clinical implications. Front Biosci. 2007;12:572–80.
134. Theoharides TC, et al. Mast cells as targets of corticotropin-releasing factor and related peptides. Trends Pharmacol Sci. 2004;25(11):563–8.
135. Asadi S, et al. Substance P (SP) induces expression of functional corticotropin-releasing hormone receptor-1 (CRHR-1) in human mast cells. J Invest Dermatol. 2012;132(2):324–9.
136. Smith EM, et al. Corticotropin releasing factor induction of leukocyte-derived immunoreactive ACTH and endorphins. Nature. 1986;321(6073):881–2.
137. Chandras C, et al. Activation of phosphatidylinositol 3-kinase/protein kinase B by corticotropin-releasing factor in human monocytes. Endocrinology. 2009;150(10):4606–14.

138. Rassouli O, et al. A novel role of peripheral corticotropin-releasing hormone (CRH) on dermal fibroblasts. PLoS One. 2011;6(7):e21654.
139. Bamberger CM, et al. Human lymphocytes produce urocortin, but not corticotropin-releasing hormone. J Clin Endocrinol Metab. 1998;83(2):708–11.
140. Sumii K, et al. Characterization of urocortin as an anti-apoptotic protein in experimental ischemia-reperfusion model of the rat testis. Biochem Biophys Res Commun. 2016;479(2):387–92.
141. Tao J, et al. Separate locations of urocortin and its receptors in mouse testis: function in male reproduction and the relevant mechanisms. Cell Physiol Biochem. 2007;19(5–6):303–12.
142. Rivier CL. Urocortin 1 inhibits rat leydig cell function. Endocrinology. 2008;149(12):6425–32.
143. Muramatsu Y, et al. Urocortin and corticotropin-releasing factor receptor expression in normal cycling human ovaries. J Clin Endocrinol Metab. 2001;86(3):1362–9.
144. Fadalti M, et al. Placental corticotropin-releasing factor. An update. Ann N Y Acad Sci. 2000;900:89–94.
145. Eskeland NL, Molineaux CJ, Schachter BS. Regulation of beta-endorphin secretion by corticotropin-releasing factor in the intact rat testis. Endocrinology. 1992;130(3):1173–9.
146. Yoon DJ, Sklar C, David R. Presence of immunoreactive corticotropin-releasing factor in rat testis. Endocrinology. 1988;122(2):759–61.
147. Rossi SP, et al. New insights into melatonin/CRH signaling in hamster Leydig cells. Gen Comp Endocrinol. 2012;178(1):153–63.
148. Huang BM, Stocco DM, Norman RL. The cellular mechanisms of corticotropin-releasing hormone (CRH)-stimulated steroidogenesis in mouse Leydig cells are similar to those for LH. J Androl. 1997;18(5):528–34.
149. Huang BM, et al. Corticotropin-releasing hormone stimulates steroidogenesis in mouse Leydig cells. Biol Reprod. 1995;53(3):620–6.
150. Tinajero JC, Fabbri A, Dufau ML. Regulation of corticotropin-releasing factor secretion from Leydig cells by serotonin. Endocrinology. 1992;130(4):1780–8.
151. Dufau ML, Tinajero JC, Fabbri A. Corticotropin-releasing factor: an antireproductive hormone of the testis. FASEB J. 1993;7(2):299–307.
152. Lee S, et al. Urocortins are present in the rat testis. Neuropeptides. 2011;45(2):131–7.
153. Jin L, et al. CRH suppressed TGFbeta1-induced epithelial-mesenchymal transition via induction of E-cadherin in breast cancer cells. Cell Signal. 2014;26(4):757–65.
154. Fang X, et al. CRH promotes human colon cancer cell proliferation via IL-6/JAK2/STAT3 signaling pathway and VEGF-induced tumor angiogenesis. Mol Carcinog. 2017;56(11):2434–45.
155. Liu Y, et al. The role of corticotropin-releasing hormone receptor 1 in the development of colitis-associated cancer in mouse model. Endocr Relat Cancer. 2014;21(4):639–51.
156. Ismail OM, El-Omar OM, Said UN. Exploring the role of Urocortin in osteoporosis. Cureus. 2023;15(5):e38978.
157. Saul D, et al. Changes in musculoskeletal system and metabolism in osteoporotic rats treated with Urocortin. Front Endocrinol (Lausanne). 2019;10:400.
158. Black DM, Rosen CJ. Postmenopausal osteoporosis. N Engl J Med. 2016;374(18):1797.
159. Sornay-Rendu E, et al. Muscle mass is associated with incident fracture in postmenopausal women: the OFELY study. Bone. 2017;94:108–13.
160. Lautherbach N, et al. Urocortin 2 promotes hypertrophy and enhances skeletal muscle function through cAMP and insulin/IGF-1 signaling pathways. Mol Metab. 2022;60:101492.
161. Hinkle RT, et al. Urocortin II treatment reduces skeletal muscle mass and function loss during atrophy and increases nonatrophying skeletal muscle mass and function. Endocrinology. 2003;144(11):4939–46.
162. Slominski AT, et al. Key role of CRF in the skin stress response system. Endocr Rev. 2013;34(6):827–84.
163. Chen A, et al. Urocortin II gene is highly expressed in mouse skin and skeletal muscle tissues: localization, basal expression in corticotropin-releasing factor receptor (CRFR) 1- and CRFR2-null mice, and regulation by glucocorticoids. Endocrinology. 2004;145(5):2445–57.

164. Slominski A, et al. Cutaneous expression of corticotropin-releasing hormone (CRH), urocortin, and CRH receptors. FASEB J. 2001;15(10):1678–93.
165. Slominski A, Wortsman J. Neuroendocrinology of the skin. Endocr Rev. 2000;21(5):457–87.
166. Papadopoulou N, et al. Corticotropin-releasing hormone receptor-1 and histidine decarboxylase expression in chronic urticaria. J Invest Dermatol. 2005;125(5):952–5.
167. Donelan J, et al. Perifollicular and perivascular mouse skin mast cells express corticotropin-releasing hormone receptor. J Invest Dermatol. 2006;126(4):929–32.

Chapter 3
The Receptors for CRF Peptides

Shengnan Li and Chao Zhu

Corticotropin-releasing hormone (factor) family peptides (CRF peptides, CRFp) act in both the brain and the periphery to coordinate the overall body response to stress. The involvement of the CRF system (including CRFp, CRF receptors (CRFr), and CRF binding protein (CRF-BP)) in a variety of both central and peripheral disease states has stimulated great interest in this system as a potential site of therapeutic intervention [1]. CRFr belong to class B1 of the super-family of G protein-coupled receptors (GPCRs) [2, 3]. CRFr are classified into two subtypes, CRF_1 and CRF_2. Both receptors are positively coupled to adenylyl cyclase (AC) but they have a distinct pharmacological feature [4]. As described in Chap. 2, mammalian CRFp include four members, corticotropin releasing hormone (CRH), Urocortin (UCN1), UCN2, and UCN3. These CRFp mediate the actions through the GPCRs, with CRH selectively on CRF_1, UCN1 on both CRF_1 and CRF_2, and UCN2,3 selectively on CRF_2 [5–7]. The cloning of multiple CRFr subtypes has precipitated a new era in CRF system research that has allowed precise molecular, pharmacological, and anatomical examination of mammalian CRFr [8]. This chapter will mainly focus on the basic features of CRFr while their distribution and functions in different peripheral systems will be summarized together with the ligands (CRFp) in the subsequent chapters (Chaps. 4, 5, 6, 7, and 8).

S. Li (✉) · C. Zhu
Department of Pharmacology, School of Basic Medical Sciences,
Nanjing Medical University, Nanjing, Jiangsu, China
e-mail: snli@njmu.edu.cn

© The Author(s), under exclusive license to Springer Nature Singapore Pte Ltd. 2025
C. Zhu et al. (eds.), *The Peripheral Existence and Effects of Corticotropin-releasing Factor Family*, https://doi.org/10.1007/978-981-96-5322-5_3

1 The Two Distinct CRF Receptors

GPCRs are a family of membrane receptors regulating physiology and pathology of various organs and function as targets of many drugs in the market [9]. Heterotrimeric G proteins, composed of α, β, and γ subunits, act as the key downstream signaling molecules of GPCRs [10]. Class B1 GPCRs (secretin-like GPCRs, SecRs) are a small family of 15 peptide-binding receptors, including attractive therapeutic targets for many diseases. A general mechanism of peptide binding for SecRs is of a two-domain model, with the C-terminal ligand region binding to the extracellular N-terminal domain (ECD) of the receptor, promoting interaction of the N-terminal ligand region with the juxtamembrane domain of the receptor [11, 12]. CRFr belong to SecRs (with stimulatory G protein, Gs) coupled with AC and CRFp binding to CRFr triggers cyclic adenosine monophosphate (cAMP) production [13, 14] (Fig. 3.1). The cryoelectron microscopy (cryo-EM) structures of B1 GPCR-peptide complex [15] and CRFr in complex with CRFp-Gs are already reported [16, 17] (Fig. 3.2). The two distinct subtypes of CRFr, CRF_1 and CRF_2, have been cloned and characterized since 1990s. CRF_1 shares 70% sequence identity with CRF_2 and has much higher affinity for rat/human CRH (r/hCRH) than CRF_2 [18]. For ligand selectivity, CRF_1 selectively respond to CRH and CRF_1 and CRF_2 have equal affinity to UCN1, while UCN2 and UCN3 are CRF_2-selective [2, 7, 19]. It is noteworthy that CRFr are mostly first cloned from the brain and related tissues and identically found widely expressed in the periphery.

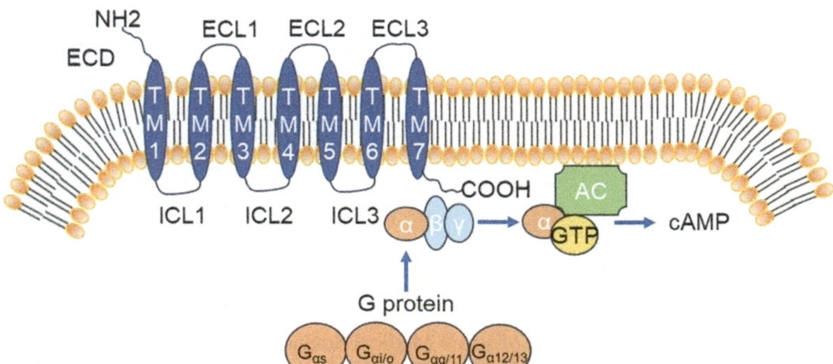

Fig. 3.1 CRFr belong to Class B1 G protein-coupled receptor associated with adenyl cyclase. *ECD* extracellular domain, *ICL* intracellular loop, *ECL* extracellular loop, *TM* transmembrane domain, *AC* adenyl cyclase

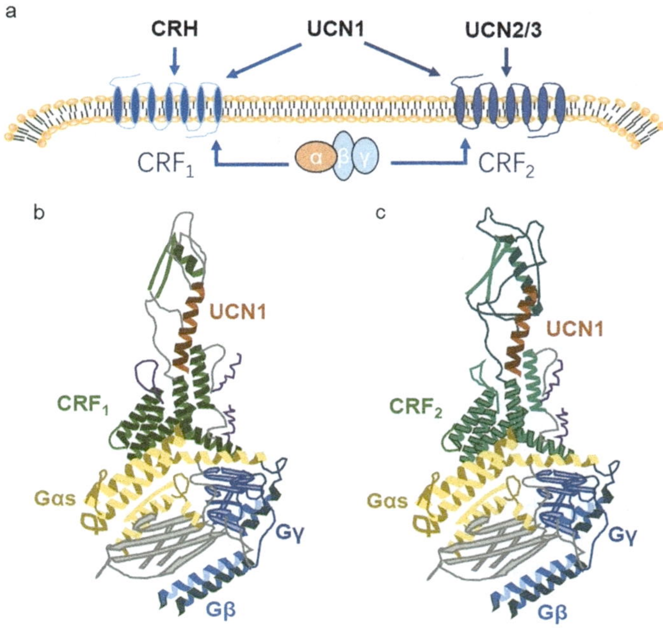

Fig. 3.2 The sketchy pictures representing CRFr-CRFp binding specificity and the cryo-EM structures of UCN-1 bound CRF_1 and CRF_2 in Gs complex. (The picture is adapted based on the original data from Ma et al. [17] (Reprinted with permission from Elsevier, open access). (**a**) Binding specificity of CRFr to CRFp; (**b**) cryo-EM density map of CRF_1-UCN1-Gs; (**c**) cryo-EM density map of CRF_2-UCN1-Gs)

1.1 The Subtype CRF_1

CRF_1 is activated endogenously by CRH and UCN1 and implicated in a lot of central and peripheral states including cardiovascular and gastrointestinal diseases, such as vasculitis and irritable bowel disease (IBS) [20–25].

1.1.1 The Primary Structure of CRF_1

Early in the 1990s, the cloning of a cDNA coding for a CRF_1 from a human corticotropic tumor library is reported by Vale and colleagues [26]. The cloned cDNA encodes a **415**-amino acid (AA) protein comprising seven putative membrane-spanning domains and is structurally related to the subfamily of class B1 GPCRs. The cloned receptor expressed in COS-7 cells binds to r/hCRH with high affinity and specificity, functionally coupled to AC stimulating cAMP formation. Correspondingly, the CRH antagonist, α-helical-CRH(9–41) (α-helCRH(9–41)), inhibits the CRH-stimulated increase in intracellular cAMP. By expressing cloning of cDNA from a human Cushing's corticotropic adenoma, identical $hCRF_1$ is characterized, confirmed by its transducing a CRH-stimulated accumulation of intracellular cAMP which is inhibited by α-helCRH(9–41) [27]. Northern blot analysis reveals that the CRF_1 is expressed in the rat pituitary and brain as well as in the mouse AtT20 corticotropic cells [26]. The mouse and human cDNAs both encode **415** AA proteins that are 97% identical, containing seven putative transmembrane (TM) domains characteristic of GPCRs. COS-7 cells transfected with the mouse CRF_1 ($mCRF_1$) cDNA bind to radiolabeled ovine CRH (oCRH) with high affinity and respond specifically to CRH resulting in intracellular cAMP increase [28]. The structure of the cDNA for a $rCRF_1$ cloned by hybridization from a rat brain cDNA library is also reported. Like $hCRF_1$, the sequence of the $rCRF_1$ encodes a **415** AA protein comprising seven TM domains as well with 97% homology to $hCRF_1$ at the AA sequence level. When expressed in COSM6 cells, the $rCRF_1$ binds to CRH with high affinity, causing increases in intracellular cAMP which is inhibited by α-helCRH(9–41) [27, 29]. The molecular cloning of a cDNA containing a 1245 bp open reading frame encoding a **415** AA sheep CRF_1 ($oCRF_1$), 94 and 95% homologous to $rCRF_1$ and $hCRF_1$, respectively, are also successful. In the transfected Cos-7 cells, $oCRF_1$ shows high affinity for oCRH, which is lowered by the non-hydrolyzable GTP analogue (GTPγS). Moreover, CRH effectively stimulates the accumulation of cAMP in Cos-7 cells transfected with $oCRF_1$ [30]. The full-length cDNA of monkey CRF_1 is isolated from a monkey amygdala cDNA library. The cloned monkey CRF_1 cDNA contains 2374 bp with an open reading frame encoding a **415** AA peptide. The sequence of the monkey CRF_1 cDNA shows a high homology with other species of CRF_1, being 99.5% identical to $hCRF_1$. When expressed into COS-7 cells, high specific binding of [^{125}I]-oCRH is observed, which is competed by h/r CRH and related peptides and inhibited by CRF_1 receptor-specific antagonists (CP-154,526, SC241, and CRA1000). Moreover, the binding is influenced by GTP and GTPγS, while ATP has a negligible effect [31], thereby also confirming that the monkey CRF_1 belongs to GPCRs [9, 32], in accordance with the result that CRH increases cAMP formation in COS-7 cells transiently expressing the monkey CRF_1 [31].

1.1.2 The Secondary Structure of CRF_1

As a class B1 GPCR, CRF_1 contains an N-terminal ECD that provides the primary ligand binding determinants [33]. The CRF_1 ECD adopts the α-β-βα fold as other class B GPCR ECDs, but the N-terminal α-helix is significantly shorter and does not contact the ligand CRH. CRH adopts a continuous α-helix that docks in a hydrophobic surface of the ECD, which is distinct from the peptide-binding site of other class B GPCRs, thereby providing a basis for the specificity of ligand recognition between CRF_1 and other class B GPCRs [34] (Fig. 3.1). The X-ray crystal structures for CRF_1 demonstrate that two unique hydrogen bonds are present in the hydrogen bond network, while the stalk region forms an α-helix and the hydrophobic network contains an antagonist binding site [35].

By using chimeric receptor constructs of $hCRF_1$ (also CRF_2, see below), followed by generating its point mutations, the interactions between r/hCRH and CRF_1 and the regions involved in receptor-ligand binding and intracellular cAMP after the chimeric and mutant receptors-ligand binding are observed by Maki and colleagues [4, 18]. It is found that three regions of the receptor are important for optimal binding of r/hCRH and/or receptor activation, the first region being mapped to the junction of the third ECD and the fifth TM domain. The substitution of three AA of CRF_1 in this region (Val266, Tyr267, and Thr268) by the corresponding CRF_2 AA (Asp266, Leu267, and Val268) increases cAMP level by approximately ten-fold. The other two regions are localized to the second ECD of the CRF_1 involving AA 175–178 and His189 residue. Substitutions in these two regions each increase cAMP level for r/hCRH by about 7 ~ 8-fold only in the presence of AA 266–268 mutation involving the first ECD, suggesting that these two regions' roles in peptide ligand binding are secondary [18].

As already described, class B1 GPCRs are important therapeutic targets for many human diseases [36, 37]. Therefore, the design of modulators targeting B1 GPCRs in drug discovery is meaningful, and more structural insights allow structure-based drug design methods targeting these receptors [16, 38]. By cryo-EM, molecular dynamics, and biochemical cross-linking, a 2.3 Å structure and interrogate dynamics of secretin bound to the receptor and Gs complex (SecR:Gs) are determined by Miller and colleagues. SecRs exhibit a unique organization of ECD relative to its 7-TM domain core, forming more extended interactions than other GPCRs. Numerous polar interactions form between Secretin and SecR extracellular loops (ECLs) and TM helices, and the interactions are dynamic [12, 39]. Structure determination of the most common spliced forms of CRF_1 and the structural features of CRF_1-ligand complex show CRF_1's character of class B1 GPCRs [40, 41]. It is observed that CRF_1 maintains the ability to signal to Gs-mediated cAMP production [40]. Moreover, in studying the structure of CRH-CRF_1-Gs complex, Wootten group report that diverse orientations of the ECD to SecR core depend, to some extent, on evolutionary conservation in the structure and nature of peptide interactions. Differences in peptide interactions to SecR core also influence the interlinked TM2-TM1-TM6/ECL3/TM7 domain, which is likely important in the diverse signaling. On the other hand, common conformational reorganization of ECL2, linked to reorganization of ICL2, modulates Gs contacts. ICL2 is revealed as a key domain forming dynamic Gs interactions in a receptor- and ligand-specific manner [42]. In addition, Ma et al. present two cryo-EM structures of UCN1-bound CRF_1 and CRF_2 with Gs. In both structures, UCN1 adopts a single straight helix with its N terminus dipped into the receptor TM bundle. The peptide-binding residues in CRF_1 and CRF_2 are found to be different from other class B GPCRs, but the residues for SecR activation and Gs coupling are conserved. Moreover, the structures reveal bound cholesterol molecules to SecR TM helices [17] (Fig. 3.2).

More and more deeper insights into the mechanism underlying stepwise conformational changes during GPCR-Gs coupling are obtained via advanced methods, such as hydrogen/deuterium exchange mass spectrometry, hydroxyl radical footprinting-mass spectrometry, X-ray crystallography, cryo-EM, and molecular dynamics simulation techniques [43]. As precedingly mentioned, cryo-EM structures allow more clear exhibition of UCN1-CRFr-Gs complex, showing the difference in the peptide-binding residues from other members of class B GPCRs, besides displaying the common conserved residues and bound cholesterol molecules to the receptor transmembrane helices, which defines the basis of ligand-binding specificity in the CRFr-ligand complex, establishing a common mechanism of class B GPCR activation and G protein coupling [17]. Moreover, it is showed that the purified N-terminal ECDs of hCRF$_1$ (and CRF$_{2\alpha}$) are sufficient to discriminate the peptides [44]. And hCRF$_1$ (and mCRF$_{2\beta}$) ECD forms the same fold as CRF$_{2\alpha}$ ECD, except the latter containing a unique N-terminal α-helix signal peptide (pseudo signal peptide, PSP) [44–47]. Importantly, different from other GPCRs having the signal anchor sequences usually in TM1, CRF$_1$ (also CRF$_{2\beta}$) possesses a conventional N-terminal signal peptide (SP) in the ECD, crucial for the functions and cleaved off during inserting into the endoplasmic reticulum (ER) membrane by the signal peptidases of the ER [45, 48], although there is inconsistent report that mutant CRF$_1$ lacking SP is also functional and displays wild-type properties as ligand binding and AC activation [49]. Also, CRF$_1$ECD peptide-binding site architecture is similar to that of CRF$_{2\alpha}$ ECD; hence CRH-CRF$_1$ binding resembles CRF$_{2\alpha}$-α-helical UCNs binding. However, based on the comparison between their electrostatic surface potentials of the ECDs, a charge compatibility mechanism may also be reasonable for the ligand discrimination since there exists a single AA difference (CRF$_1$ Glu104/ CRF$_{2\alpha}$ Pro-100) near residue 35 (Arg in CRH/UCN1, Ala in UCN2/3). Therefore, CRF$_1$ Glu-104 may act as a selectivity filter preventing UCN2/3 (CRF$_2$ selective agonist) binding, with Ala-35 being nonpolar, incompatible with the negatively charged Glu-104 [44]. Functionally, cell surface expression of CRF$_1$ is higher than that of CRF$_{2\alpha}$ due to the presence of PSP. And it is interesting to find out that PSP does not affect CRF$_{2\alpha}$ coupling to the Gs but abolishes the Gi-mediated inhibition of AC. Moreover, it is observed that the properties mediated by PSP are entirely transferable to the CRF$_1$ [47]. Collectively, the structures' difference explains the distinctness of the two CRFr and provides a molecular basis for designing therapeutic agents selectively targeting the specific receptor (see below).

Adding to the profile of CRF$_1$, it is observed to interact with receptor activity modifying proteins (PAMPs). By co-transfecting CRF$_1$ and RAMPs in HEK 293S and CHO-K1 cells, it is found that CRF$_1$ enhances the cell surface expression of RAMP2; and an enhanced G protein coupling in a receptor and agonist-dependent manner is discovered. The CRF$_1$- RAMP2 complex results in enhanced elevation of intracellular calcium to CRH and UCN1 [50].

1.2 The Subtype CRF$_2$

Three isoforms belonging to the CRF$_2$ subtype receptors, CRF$_{2\alpha}$, CRF$_{2\beta}$, and CRF$_{2\gamma}$, which differ in their ECDs, have been identified in rodents and humans [51–55]. Difference in their N-terminal coding sequence results in the production of distinct receptors. $CRF_{2\alpha}$ is found almost exclusively in the brain, whereas $CRF_{2\beta}$ appears to be both in the brain and in the periphery, especially in the heart and skeletal muscle [56]. As already mentioned above, CRF_2 is also a B1 class GPCR, having distinct feature from CRF_1 and the cryo-EM structure in complex with CRFp-Gs being reported [4, 17] (Fig. 3.2).

1.2.1 The Structure of CRF_2

In 1990s after the cloning of CRF_1, a second member of the CRFr encoding a **411** AA rat brain protein with approximately 70% homology to CRF_1 is identified (designated as CRF_2) [29]. Then Souza and colleagues report the genomic structure and the corresponding cDNA sequence of the $hCRF_2$, consisting of at least 12 exons and spans approximately 30 kilobases. The cDNA sequence in the protein-coding region is 94% identical to that of the reported $rCRF_{2\alpha}$, **411** AA in length and 70% identical to the $hCRF_1$, with least sequence homology in the ECD (47% identical). Functionally, cells transfected with the full-length $hCRF_2$ cDNA respond to r/hCRH and Sauvagine (Svg) by increasing the intracellular cAMP level, which is competitively inhibited by the CRFr antagonist D-Phe-CRH. This pharmacological profile is also comparable to that of $rCRF_{2\alpha}$ [52]. Consistently, Lovenberg et al. also report the isolation of a cDNA clone encoding this distinct $rCRF_2$. A PCR fragment obtained from rat brain is utilized to isolate a full-length cDNA encoding a **411**-AA protein with approximately 70% identity to the known CRF_1, which stimulates cAMP production in response to CRH and known CRH-like agonists when expressed in mouse Ltk-cells [57]. $CRF_{2\alpha}$ possesses a putative N-terminal signal peptide (pseudo signal peptide, PSP, as described above) [46], the PSP being observed completely incapable of mediating ER targeting and un-cleaved forming part of the mature receptor protein, different from the corresponding conventional sequence of CRF_1 and $CRF_{2\beta}$ being cleaved-off after mediating the ER targeting process [58]. Interestingly, replacing the residue Asn13 by hydrophobic residues converts the sequence into a fully functional and cleaved SP demonstrating that conventional SP functions are inhibited by a single AA residue (Asn) [58], supporting the transferability between PSP and SP [47]. These results suggest that the extreme N termini of the individual CRFr subtypes differ substantially. Moreover, rat and human $CRF_{2\alpha}$ comparison is done by Hall group through expressing them in CHO-pro5 cells and stable cell lines and using [^{125}I][tyr0]Svg for characterization. No pharmacological differences are found between rat and human $CRF_{2\alpha}$, except that α-helCRH(9–41) exhibits ten-fold higher affinity for $rCRF_{2\alpha}$ than for $hCRF_{2\alpha}$ [59]. Moreover, Gysling group observe $CRF_{2\alpha}$/dopamine1 receptor (D1R) heteromers in HEK293T cells. Co-expression of both receptors is found to promote D1R intracellular and $CRF_{2\alpha}$ cell surface targeting. The heteromerization of D1R / $CRF_{2\alpha}$ maintains the signaling through cAMP of both receptors and switches D1R signaling properties, with the heteromeric D1R being able to mobilize intracellular calcium upon stimulation by a D1R agonist [60, 61]. Interestingly, Vale group identify a cDNA from mouse brain encoding a splice variant, soluble $CRF_{2\alpha}$ ($sCRF_{2\alpha}$), in which exon 6 is deleted from the gene encoding $CRFR_{2\alpha}$. Translation of $sCRF_{2\alpha}$ produces a predicted 143-AA soluble protein, which includes a majority of ECD1 of $CRF_{2\alpha}$ followed by a unique 38-AA hydrophilic C terminus resulting from exon 6 deletion. By using RT-PCR and Southern hybridization, the relative mRNA expression levels of $CRF_{2\alpha}$ and $sCRF_{2\alpha}$ in the mouse brain are measured with results showing high levels of $sCRF_{2\alpha}$ in the olfactory bulb, cortex, and mid-brain regions and interestingly, its close approximation of distribution to CRF_1 [62].

Moreover, an additional splice variant of CRF_2 ($CRF_{2\beta}$) with a different N-terminal domain encoding a protein of **431** AA is also cloned [29]. Vale and colleagues first report the cloning of a second CRFr cDNA, which encodes a protein of **431** AA, being 16 AA longer and 68% similar to their previously cloned CRF_1 [26]. Comparison between the AA sequence of $CRF_{2\beta}$ and that of CRF_1 reveals major differences in their N-terminal domain and in the ECLs, whereas the sequences of the ICLs are nearly identical. $CRF_{2\beta}$ are expressed in the heart, as well as in other peripheral tissues, including the gastrointestinal tract and epididymis, also in brain

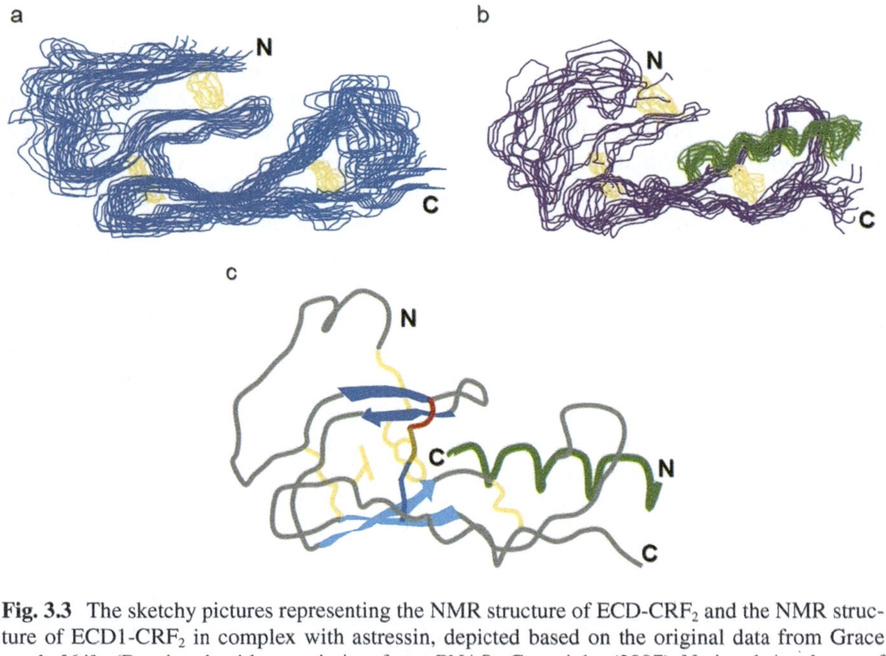

Fig. 3.3 The sketchy pictures representing the NMR structure of ECD-CRF_2 and the NMR structure of ECD1-CRF_2 in complex with astressin, depicted based on the original data from Grace et al. [64]. (Reprinted with permission from PNAS; Copyright (2007) National Academy of Sciences, U.S.A. Methods used for the original images obtaining are similar to those for the ligands (Chap. 2, Figs. 2.1 and 2.2); (**a**) Superposition of 20 lowest energy conformers representing the 3D-NMR structure of free ECD1-CRF_2; (**b**) superposition of 20 lowest energy conformers ECD1-CRF_2 in complex with astressin (The backbone of astressin is in green); (**c**) ribbon diagram of the lowest energy conformer representing the 3D-NMR structure of the ECD-CRF_2-astressin complex. The backbone of astressin is shown in green. Other parts in different colors include the side chains, the disulfide bonds, and the salt bridge [64])

[63]. In rat brain, a splice variant of CRF_2 mRNA is also identified encoding a protein of **431** AA [57]. The short-consensus-repeat fold (SCR) within ECD1 of this CRF_2 comprises the major ligand binding site docking a peptide ligand (or antagonist) via its C-terminal segment, thus positioning the N-terminal segment to interact with the receptor for its activation (or inactivation) [2, 64]. And the three-dimensional (3D)-nuclear magnetic resonance (NMR) structure of the $CRF_{2\beta}$'s ECD1in complex with the unselective CRFr antagonist, astressin, is presented by Grace and colleagues (Fig. 3.3), the C-terminal segment of astressin forming an amphipathic helix, with the hydrophobic face interacting with the SCR motif, covering a large intermolecular interface. In addition, the complex is characterized and stabilized by three disulfide bridges, two tryptophan residues, and an internal salt bridge (Asp65-Arg101) [2, 64], disruption of which by D65A mutation damages ligand recognition, losing the well-defined disulfide pattern and SCR structure [2]. These structural studies identify the major determinants for CRFp specificity and selectivity (such as key residues involved in ligand recognition and G coupling) and support a two-step model for receptor activation [11, 17, 64]. The results are strongly in agreement with the structure-based sequence comparison showing the importance of key AA conservation in the GPCRs, suggesting a corresponding conservation of a Sushi domain/SCR of their ECD [2, 65, 66]. Furthermore, similar to $CRF_{2\alpha}$ [60, 61], $CRF_{2\beta}$ is also found to heteromerize with D1R in A7r5 cells, which endogenously express $CRF_{2\beta}$ and D1R. By comparing the expression and localization of both isoforms, it is observed that the immunoreactivity for $CRF_{2\beta}$ is similar to that of $CRF_{2\alpha}$ in the endoplasmic compartment but significantly higher in the Golgi compartment. Immunoprecipitation analysis shows that $CRF_{2\beta}$ forms a heteromeric protein complex with D1R. Furthermore, the protein complex formed by $CRF_{2\beta}$ and D1R is stable enough to change the sub-cellular localization of $CRF_{2\beta}$ when co-expressed with a construct of D1R bearing a nuclear localization signal. Immunofluorescence in A7r5 cells shows significant colocalization of $CRF_{2\beta}$ with D1R [55]. These results imply that $CRF_{2\beta}$-D1R complex may be a potential therapeutic target in tissues where both receptors are co-expressed, such as the septum in the brain and the heart, kidney, and skeletal muscle in the periphery [55, 67], contrary to the report that D1R/D2R receptors do not participate in CRH-induced effects, eliminating its influence on CRF_1 [68].

Largent group report the discovery of another CRF_2 isoform, $CRF_{2\gamma}$, in human brain. The $CRF_{2\gamma}$ cDNA encodes for a **397**AA protein that has an amino terminus with no significant homology to the already reported *alpha*- and *beta*-termini [54]. Relatively less investigations are presented on the structure features of $CRF_{2\gamma}$.

1.2.2 Supplement to Pharmacological Characterization of CRF_2

The pharmacological profiles of the $CRF_{2\alpha}$ and $CRF_{2\beta}$ splice variants are observed to be identical, suggesting that the region of the N-terminus that varies between them is probably not critical in their binding of peptide ligands or functional activation [51]. By using radioligand binding with [^{125}I]-tyr0-Svg and a gene expression assay in which the firefly luciferase gene expression is under the control of cAMP responsive elements, for pharmacological characterization of $hCRF_2$, it is found that association kinetics of [^{125}I]-tyr0-Svg binding to $hCRF_{2β}$ and $hCRF_{2α}$ are monophasic while dissociation kinetics are biphasic. A non-hydrolysable GTP analogue, Gpp(NH)p, reduces the high affinity binding of [^{125}I]-tyr0-Svg to both $hCRF_2$ isoforms. The rank order of potency of CRFp in competition experiments and the luciferase gene reporter system is identical for both $hCRF_2$ isoforms (UCN1 > Svg > r/hCRH > oCRH). Also, the peptide antagonist α-helCRH(9–41) is observed to exhibit a non-competitive antagonism of UCN1-stimulated luciferase expression with both isoforms of $hCRF_2$ [51].

$CRF_{2β}$ is positively coupled to adenylate cyclase and is bound preferentially by UCNs. In the rodent, $CRF_{2β}$ mRNA is found expressed in the cardiovascular system, where its levels are associated with UCN1 [69, 70]. Regulation of $CRF_{2β}$ levels by UCN1 in A7r5 aortic smooth muscle cells is also observed. Ribonuclease protection assays show that A7r5 cells express $CRF_{2β}$, via which UCN1 induces accumulation of intracellular cAMP, causing a significant decrease in $CRF_{2β}$ mRNA levels as cAMP agonists or analogues. H7, a broad protein kinase (PKA) inhibitor, blocks the UCN1- or cAMP-induced decreases in $CRF_{2β}$ mRNA, and consistently, the PKA inhibitor, H89, also partially reduces the UCN1- or cAMP-induced decreases in $CRF_{2β}$ mRNA levels [71], suggests that a protein kinase pathway is involved in this regulation in A7r5 cells.

$CRF_{2γ}$ has relatively less been researched and rare evidence is presented on the pharmacological profile. When expressed in 293-EBNA (Epstein-Barr nuclear antigen) cells, $CRF_{2γ}$ responds in a dose-dependent manner to CRH and related peptides with a rank order of potency as UCN1 > or = Svg > r/hCRH, with EC_{50} more similar to $CRF_{2α}$ than $CRF_{2β}$. Equilibrium saturation isotherm analysis with radiolabeled Svg reveals that the binding to $CRF_{2γ}$ is a two-site model, with a 60 pM Kd high-affinity site and a 5 nM Kd low-affinity site [54].

Finally, GPCRs coupled with G proteins are well studied and the cryo-EM structures for class B1 GPCRs in complex with Gs protein have been determined [11, 72, 73]. Most recently, structure of class B GPCRs with Gq/11 has been solved, by demonstrating CRF_2 bound to UCN1 coupled with G11 and comparing these structures with the structure of CRF_2 in complex with Gs, providing important insights into the structural basis for the ability of CRF_2 to couple with multiple G protein subtypes [74].

2 CRFr Agonists and Antagonists

CRFp and CRFr present in the central nervous system and a wide variety of peripheral tissues are associated with the pathophysiology of many disease states, leading to the development of CRFr agonists and antagonists to further elucidate the role of CRFp in physiological and disease processes [75–78]. The successful cloning of

CRFr as well as the discovery of their peptide and non-peptide antagonists preludes a new era of CRF-system study.

2.1 CRFr Agonists

As described in Chap. 2, the nature peptide ligands, CRFp, are CRFr agonists, CRH being selective CRF_1 agonist, UCN1 CRF_1&$_2$ agonist, and UCN2&3 selective CRF_2 agonist. Moreover, a lot of synthetized CRH analogues have CRFr-activating potency. By modifications, such as substitution or deletion of residues (residue1-7) and introduction of lactam rings at N-terminus of CRH, many CRH-derived CRFr agonists are obtained, which may vary in the potencies [79–83]. Substitution of each amino acid by its corresponding D-isomer in oCRH results in agonist-analogues with varying potencies, some found to be equipotent to, or twice as potent as, oCRH, and some less potent than oCRH [82]. Deletion of the first 1–7 residues in CRH results in partial agonists because of the gradual loss of intrinsic activity [80]. Moreover, the lactam ring introduced at the N-terminus of CRH fragments (of residue 1-7 deletion) may result in the production of CRFr agonist, such as cyclo(30–33)[Ac-Leu8,DPhe12,Nle21, Glu30,Lys33,Nle38]hCRH(8–41), being equipotent to CRH [80].

2.2 CRFr Antagonists

2.2.1 Unselective CRFr Antagonists

The frequently research-used unselective CRFr antagonists include α-helCRH(9–41) (and analogues) and astressin (and analogues), exerting blocking effects on both CRF_1 and CRF_2. As precedingly described, CRFp assume an α-helical conformation upon binding and interacting with to CRFr, based on which Vale and colleagues report their studies in the synthesis of the agonists and antagonists in 1990s [81, 84, 85]. Similar to agonists' synthesis, deletion or substitution of AA residues of CRH and introduction of covalent constraints such as lactam rings in CRH lead to the discovery of useful CRFr antagonists, such as α-helCRH(9–41) and astressin [83, 84, 86]. It is well recognized that deletions of residues (residues 1–7) in the CRH lead to agonists (of less potency), but further deletions (residues 8–14) help produce antagonists such as astressin [80, 87].

In both oCRH and α-helCRH, deletion of residues 1-6, 1-7, and 1-8 leads to gradual loss of intrinsic activity, resulting in the synthesis of [Met18,Lys23,Glu27 ,29,40,Ala32,41,-Leu33,3 6,38]h/rCRH, α-helCRH(9–41), a potent competitive antagonist [80, 88, 89]. And after the finding that antagonists can be generated by deletion of the first 8–14 residues, a series of CRFr antagonists exhibiting significantly higher in vitro and in vivo biological potency than α-helCRH(9–41) have been reported [82, 87]. Moreover, the lactam rings introduced in CRH result in the production of two potent CRFr antagonists, cyclo(20–23) [DPhe12,Glu20,Lys23,Nle21,38] hCRH(12–41) and astressin [80, 81]. As in the cases of agonists, lactam ring-introductions are useful for stabilizing α-helical conformation of the molecule, with the cyclo(Glu30-Lys33) introduction being favored in the synthesis, suggesting that the lactam cyclization at residues 30–33 favors a structural constraint (α-helix) stabilizing an α-helical conformation in both the agonists and the antagonists, astressin family [80, 81]. Furthermore, the role of residues 4–8 on CRFr activation using successive deletions is investigated, with results showing that residue 8 (Leu or Iso) bears the *sole* responsibility for CRFr activation since deletion of the residue leads to potent antagonists [80]. In addition, two series of CRFr antagonists with N-α- and C-α-methylated Ala and Leu are evaluated for their biological activities in vitro and in vivo [90, 91]. The poly-N-methylated analogue of α-helCRH(9–41), [N-α-MeLeu10,15,27,37, N-α-MeAla22,32,41]-α-helCRH(9–41), is found to be considerably less potent than the parent non-N-methylated analogue, being interpreted by the basis that backbone substitutions on the nitrogen break α-helices. On the other hand, with C-α-MeLeu and/or C-α-MeAla residues at selected positions, [DPhe12,Nle21,38]h/rCRH(12–41), is a potent CRFr antagonist, since C-α-methylation is recognized to increase α-helicity. Also, in vitro potency measurement shows that monosubstituted analogues vary (twice to one fourth as the parent compound) in potency, while the pluri-substituted peptides are slightly less potent, being likely due to an unexpected reduction in the helical content. Interestingly, beside its increased potency, the C-α-MeLeu analogue, [DPhe12,Nle21,38, C-α-MeLeu37]h/rCRH(12–41), is found to be longer acting than the parent compound in two in vivo assays in the rat [91]. More modifications include elongation of CRH chain by three residues at the N-terminus, its acetylation, and the [C-αMeLeu27] substitution to yield cyclo(30–33)[DPhe12, Nle21,C-αMeLeu27,Glu30, Lys33,Nle38]Ac-hCRH(9–41), which is found to be longer acting than astressin [90, 92]. To further increase the efficiency of the antagonists, two or more C-αMe-Leu residues at favorable positions are introduced. The introduction of C-αMe-Leu residues at positions 27 and either 18, 37, or 40 results in significant increases in action duration while the same substitution at positions 27 and either 15, 17, 19, or 41 leads to short acting analogues. Other substitutions by C-αMeLeu at positions 27 and either 10, 13, 14, 21, 24, 36, or 38 yield analogues with intermediate duration of action. Cyclo(30–33)[DPhe12, Nle21, C-αMeLeu27,Glu30,Lys33,Nle38, C-αMeLeu40]Ac-hCRH(9–41) is one of the most efficacious analogues of this series, being even longer acting in rats [90].

Specific for the often-used astressin, cyclo(30–33) [DPhe12,Nle21,Glu30,Lys33,Nle38]hCRH(12–41), the synthesis comprises residues' replacement/deletion and lactam ring introduction in rCRH structure [92, 93]. Both the ligand CRFp and astressin assume an α-helical conformation when interacting with CRFr. And it is suggested that the possibility of a helix-turn-helix motif around a turn encompassing residues 30–33 would confer high affinity for both CRF_1 and CRF_2 in agonists and antagonists [80, 81, 92]. Astressin is C-terminally amidated and exhibits a similar affinity to CRF_1 and CRF_2, in accordance with the structure of astressin-amide having a well-defined helical structure from Leu(27) to Ile(41) [94]. As precedingly described, ECD1 is important for CRFr (class B1 GPCRs) ligand recognition [95], and consistent experimental data supporting the un-selectivity of astressin and ECD1 significance are obtained. A bacterially expressed soluble protein, ECD1-$CRF_{2β}$, corresponding to the ECD1 of mouse $CRF_{2β}$, is characterized. Astressin binds to ECD1-$CRF_{2β}$, with high affinity to UCN1, UCN2,3, and CRH, similar to that for binding to CRF_1 [5].

The synthesis of N-terminally modified astressin analogues and their biochemical evaluation as CRFr antagonists are also reported. It is found that the N-terminal lipidated astressin derivatives are active as CRF_1 and CRF_2 antagonists with nearly equal activities as compared to unmodified Astressin [96]. As described above, Keorber and colleagues test the hypothesis that the lactam ring promotes conformational stability to yield analogues with increased potency both in vitro and in vivo as compared to that of their linear counterparts [81]. Results from the same group show that ***cyclo***(30–33)[DPhe12,Nle21,38, Glu30,DHis32,Lys33]hCRH(12–41) and ***dicyclo***(26–36,30–33)[Ac-Asp9,DPhe12,Nle21,38, Cys26, Glu30,Lys33, Cys36]hCRH(9–41) are twice and 1/100 as potent as astressin, respectively, confirming the role of lactam rings and suggesting a putative turn that encompasses residues 30–33 [87]. Moreover, through extending the astressin chain length by different number of residues at the N-terminus and acetylation, the potency is observed in vivo, with results demonstrating that three-residues longer peptides are longer acting than astressin. In addition, C-αMe-Leu residues in lieu of Leu at positions 14, 15, 19, 27, and 37 in [DHis32]astressin are introduced, with the product [C-αMe-Leu27,DHis32]astressin being more potent than the other analogues in vitro [87].

Furthermore, the discovery of small and potent peptide antagonists of CRFr is reported. Through the structure-activity relationship studies of 12-AA peptide corresponding to the C-terminal residues of astressin, it is assumed that a particular surface of the α-helix is important for binding to the receptor. The small peptide containing d-Ala31 and cyclohexylalanine38 on the surface is observed to be as potent as astressin in binding to CRFr and shows significant effect in rats [97].

Non-peptide unselective CRFr antagonists have not been reported as much in research-use, instead, non-peptide CRF_1 antagonists are developed and used frequently [98, 99] (see below).

2.2.2 Selective CRF_1 Antagonists

Frequently research-used CRF_1 antagonists, such as CP-154,526, antalarmin and NBI-27914, are small non-peptide molecules [4, 100–104]. These compounds have selective CRF_1-antagonizing effects, inhibiting CRH-stimulated cAMP, and hence CRH-stimulated ACTH release from cultured rat anterior pituitary cells or other related outcomes [105–108]. Moreover, when administered peripherally, they compete for ex vivo [^{125}I]Svg binding to CRF_1 in brain sections demonstrating their ability to cross the blood-brain barrier (BBB), which may be favorably taken use of when needed, being an advantage as compared to the peptide antagonists. In in vivo studies, peripheral administration of these compounds attenuates stress-induced elevations in plasma ACTH levels in rats. Furthermore, peripherally administered non-peptide CRF_1 antagonists are demonstrated to inhibit CRH-induced seizure activity [105]. These results demonstrate that the non-peptide antagonists will prove useful in the discovery and development of potential orally active therapeutics for CRF system-related disorders. In addition, CRF_1 antagonists are commonly used as competitive antagonists due to their competence with agonists as described above. However, varying degrees of insurmountable and non-competitive behavior of some antagonists are also reported [109].

Many small-molecule non-peptide CRF_1 antagonists are developed, which are in various stages in clinical trials with some showing great promise in treatment of anxiety, depression, peptic ulcers, inflammation, and IBS [100, 110]. The structure of CP-154,526 is 2 butylethyl[2,5-dimethyl-7-(2,4,6-trimethylphenyl)-7H-pyrrolo [2,3-d]pyrimidin-4-yl]amine [111]. Antalarmin, a close analogue of CP-154,526, is also synthesized by pyrimidine substitution [93, 101, 112] and frequently used as a standard CRF_1 antagonist [93]. And many related compounds are discovered. The binding affinities of selected compounds for CRF_1 are determined showing similar property as compared to a standard CRF_1 antagonist antalarmin [93]. Most recently, the synthesis and biological evaluation of a new series of pyrimidine-substitute CRF_1 antagonists, thiazolo[4,5-d]pyrimidine CRF_1 antagonists, is reported. Several compounds showing promising binding affinity are obtained, as compared with the standard CRF_1 antagonist antalarmin [113].

NBI27914 is obtained by pyridine substitution, i.e., [5-chloro-4-(N-(cyclopropyl) methyl-N-propylamino)-2-methyl-6-(2,4,6-trichlorophenyl)]) amino-pyridine. NBI27914 binds selectively to CRF_1 with a very high affinity [114]. Like antalarmin, pretreatment with NBI 27914 increases the latency and decreases the duration of CRH-induced seizures in rats, supporting its ability to penetrate BBB [115]. Several mutations in the chain of CRF_1 have been identified reducing the binding affinity of the non-peptide antagonist, NBI 27914 [4, 116]. It is observed that the Met276 to Ile (or Val) mutation reduces binding affinity of standard non-peptide antagonists drastically while having no effect on peptide ligand binding. Mutation of Met276 to the rotationally constrained Val produces similar reductions of affinity as Ile mutation. And investigations suggest that these Met276 mutations interfere with binding of the heterocyclic core of the compounds [116]. These findings imply that non-peptide antagonists, and specifically their heterocyclic core, bind in the vicinity of Met276 of CRF_1 instead of the ECD, to which peptide ligands bind. Moreover, mutations of His199 also interfere with the binding for the non-peptide antagonist [4].

Another in vitro pharmacological profile of a small molecule CRF_1 antagonist, (+/−)-N-[2-methyl-4-methoxyphenyl]-1-(1-(methoxymethyl)propyl)-6-methyl-1H-1,2,3-triazolo[4,5-c]pyridin-4-amine (SN003) is reported. SN003 has high affinity and selectivity for CRF_1 expressed in rat and HEK293EBNA cells. It is shown to inhibit CRH-induced cAMP accumulation in human CRF_1-HEK293e cells and CRH-stimulated adrenocorticotropin hormone release from rat pituitary cells without agonist activities. Binding kinetic analysis demonstrates that SN003 is not a simply competitive antagonist [117]. Also, benzazole derivatives with a flexible aryl group bonded through a one-atom linker as a new scaffold for a CRF_1 antagonist are designed, synthesized, and evaluated. In a structure-activity relationship study by Aso group, 4-chloro-N^2-(4-chloro-2-methoxy-6-methylphenyl)-1-methyl-N^7,N^7-dipropyl-1H-benzimidazole-2,7-diamine is found to have the most potent binding activity against $hCRF_1$. Its potent CRF_1-binding activity in brain in ex vivo test and in vivo hypothalamic-pituitary-adrenal (HPA) axis-suppressing effects are observed after oral administration in mice [118]. The results demonstrate that benzimidazole shows in vivo CRF_1 antagonistic activity and good brain penetration, indicating that it is a promising lead for drug discovery of CRF_1 antagonist relevance. Interestingly, a series of derivatives of oxo-7H-benzo[e]perimidine-4-carboxylic acid potently displace radioligand binding of ^{125}I-CRH to both CRF_1 and CRF_2, which antagonize CRH-stimulated cAMP formation and CRH-stimulated corticotropin release from rat pituitary in vivo. These compounds are the first non-peptide antagonists to show activity at both CRF_1 and CRF_2 [119].

Taken together, several classes of small molecule CRF_1 antagonists which belong to the non-peptide class have been developed with many being widely used for research purposes and some pharmaceutical companies are pursuing development of the small non-peptide CRF_1 antagonists [99]. Most recently, Hyun-Soo Cho and colleagues elucidate the crystal structure of CRF_1 by using X-ray free-electron lasers, revealing that two unique hydrogen bonds are present in the hydrogen bond network and the stalk region forms an α-helix and the hydrophobic network contains an antagonist binding site, based on which they develop two CRF_1 antagonists—BMK-C203 and BMK-C205, the latter exerting significant antidepressant effects in mice [35].

2.2.3 Selective CRF_2 Antagonists

As already described, CRF_2 exists as three splice variants of the same gene and have been designated as $CRF_{2\alpha}$, $CRF_{2\beta}$ and $CRF_{2\gamma}$. Anti-sauvagine-30 (aSvg30) and Astressin2B are commonly research-used CRF_2 selective peptide antagonists. Respectively selective antagonists for the three isoforms are not reported yet.

As described by Rivier and colleagues, a Glu32-Lys35 side chain to side chain covalent lactam constraint in hCRH and the corresponding Glu31-Lys34 side chain to side chain covalent lactam constraint in Svg yield potent ligands that are selective for CRF_2 [92]. And discovery of the CRF_2 selective peptide agonists, UCN2 and UCN3, prompt investigations into the structural source of CRF_1 versus CRF_2 selectivity of CRFp. Data from chimeric peptides demonstrate that AA in both the N-terminus and C-terminus of CRH, UCN1, UCN2, and Svg influence CRFr selectivity [120]. Analysis of specific AA residues in the N-terminus and C-terminus indicates that the presence of a Pro11 and Ala35&39 (hCRH numbering) in CRH,

UCN1, and Svg decreases CRF_1 activity and increases CRF_2 selectivity [120]. Accordingly, [^{125}I]Svg has a high affinity for both CRF_1 and CRF_2 and is used in both radioligand binding and receptor autoradiographic studies as a tool to aid in the discovery of selective CRFr antagonists [105]. Furthermore, CRF_2 encodes an arginine residue at the junction between ECD2 and TM3, which plays a role for the discrimination of different CRFp [121] and hence relevant CRFr antagonists.

Taken together with the abovementioned knowledge, a huge series of work are presented in the synthetizing analogues of CRFp and CRFr antagonists [122–124]. aSvg30, an N-terminally truncated version of the CRH analogue, [D-Phe11, His12]Svg(11–40), is characterized as a specific antagonist to mouse $CRF_{2β}$, suppressing agonist-induced adenylate cyclase activity in HEK cells expressing $mCRF_{2β}$ [125]. Then, a photoactivatable analogue of aSvg30, with the N-terminal AA, D-Phe in aSvg30 replaced by a phenyldiazirine, the 4-(1-azi-2,2,2-trifluoroethyl) benzoyl (ATB) residue, resulting in ATB-[His12]Svg, based on which ATB-[His12]Svg(12–40) is synthesized, showing high selective binding to $mCRF_{2β}$ but not $rCRF_1$ (as tested in HEK 293 cells expressing either $rCRF_1$ or $mCRF_{2β}$) and decreasing Svg-stimulated cAMP activity in $mCRF_{2β}$-expressing cells [126].

More analogues of aSvg30 are synthesized and characterized in vitro and in vivo. The synthesized aSvg30 analogues are N-terminally extended by one or two residues or contain the Ala22Arg23Ala24 (ARA motif) of CRH, some also with the introduction of a lactam bridge between positions 29 and 32. N-terminal prolongation and replacement of D-Phe11 by Tyr11 increases the affinity for CRF_2 (aSvg30 (10–40) > aSvg30 (11–40)), while the introduction of the ARA motif or the lactam bridge results in a favor for CRF_1 selectivity [124]. In addition, the radiolabeled ^{125}I-aSvg30 is synthesized and observed exclusively binding to $hCRF_{2α}$ but not to $hCRF_1$. The binding to $hCRF_{2α}$ is saturable and happens specifically to brain areas expressing CRF_2. Also, with the N-terminal AA D-Phe replaced by a D-Tyr residue for specific radioactive labeling with ^{123}I, Met17 substituted by norleucine, and the N-terminus acetylation in aSvg30, different aSvg30 analogues are produced, of which Ac-[D-Tyr11, His12, Nle17]Svg(11–40), named **K31440**, shows high specific binding to $hCRF_{2α}$ and $hCRF_{2β}$ but not the $hCRF_1$ while decreasing Svg-stimulated cAMP activity similarly to aSvg30 in HEK 293 cells transfected with $hCRF_1$, $hCRF_{2α}$, and $hCRF_{2β}$. In the in vivo experiment, ^{123}I-K31440 is detected in small intestine of nude mice [127], demonstrating that ^{123}I-K31440 may serve as a useful tool to detect native CRF_2 and elucidate its role in gastrointestinal disorders and diseases such as IBS. Lawrence et al. test more analogues for their ability to compete for [^{125}I-Tyr0]Svg binding and inhibit Svg-stimulated AC activity in human embryonic kidney HEK 293 cells, permanently transfected with cDNA coding for the $hCRF_1$, $hCRF_{2α}$, and $hCRF_{2β}$. One analogue [D-Phe11, His12, Nle17]Svg(11–40), named **K41498**, is observed to show high affinity binding to $hCRF_{2α}$ and $hCRF_{2β}$ but not the $hCRF_1$ and decrease Svg-stimulated cAMP accumulation in $hCRF_2$ expressing cells. In conscious Wistar-Kyoto rats, K41498 antagonizes the hypotensive response to systemic urocortin [123].

Another often used CRF_2 antagonist, astressin2B, [Lys34]Ac-Svg(8–40), is obtained by deletions and substitutions known to increase duration of action with

CRF_2 selectivity, similar to cyclo31–34[D-Phe11, His12, C-αMeLeu13,39, Nle17,Glu31. CRFr autoradiography is performed in rat tissue expressing CRF_2 and CRF_1 to confirm astressin2B affinity. It is found that astressin2B binds to established CRF_2 but not CRF_1 [92], supported by its in vivo use blocking UCN2 effect [92, 128, 129]. Extended duration of action of astressin2B vs that of aSvg30 is similar, also demonstrated in the CRF_2-mediated mouse model [92].

The development of non-peptide selective CRF_2 antagonists has up-to-date rare reports about [99].

2.2.4 CRF-Binding Protein Functioning Like a CRFr Antagonist

In addition to the CRFr antagonists, the actions of CRFp can also be modulated by a binding protein of **322** AA, namely, CRF-binding protein (CRF-BP) [130–132]. CRF-BP is a 37-kDa protein first purified from human plasma and subsequently cloned. CRF-BP is observed to be expressed in the brains of all species but is uniquely expressed in human liver and placenta [130, 133]. And wide existence in other peripheral organs/tissues, such as the pituitary, the plasma, and adrenal gland, is also observed mediating local functions of CRFp [134–136], as CRF-BP being observed to inhibit ACTH release by CRH in vitro [136]. CRF-BP binds to CRFp, forming complex and decreasing free CRFp level, functioning similarly to CRFr antagonist. Correspondingly, some ligands of CRF-BP, like CRH(6–33), can elevate levels of free CRFp resulting in similar effects of CRFr agonists [137]. Both UCN1 and CRH are found to interact with CRF-BP [138, 139]. These reports indicate that by controlling the amount of free CRFp, it is likely that the CRF-BP is an important modulator of CRFp both in the CNS and in the periphery and ligand inhibitors of CRF-BP may have a therapeutic meaning [130, 140].

3 Summary

CRF receptors belong to secretin-like (class B1) GPCRs, mostly linked to Gs associated with AC. They include two distinct subtypes, CRF_1 and CRF_2, the latter having three isoforms, $CRF_{2\alpha}$, $CRF_{2\beta}$, and $CRF_{2\gamma}$, which are all successfully cloned from their cDNAs encoding **415**, **411**, **431**, and **397** amino acid protein, respectively. Structure features such as α-helices and distinct ECDs are critical for the activity of CRFr. Modifications of their ligands (CRH, sauvagine) lead to synthesis of peptide CRFr antagonists, including the CRFr unselective (α-helCRH(9–41), astressin, and analogues) and CRF_2-selective antagonists (astressin2B and aSvg30 and analogues). The most used selective CRF_1 antagonists are non-peptide antagonists (CP-154526, antalarmin, and NBI-27914), which may have advantages such as being more likely to penetrate BBB when compared to peptide antagonists. Moreover, CRF-BP, a **322**AA protein, binds to CRFp reducing free CRFp levels, having similar inhibitory effects to those of CRFr antagonists. Knowing the characteristics of CRFr is important for understanding their interactions with CRFp and will facilitate the development of CRF system-related drugs.

References

1. Perrin MH, Vale WW. Corticotropin releasing factor receptors and their ligand family. Ann N Y Acad Sci. 1999;885:312–28.
2. Perrin MH, et al. The three-dimensional structure of the N-terminal domain of corticotropin-releasing factor receptors: sushi domains and the B1 family of G protein-coupled receptors. Ann N Y Acad Sci. 2006;1070:105–19.
3. Perrin MH, et al. Distinct structural and functional roles of conserved residues in the first extracellular domain of receptors for corticotropin-releasing factor and related G-protein-coupled receptors. J Biol Chem. 2007;282(52):37529–36.
4. Liaw CW, et al. Localization of agonist- and antagonist-binding domains of human corticotropin-releasing factor receptors. Mol Endocrinol. 1997;11(13):2048–53.
5. Perrin MH, et al. A soluble form of the first extracellular domain of mouse type 2beta corticotropin-releasing factor receptor reveals differential ligand specificity. J Biol Chem. 2003;278(18):15595–600.
6. Liapakis G, et al. Members of CRF family and their receptors: from past to future. Curr Med Chem. 2011;18(17):2583–600.
7. Bale TL, Vale WW. CRF and CRF receptors: role in stress responsivity and other behaviors. Annu Rev Pharmacol Toxicol. 2004;44:525–57.
8. Chalmers DT, et al. Corticotrophin-releasing factor receptors: from molecular biology to drug design. Trends Pharmacol Sci. 1996;17(4):166–72.
9. Vasudevan NT. cAMP assays in GPCR drug discovery. Methods Cell Biol. 2017;142:51–7.
10. Duc NM, Kim HR, Chung KY. Structural mechanism of G protein activation by G protein-coupled receptor. Eur J Pharmacol. 2015;763(Pt B):214–22.
11. Hoare SR. Mechanisms of peptide and nonpeptide ligand binding to class B G-protein-coupled receptors. Drug Discov Today. 2005;10(6):417–27.
12. Cary BP, et al. New insights into the structure and function of class B1 GPCRs. Endocr Rev. 2023;44(3):492–517.
13. Dos Santos Claro PA, et al. Assessing real-time signaling and agonist-induced CRHR1 internalization by optical methods. Methods Cell Biol. 2019;149:239–57.
14. Wu SV, et al. Identification and characterization of multiple corticotropin-releasing factor type 2 receptor isoforms in the rat esophagus. Endocrinology. 2007;148(4):1675–87.
15. Josephs TM, et al. Structure and dynamics of the CGRP receptor in apo and peptide-bound forms. Science. 2021;372(6538)
16. Bortolato A, et al. Structure of class B GPCRs: new horizons for drug discovery. Br J Pharmacol. 2014;171(13):3132–45.
17. Ma S, et al. Molecular basis for hormone recognition and activation of corticotropin-releasing factor receptors. Mol Cell. 2020;77(3):669–680 e4.
18. Liaw CW, et al. Localization of ligand-binding domains of human corticotropin-releasing factor receptor: a chimeric receptor approach. Mol Endocrinol. 1997;11(7):980–5.
19. Grace CR, et al. Common and divergent structural features of a series of corticotropin releasing factor-related peptides. J Am Chem Soc. 2007;129(51):16102–14.
20. Deussing JM, Chen A. The corticotropin-releasing factor family: physiology of the stress response. Physiol Rev. 2018;98(4):2225–86.
21. Nazarloo HP, et al. The roles of corticotropin-releasing factor-related peptides and their receptors in the cardiovascular system. Curr Protein Pept Sci. 2006;7(3):229–39.
22. Zhu C, Li S. The peripheral corticotropin releasing factor family's role in vasculitis. Vasc Pharmacol. 2024;154:107275.
23. Zhu C, Li S. Role of CRH in colitis and colitis-associated cancer: a combinative result of central and peripheral effects? Front Endocrinol (Lausanne). 2024;15:1363748.
24. Tache Y, et al. Brain and gut CRF signaling: biological actions and role in the gastrointestinal tract. Curr Mol Pharmacol. 2018;11(1):51–71.

25. Tache Y, Brunnhuber S. From Hans Selye's discovery of biological stress to the identification of corticotropin-releasing factor signaling pathways: implication in stress-related functional bowel diseases. Ann N Y Acad Sci. 2008;1148:29–41.
26. Chen R, et al. Expression cloning of a human corticotropin-releasing-factor receptor. Proc Natl Acad Sci USA. 1993;90(19):8967–71.
27. Perrin MH, et al. Cloning and functional expression of a rat brain corticotropin releasing factor (CRF) receptor. Endocrinology. 1993;133(6):3058–61.
28. Vita N, et al. Primary structure and functional expression of mouse pituitary and human brain corticotrophin releasing factor receptors. FEBS Lett. 1993;335(1):1–5.
29. De Souza EB. Corticotropin-releasing factor receptors: physiology, pharmacology, biochemistry and role in central nervous system and immune disorders. Psychoneuroendocrinology. 1995;20(8):789–819.
30. Myers DA, Trinh JV, Myers TR. Structure and function of the ovine type 1 corticotropin releasing factor receptor (CRF1) and a carboxyl-terminal variant. Mol Cell Endocrinol. 1998;144(1–2):21–35.
31. Oshida Y, et al. Monkey corticotropin-releasing factor1 receptor: complementary DNA cloning and pharmacological characterization. Life Sci. 2004;74(15):1911–24.
32. Schuster D, et al. Structural insights into membrane adenylyl cyclases, initiators of cAMP signaling. Trends Biochem Sci. 2024;49(2):156–68.
33. Zhao LH, et al. Differential requirement of the extracellular domain in activation of class B G protein-coupled receptors. J Biol Chem. 2016;291(29):15119–30.
34. Pioszak AA, et al. Molecular recognition of corticotropin-releasing factor by its G-protein-coupled receptor CRFR1. J Biol Chem. 2008;283(47):32900–12.
35. Kim H, et al. Structure-based drug discovery of a corticotropin-releasing hormone receptor 1 antagonist using an X-ray free-electron laser. Exp Mol Med. 2023;55(9):2039–50.
36. Wootten D, et al. Allostery and biased Agonism at class B G protein-coupled receptors. Chem Rev. 2017;117(1):111–38.
37. Sangwung P, et al. Class B1 GPCRs: insights into multi-receptor pharmacology for the treatment of metabolic disease. Am J Physiol Endocrinol Metab. 2024;
38. Hollenstein K, et al. Structure of class B GPCR corticotropin-releasing factor receptor 1. Nature. 2013;499(7459):438–43.
39. Dong M, et al. Structure and dynamics of the active Gs-coupled human secretin receptor. Nat Commun. 2020;11(1):4137.
40. Pal K, Melcher K, Xu HE. Structure modeling using genetically engineered crosslinking. Cell. 2013;155(6):1207–8.
41. Coin I, et al. Genetically encoded chemical probes in cells reveal the binding path of urocortin-I to CRF class B GPCR. Cell. 2013;155(6):1258–69.
42. Liang YL, et al. Toward a structural understanding of class B GPCR peptide binding and activation. Mol Cell. 2020;77(3):656–668 e5.
43. Ahn D, Ham D, Chung KY. The conformational transition during G protein-coupled receptor (GPCR) and G protein interaction. Curr Opin Struct Biol. 2021;69:117–23.
44. Pal K, et al. Structural basis for hormone recognition by the human CRFR2alpha G protein-coupled receptor. J Biol Chem. 2010;285(51):40351–61.
45. Schulein R, Gibert A, Rutz C. Functional significance of the signal peptides of corticotropin-releasing factor receptors. Curr Mol Pharmacol. 2017;10(4):311–7.
46. Teichmann A, et al. The pseudo signal peptide of the corticotropin-releasing factor receptor type 2A prevents receptor oligomerization. J Biol Chem. 2012;287(32):27265–74.
47. Schulz K, et al. The pseudo signal peptide of the corticotropin-releasing factor receptor type 2a decreases receptor expression and prevents Gi-mediated inhibition of adenylyl cyclase activity. J Biol Chem. 2010;285(43):32878–87.
48. Perrin MH, et al. Expression, purification, and characterization of a soluble form of the first extracellular domain of the human type 1 corticotropin releasing factor receptor. J Biol Chem. 2001;276(34):31528–34.

49. Alken M, et al. The signal peptide of the rat corticotropin-releasing factor receptor 1 promotes receptor expression but is not essential for establishing a functional receptor. Biochem J. 2005;390(Pt 2):455–64.
50. Wootten D, et al. Receptor activity modifying proteins (RAMPs) interact with the VPAC2 receptor and CRF1 receptors and modulate their function. Br J Pharmacol. 2013;168(4):822–34.
51. Ardati A, et al. Human CRF2 alpha and beta splice variants: pharmacological characterization using radioligand binding and a luciferase gene expression assay. Neuropharmacology. 1999;38(3):441–8.
52. Liaw CW, et al. Cloning and characterization of the human corticotropin-releasing factor-2 receptor complementary deoxyribonucleic acid. Endocrinology. 1996;137(1):72–7.
53. Valdenaire O, et al. A new functional isoform of the human CRF2 receptor for corticotropin-releasing factor. Biochim Biophys Acta. 1997;1352(2):129–32.
54. Kostich WA, et al. Molecular identification and analysis of a novel human corticotropin-releasing factor (CRF) receptor: the CRF2gamma receptor. Mol Endocrinol. 1998;12(8):1077–85.
55. Yarur HE, Andres ME, Gysling K. Type 2beta corticotrophin releasing factor receptor forms a Heteromeric complex with dopamine D1 receptor in living cells. Front Pharmacol. 2019;10:1501.
56. Lovenberg TW, et al. CRF2 alpha and CRF2 beta receptor mRNAs are differentially distributed between the rat central nervous system and peripheral tissues. Endocrinology. 1995;136(9):4139–42.
57. Lovenberg TW, et al. Cloning and characterization of a functionally distinct corticotropin-releasing factor receptor subtype from rat brain. Proc Natl Acad Sci USA. 1995;92(3):836–40.
58. Rutz C, et al. The corticotropin-releasing factor receptor type 2a contains an N-terminal pseudo signal peptide. J Biol Chem. 2006;281(34):24910–21.
59. Suman-Chauhan N, et al. Expression and characterisation of human and rat CRF2alpha receptors. Eur J Pharmacol. 1999;379(2–3):219–27.
60. Yarur HE, et al. Cross-talk between dopamine D1 and corticotropin releasing factor type 2 receptors leads to occlusion of their ERK1/2 signaling. J Neurochem. 2020;155(3):264–73.
61. Fuenzalida J, et al. Dopamine D1 and corticotrophin-releasing hormone type-2alpha receptors assemble into functionally interacting complexes in living cells. Br J Pharmacol. 2014;171(24):5650–64.
62. Chen AM, et al. A soluble mouse brain splice variant of type 2alpha corticotropin-releasing factor (CRF) receptor binds ligands and modulates their activity. Proc Natl Acad Sci USA. 2005;102(7):2620–5.
63. Perrin M, et al. Identification of a second corticotropin-releasing factor receptor gene and characterization of a cDNA expressed in heart. Proc Natl Acad Sci USA. 1995;92(7):2969–73.
64. Grace CR, et al. Structure of the N-terminal domain of a type B1 G protein-coupled receptor in complex with a peptide ligand. Proc Natl Acad Sci USA. 2007;104(12):4858–63.
65. Sato T. Conserved 2nd residue of helix 8 of GPCR may confer the subclass-characteristic and distinct roles through a rapid initial interaction with specific G proteins. Int J Mol Sci. 2019;20(7)
66. Langer I, Langlet C, Robberecht P. Effect of inactivating mutations on phosphorylation and internalization of the human VPAC2 receptor. J Mol Endocrinol. 2005;34(2):405–14.
67. Yarur HE, et al. Functional interplay of Type-2 corticotrophin releasing factor and dopamine receptors in the basolateral amygdala-medial prefrontal cortex circuitry. Int J Neuropsychopharmacol. 2021;24(3):221–8.
68. Vinkers CH, et al. Role of dopamine D1 and D2 receptors in CRF-induced disruption of sensorimotor gating. Pharmacol Biochem Behav. 2007;86(3):550–8.
69. Nazarloo HP, et al. Down-regulation of corticotropin-releasing hormone receptor type 2beta mRNA expression in the rat cardiovascular system following food deprivation. Regul Pept. 2002;105(2):121–9.

70. Kageyama K, et al. Regulation of corticotropin-releasing factor receptor type 2 beta messenger ribonucleic acid in the rat cardiovascular system by urocortin, glucocorticoids, and cytokines. Endocrinology. 2000;141(7):2285–93.
71. Kageyama K, et al. Regulation of corticotropin-releasing factor receptor type 2beta mRNA via cyclic AMP pathway in A7r5 aortic smooth muscle cells. Cell Signal. 2003;15(1):17–25.
72. Flock T, et al. Selectivity determinants of GPCR-G-protein binding. Nature. 2017;545(7654):317–22.
73. Garcia-Nafria J, Tate CG. Cryo-EM structures of GPCRs coupled to G(s), G(i) and G(o). Mol Cell Endocrinol. 2019;488:1–13.
74. Zhao LH, et al. Structure insights into selective coupling of G protein subtypes by a class B G protein-coupled receptor. Nat Commun. 2022;13(1):6670.
75. Grammatopoulos DK, Chrousos GP. Functional characteristics of CRH receptors and potential clinical applications of CRH-receptor antagonists. Trends Endocrinol Metab. 2002;13(10):436–44.
76. Liapakis G. Editorial: Corticotropin releasing factor (CRF) and its receptors: from structure to function in health and disease (part I). Curr Mol Pharmacol. 2017;10(4):257–8.
77. Liapakis G. Editorial: Corticotropin releasing factor (CRF) and its receptors: from structure to function in health and disease (part II). Curr Mol Pharmacol. 2018;11(1):2–3.
78. Sanders J, Nemeroff C. The CRF system as a therapeutic target for neuropsychiatric disorders. Trends Pharmacol Sci. 2016;37(12):1045–54.
79. Papazacharias S, et al. Synthesis and biological evaluation of new CRH analogues. Bioinorg Chem Appl. 2010;2010
80. Rivier J, et al. Minimal-size, constrained corticotropin-releasing factor agonists with i-(i+3) Glu-Lys and Lys-Glu bridges. J Med Chem. 1998;41(14):2614–20.
81. Koerber SC, et al. Constrained corticotropin-releasing factor (CRF) agonists and antagonists with i-(i+3) Glu-Xaa-DXbb-Lys bridges. J Med Chem. 1998;41(25):5002–11.
82. Rivier J, et al. Single point D-substituted corticotropin-releasing factor analogues: effects on potency and physicochemical characteristics. J Med Chem. 1993;36(20):2851–9.
83. Gulyas J, et al. Potent, structurally constrained agonists and competitive antagonists of corticotropin-releasing factor. Proc Natl Acad Sci USA. 1995;92(23):10575–9.
84. Miranda A, et al. Constrained corticotropin-releasing factor antagonists with i-(i + 3) Glu-Lys bridges. J Med Chem. 1997;40(22):3651–8.
85. Cervini L, et al. Corticotropin releasing factor (CRF) agonists with reduced amide bonds and Ser7 substitutions. J Med Chem. 1999;42(4):761–8.
86. Miranda A, et al. Conformationally restricted competitive antagonists of human/rat corticotropin-releasing factor. J Med Chem. 1994;37(10):1450–9.
87. Rivier J, et al. Astressin analogues (corticotropin-releasing factor antagonists) with extended duration of action in the rat. J Med Chem. 1998;41(25):5012–9.
88. Fisher L, et al. Differential antagonist activity of alpha-helical corticotropin-releasing factor9-41 in three bioassay systems. Endocrinology. 1991;129(3):1312–6.
89. Rivier JE, Rivier CL. Corticotropin-releasing factor peptide antagonists: design, characterization and potential clinical relevance. Front Neuroendocrinol. 2014;35(2):161–70.
90. Rivier JE, et al. Constrained corticotropin releasing factor antagonists (astressin analogues) with long duration of action in the rat. J Med Chem. 1999;42(16):3175–82.
91. Hernandez JF, et al. Synthesis and relative potencies of new constrained CRF antagonists. J Med Chem. 1993;36(20):2860–7.
92. Rivier J, et al. Potent and long-acting corticotropin releasing factor (CRF) receptor 2 selective peptide competitive antagonists. J Med Chem. 2002;45(21):4737–47.
93. Teleb M, et al. Synthesis of 2-imino and 2-hydrazono thiazolo[4,5-d]pyrimidines as corticotropin releasing factor (CRF) antagonists. Eur J Med Chem. 2017;138:900–8.
94. Grace CR, et al. Astressin-amide and astressin-acid are structurally different in dimethylsulfoxide. Biopolymers. 2007;87(2–3):196–205.

95. Grace CR, et al. NMR structure and peptide hormone binding site of the first extracellular domain of a type B1 G protein-coupled receptor. Proc Natl Acad Sci USA. 2004;101(35):12836–41.
96. Rijkers DT, den Hartog JA, Liskamp RM. Synthesis and biological activity of N-terminal lipidated and/or fluorescently labeled conjugates of astressin as corticotropin releasing factor antagonists. Bioorg Med Chem. 2004;12(19):5099–106.
97. Yamada Y, et al. New class of corticotropin-releasing factor (CRF) antagonists: small peptides having high binding affinity for CRF receptor. J Med Chem. 2004;47(5):1075–8.
98. Hoare SRJ, Grigoriadis DE. Non-peptide CRF-receptor antagonists: Allosterism, kinetics and translation to efficacy in human disease. Curr Mol Pharmacol. 2017;10(4):282–95.
99. Fahmy H, Kuppast B, Ismail MT. Structure and function of small non-peptide CRF antagonists and their potential clinical use. Curr Mol Pharmacol. 2017;10(4):270–81.
100. Seymour PA, Schmidt AW, Schulz DW. The pharmacology of CP-154,526, a non-peptide antagonist of the CRH1 receptor: a review. CNS Drug Rev. 2003;9(1):57–96.
101. Sakellaris S, et al. Selective antagonism of CRF1 receptor by a substituted pyrimidine. Hormones (Athens). 2019;18(2):215–21.
102. Schulz DW, et al. CP-154,526: a potent and selective nonpeptide antagonist of corticotropin releasing factor receptors. Proc Natl Acad Sci USA. 1996;93(19):10477–82.
103. Zorrilla EP, et al. Effects of antalarmin, a CRF type 1 receptor antagonist, on anxiety-like behavior and motor activation in the rat. Brain Res. 2002;952(2):188–99.
104. Chen C. Recent advances in small molecule antagonists of the corticotropin-releasing factor type-1 receptor-focus on pharmacology and pharmacokinetics. Curr Med Chem. 2006;13(11):1261–82.
105. McCarthy JR, Heinrichs SC, Grigoriadis DE. Recent advances with the CRF1 receptor: design of small molecule inhibitors, receptor subtypes and clinical indications. Curr Pharm Des. 1999;5(5):289–315.
106. Hao K, et al. Inactivation of corticotropin-releasing hormone-induced insulinotropic role by high-altitude hypoxia. Diabetes. 2015;64(3):785–95.
107. Cao J, et al. Human mast cells express corticotropin-releasing hormone (CRH) receptors and CRH leads to selective secretion of vascular endothelial growth factor. J Immunol. 2005;174(12):7665–75.
108. Hoare SR, et al. Ligand affinity for amino-terminal and juxtamembrane domains of the corticotropin releasing factor type I receptor: regulation by G-protein and nonpeptide antagonists. Biochemistry. 2004;43(13):3996–4011.
109. Ramsey SJ, et al. Quantitative pharmacological analysis of antagonist binding kinetics at CRF1 receptors in vitro and in vivo. Br J Pharmacol. 2011;164(3):992–1007.
110. Kohman RA, et al. Alleviation of the effects of endotoxin exposure on behavior and hippocampal IL-1beta by a selective non-peptide antagonist of corticotropin-releasing factor receptors. Brain Behav Immun. 2007;21(6):824–35.
111. Chen YL, et al. Synthesis and oral efficacy of a 4-(butylethylamino)pyrrolo[2,3-d]pyrimidine: a centrally active corticotropin-releasing factor1 receptor antagonist. J Med Chem. 1997;40(11):1749–54.
112. Kuppast B, et al. Synthesis of substituted pyrimidines as corticotropin releasing factor (CRF) receptor ligands. Eur J Med Chem. 2014;78:1–9.
113. Islam MR, et al. Design, synthesis, structural optimization, SAR, in silico prediction of physicochemical properties and pharmacological evaluation of novel & potent thiazolo[4,5-d]pyrimidine corticotropin releasing factor (CRF) receptor antagonists. Eur J Pharm Sci. 2022;169:106084.
114. Bhattacharya S, et al. Allosteric antagonist binding sites in class B GPCRs: corticotropin receptor 1. J Comput Aided Mol Des. 2010;24(8):659–74.
115. Baram TZ, et al. The CRF1 receptor mediates the excitatory actions of corticotropin releasing factor (CRF) in the developing rat brain: in vivo evidence using a novel, selective, nonpeptide CRF receptor antagonist. Brain Res. 1997;770(1–2):89–95.

116. Hoare SR, et al. Single amino acid residue determinants of non-peptide antagonist binding to the corticotropin-releasing factor1 (CRF1) receptor. Biochem Pharmacol. 2006;72(2):244–55.
117. Zhang G, et al. Pharmacological characterization of a novel nonpeptide antagonist radioligand, (+/−)-N-[2-methyl-4-methoxyphenyl]-1-(1-(methoxymethyl) propyl)-6-methyl-1H-1,2,3-triazolo[4,5-c]pyridin-4-amine ([3H]SN003) for corticotropin-releasing factor1 receptors. J Pharmacol Exp Ther. 2003;305(1):57–69.
118. Mochizuki M, et al. Design and synthesis of Benzimidazoles as novel Corticotropin-releasing factor 1 receptor antagonists. J Med Chem. 2016;59(6):2551–66.
119. Luthin DR, et al. Synthesis and biological activity of oxo-7H-benzo[e]perimidine-4-carboxylic acid derivatives as potent, nonpeptide corticotropin releasing factor (CRF) receptor antagonists. Bioorg Med Chem Lett. 1999;9(5):765–70.
120. Mazur AW, et al. Determinants of corticotropin releasing factor. Receptor selectivity of corticotropin releasing factor related peptides. J Med Chem. 2004;47(13):3450–4.
121. Dautzenberg FM, et al. Evidence for the abundant expression of arginine 185 containing human CRF(2alpha) receptors and the role of position 185 for receptor-ligand selectivity. Neuropharmacology. 2000;39(8):1368–76.
122. Higelin J, et al. 125I-Antisauvagine-30: a novel and specific high-affinity radioligand for the characterization of corticotropin-releasing factor type 2 receptors. Neuropharmacology. 2001;40(1):114–22.
123. Lawrence AJ, et al. The highly selective CRF(2) receptor antagonist K41498 binds to presynaptic CRF(2) receptors in rat brain. Br J Pharmacol. 2002;136(6):896–904.
124. Brauns O, et al. Secondary structure of antisauvagine analogues is important for CRF receptor antagonism: development of antagonists with increased potency and receptor selectivity. Peptides. 2002;23(10):1817–27.
125. Ruhmann A, et al. Structural requirements for peptidic antagonists of the corticotropin-releasing factor receptor (CRFR): development of CRFR2beta-selective antisauvagine-30. Proc Natl Acad Sci USA. 1998;95(26):15264–9.
126. Bonk I, Ruhmann A. Development of a selective photoactivatable antagonist for corticotropin-releasing factor receptor, type 2 (CRF2). Eur J Biochem. 2002;269(21):5288–94.
127. Ruhmann A, et al. Design, synthesis and pharmacological characterization of new highly selective CRF(2) antagonists: development of 123I-K31440 as a potential SPECT ligand. Peptides. 2002;23(3):453–60.
128. Henry B, Vale W, Markou A. The effect of lateral septum corticotropin-releasing factor receptor 2 activation on anxiety is modulated by stress. J Neurosci. 2006;26(36):9142–52.
129. Takeuchi K, et al. Involvement of corticotropin-releasing factor and corticotropin-releasing factor 2 receptors in pathogenesis of ischemia/reperfusion-induced enteritis in rats. J Physiol Pharmacol. 2016;67(5):697–707.
130. Behan DP, et al. Corticotropin releasing factor (CRF) binding protein: a novel regulator of CRF and related peptides. Front Neuroendocrinol. 1995;16(4):362–82.
131. Petraglia F, et al. Corticotropin-releasing factor-binding protein: origins and possible functions. Horm Res. 1996;45(3–5):187–91.
132. Sanson A, et al. CRF binding protein activity in the hypothalamic paraventricular nucleus is essential for stress adaptations and normal maternal behaviour in lactating rats. Neurobiol Stress. 2024;30:100631.
133. Baigent SM, Lowry PJ. mRNA expression profiles for corticotrophin-releasing factor (CRF), urocortin, CRF receptors and CRF-binding protein in peripheral rat tissues. J Mol Endocrinol. 2000;25(1):43–52.
134. Chatzaki E, Margioris AN, Gravanis A. Expression and regulation of corticotropin-releasing hormone binding protein (CRH-BP) in rat adrenals. J Neurochem. 2002;80(1):81–90.
135. Potter E, et al. Cloning and characterization of the cDNAs for human and rat corticotropin releasing factor-binding proteins. Nature. 1991;349(6308):423–6.
136. Stinnett GS, Westphal NJ, Seasholtz AF. Pituitary CRH-binding protein and stress in female mice. Physiol Behav. 2015;150:16–23.

137. Slater PG, et al. CRF binding protein facilitates the presence of CRF type 2alpha receptor on the cell surface. Proc Natl Acad Sci USA. 2016;113(15):4075–80.
138. Behan DP, et al. Urocortin interaction with corticotropin-releasing factor (CRF) binding protein (CRF-BP): a novel mechanism for elevating 'free' CRF levels in human brain. Brain Res. 1996;725(2):263–7.
139. Westphal NJ, Seasholtz AF. CRH-BP: the regulation and function of a phylogenetically conserved binding protein. Front Biosci. 2006;11:1878–91.
140. Behan DP, et al. Neurobiology of corticotropin releasing factor (CRF) receptors and CRF-binding protein: implications for the treatment of CNS disorders. Mol Psychiatry. 1996;1(4):265–77.

Chapter 4
CRF Peptides in the Digestive System

Shengnan Li and Chao Zhu

Corticotropin-releasing hormone (factor) family peptides (CRF peptides, CRFp) comprise four members, corticotropin-releasing hormone (CRH), urocortin (UCN1), UCN2, and UCN3, with CRH selectively acting on type 1 CRF receptors (CRFr)—CRF_1, UCN1 on CRF_1 and CRF_2 (type 2 CRFr), and UCN2 and UCN3 on CRF_2 (see Chaps. 2 and 3). After the finding of CRH in the brain by River and colleagues [1], CRH and UCNs are also found widely distributed in peripheral cells/tissues, including the digestive system [2, 3]. All these CRFp (CRH, UCN1, UCN2, UCN3) and their two distinct CRFr, CRF_1 and CRF_2, are observed to exist in the gastrointestinal tract (GI), both the upper and the lower part, and other digestive organs. Moreover, CRFp's roles in GI have been well documented and the mechanisms may be complicated, sometimes difficult to differentiate between central and peripheral actions [4, 5]. For instance, peripheral use of UCN1 reduces feeding and induces interoceptive stress with increased cortisol level, while UCN2,3 suppresses feeding without inducing malaise in fasted and fed rats [6], suggesting the combined UCNs work on CRF_1 and CRF_2 in both central and peripheral ways, since central CRF_1 activation is associated with stress and CRF_2 activation suppresses feeding, and meanwhile, peripheral CRF_2 activation also inhibits feeding by reducing GI motility [7]. This chapter will mainly focus on the peripheral distribution and effects of CRFp in digestive system, including actions directly on the digestive organs (GI tract, pancreas, and liver) and via the immune/inflammatory cells and enteric nervous system (ENS) influencing digestive functions.

S. Li (✉) · C. Zhu
Department of Pharmacology, School of Basic Medical Sciences,
Nanjing Medical University, Nanjing, Jiangsu, China
e-mail: snli@njmu.edu.cn

© The Author(s), under exclusive license to Springer Nature Singapore Pte Ltd. 2025

C. Zhu et al. (eds.), *The Peripheral Existence and Effects of Corticotropin-releasing Factor Family*, https://doi.org/10.1007/978-981-96-5322-5_4

1 The Existence and Role of CRFp in Digestive System

CRH and UCNs are observed existing in both the upper and lower GI tract, and their roles in GI and other digestive organs are widely studied. As described in Chap. 1, CRH is a central regulator of the hormonal stress response, being able to influence GI functions. On the other hand, peripheral CRFp-related mechanisms also contribute to stress-induced changes in gut motility and intestinal mucosal function, and intraperitoneal CRH increases ion secretion and mucosal permeability to macromolecules, which mimics the results induced by acute stress prevented by CRFr antagonists given peripherally [4]. Similarly, early trauma enhances intestinal mucosal dysfunction to an acute stressor in adult rats, which is prevented by peripheral injection of CRFr antagonist [8]. A clinic study reveals that in patients with traumatic shock or undergoing elective abdominal surgery, GI dysfunction occurs, i.e., gastric emptying is retarded and intestinal permeability is increased, in which peripheral CRH is found to be implicated since CRH levels change significantly in the plasma and small bowel of the patients [9]. Collectively, these results support that peripheral CRFp are associated with stress-related alterations of gut motor function, and the role of CRFr in both the brain and the gut are key mechanisms through which various stressors impact the activity of the digestive system [10]. The direct peripheral effects of CRFp on digestive system have been well documented, detailed as follows.

1.1 CRFp in the Upper GI Tract

1.1.1 CRFp in the Stomach

Examinations on human gastric biopsies indicate that CRH is absent in the stomach tissues from healthy controls and patients with active gastritis before and after *Helicobacter pylori* eradication treatment whereas UCN1 is present, suggesting that UCN1 instead of CRH plays critical roles in human gastric functions [11]. However, there are also reports that CRH is associated with gastric activities [12, 13].

A most recent investigation in healthy volunteers confirms that peripheral CRH infusion significantly promotes gastric emptying, decreasing the gastric emptying half time [14]. However, opposite effects are also observed, i.e., peripheral injection of CRH inhibits rat gastric emptying and motility through interaction with CRF_2 [13]. Moreover, it is reported that gastric suction in premature infants may play a role in the development of intestinal disorders [15]. In accordance, neonatal rats subjected to repeated orogastric suction are found to result in global chronic somatic and visceral hyperalgesia in adulthood, which is via a CRH-mediated mechanism, being prevented by peripheral pretreatment of the CRF_1 receptor antagonist, antalarmin [16].

In rat stomach, UCN1 and CRF_2 are widely distributed, the expression of which in the mucosa and submucosa plus muscle (S + M) are detected [17]. It is observed that transcripts of UCN1 and $CRF_{2\beta}$ are expressed in all layers. In the presence of LPS, UCN1 mRNA level significantly increases in both mucosa and S + M, while $CRF_{2\beta}$ mRNA level is significantly decreased in the mucosa and M + S. In addition, $CRF_{2\alpha}$ is also detected in the gastric corpus, antrum, and pylorus, also regulated by LPS. Blockade of CRF_2 by astressin2B exacerbates LPS-delayed gastric emptying, indicating that UCN1 stimulates gastric emptying via CRF_2 [17], which is opposite to the finding that UCN1 (and UCN2,3) is also observed to inhibit rat gastric emptying and motility through interaction with CRF_2 [13]. Moreover, endogenous UCN1 is found expressed abundantly in the rat stomach parietal cells by using an immunofluorescence histochemical technique [18]. In addition, a recent study by Chatzaki et al. reveals a specific mapping of CRF_1 and CRF_2 in rat upper GI tract by using polyclonal antisera and characterization in CRF_1- and CRF_2-transfected cell lines [19]. It is found that CRF_1 is located in a narrow zone in the upper oxyntic gland within gastric corpus binding to the selective anti-CRF_1 serum (4467a-CRF_1) while the unselective anti-CRFr serum (4392a-CRFr) labels cells throughout the oxyntic gland and submucosal blood vessels. Also, colocalization of UCN1 and CRF_2 in the rat gastric glands is observed [19]. Moreover, by recording rat intraluminal gastric pressure waves, it is found that peripherally used astressin, a nonselective CRFr antagonist, blocks the response to WAS while UCN2 and astressin2B has no effect, demonstrating that WAS activates peripheral CRF_1 signaling and enhances gastric motility [20], which is opposite to the central CRH/CRF_1's influence on the stomach inhibiting gastric activity induced by pentagastrin in dogs [21].

1.1.2 CRFp in the Duodenum

High concentration of CRH is observed in rat duodenum [22]. Immunofluorescence microscopic studies reveal a CRH staining within both myenteric plexus perikaryal and nerve fibers of the rat duodenum [23]. It is observed that CRH impairs rat duodenal contractions, which is completely abolished by the unselective CRFr antagonist, astressin [24]. Moreover, CRH significantly stimulates duodenal bicarbonate secretion, which is an important factor in the pathogenesis of duodenal ulcer disease, and the effect is reversed by pretreatment of the animals with the CRFr antagonist, α-helical CRH(9–41) [25]. Interestingly, a classical Chinese medicine used for dyspepsia, Sini San (SNS), is found to downregulate the expression of CRH and modulate the expression of both CRF_1 and CRF_2 in the rat duodenum [26]. In addition, rats' maternal deprivation induces a sustained decrease in Paneth and goblet cells but an increase in endocrine cells, associated with an enhancement of CRH, UCN2, and CRF_2, but a decrease in CRF_1 expression in the duodenum [27]. In C57BL6 mice, a recent work demonstrates a signaling link between CRH and the innate epithelial immune protein NLRP6, an inflammasome shown to participate in regulating GI mucus secretion [28]. Inhibition of NLRP6 is found in water avoidance stress (WAS)-induced small-bowel inflammation, which can be prevented by the peroxisome proliferator-activated receptor-γ agonist, rosiglitazone, which induces epithelial expression of NLRP6. Importantly, higher serum level of CRH, inversely correlated with NLRP6 expression in the small intestine, is observed during WAS. Furthermore, exogenous CRH is found to inhibit NLRP6 expression. The results suggest that WAS induces CRH release, which subsequently inhibits NLRP6 leading to intestinal inflammation [28]. Consistently, functional dyspepsia (FD) patients exhibit reduced duodenal CRF_2, which is observed to be associated with reduced NLRP6 expression and autophagy function in the duodenum. This reduction causes loss of duodenal goblet cell homeostasis, with reduced cell numbers and cell function (mucin exocytosis) in PD patients. In the HT29-MTX-E12 cell line, results of studies demonstrate that CRH reduces NLRP6 expression in duodenal spheroids and functionally promotes mucus secretion [29]. Since CRH acts selectively on CRF_1, these results suggest that FD patients exhibit dysregulations in the NLRP6-autophagy axis and hence have lower goblet cell function, involving enhanced activity of CRF_1 and loss of CRF_2 in the duodenum [15].

1.2 CRFp in the Lower GI Tract

1.2.1 CRFp in the Small Intestine

Local CRH synthesis is almost undetectable in normal rat intestine tissue but observed to considerably increase in intestinal inflammation (chronic enterocolitis), located in inflammatory cells, mesenchymal cells, and myenteric plexi [30]. In contraction studies in vitro, CRH is found to relax guinea pig ileal but not gastric and jejunal smooth muscles by activating Ca^{2+}-sensitive K^+ currents (IK), causing significant hyperpolarization of the cell membranes, which is effectively antagonized by blockers of protein kinase A (PKA) or adenylyl cyclase. However, neither forskolin nor the catalytic subunit of PKA can mimic the effect of CRH on IK, suggesting that CRH exerts its relaxing activity on ileal smooth muscle cells via PKA-dependent phosphorylation related to intracellular Ca^{2+} storage mechanism [31].

In the rat small intestine (besides stomach and ENS), UCN1 expression is detected [18], and the gene expression of CRF_1 and CRF_2 is observed [32]. It is showed that the mesenteric artery undergoing ischemia/reperfusion (I/R) develops hemorrhagic lesions in ampicillin- and aminoguanidine-inhibitable manners, accompanied by enterobacterial invasion and upregulation of the inducible nitric oxide synthase (iNOS) expression, which is significantly reduced by astressin (unselective CRFr antagonist) and astressin2B (selective CRF_2 antagonist), but not by the selective CRF_1 antagonist, NBI27914. Moreover, UCN1 markedly exacerbates the I/R lesions, which is completely abrogated by astressin 2B, but not NBI27914 [32]. These results demonstrate that UCN1 plays a role in the I/R hemorrhagic lesions via CRF_2, involving enterobacteria and iNOS-NO.

1.2.2 CRFp in the Colon

The expression of CRFp and CRFr and their effects in the colorectal tissues have been well documented [33–36]. CRH and UCNs are detected in the colon of human and other species [37–39]. Also, the expression of both CRF_1 and CRF_2 is reported at the mRNA and protein levels in the colon of human and other species [33, 36, 40, 41]. In normal human colonic tissues obtained by endoscopic biopsy, immunoreactive (IR) CRH and CRH mRNA are detected in the colonic mucosal cells in the neighborhood of the base of the crypts. And it is found that normal human colonic mucosal enterochromaffin cells also produce CRH [37]. Sasano group observe that in non-pathologic sections of adult colorectal tissues from patients with colorectal cancer, UCN1 expression is predominantly detected in lamina propria macrophages. UCN1, CRF_1, and $CRF_{2\alpha}$ mRNA are detected in isolated lamina propria mononuclear cells (LPMC) and UCN1 is found to be locally synthesized in lamina propria macrophages acting on lamina propria inflammatory cells as a local regulator of the mucosal immune system [33]. Using a specific antiserum against the C-terminus of CRF_2 (2064a-CRF_2) and a selective anti-CRF_1 antiserum (4467a-CRF_1) in immunofluorescent staining, the anatomical distribution of receptor protein expression in rat colon is mapped by Chatzaki and colleagues. CRF_1 is found in the goblet and stem cells of the colonic crypts and in scattered cells of the surface epithelium and the lamina propria of the proximal colonic mucosa while CRF_2 in the luminal surface of the crypts and in blood vessels of the submucosal layer [40].

UCN3 is also expressed in the colon in human and other species [42, 43]. It is abundant in rat colon epithelial cells and myenteric neurons [42]. In the normal human large intestine, UCN3 expression is observed widely in myenteric and submucosal nervous plexus, vascular endothelial cells, vascular smooth muscle cells in subserosa, smooth muscle layers, and enterochromaffin cells while it is hardly detected in lamina propria inflammatory cells in colonic mucosa. Parallelly, CRF_2 expression is distributed similarly, but also in lamina propria inflammatory cells. By radioimmunoassay, UCN3 is also detected in the large intestine, with high concentrations in the rectum and sigmoid colon [43].

1.2.3 The Role of CRFp in Colitis and Colitis-Associated Colon Cancer

Peripheral CRFp, via CRFr, play an important role in the process of colitis [35, 44] and hence colorectal cancer (CRC), i.e., colitis-associated colon cancer (CAC) [45, 46], since colitis is a high risk for CAC [47, 48], as is recently reviewed by our group [49].

The Role of CRFp in Colitis

As described at the chapter beginning, peripheral use of CRH and UCN1 may influence GI functions both centrally (mimicking stress) and peripherally. In case of colitis, there is also no clearcut between the central and local influence of CRFp [49]. For example, evaluation on rat colonic response to CRH and hyperalgesia after ending stress exposure shows that colon epithelial permeability and conductance are increased, and visceral hypersensitivity persists for a long time. Moreover, abnormal colonic response to exogenous CRH (*which may act centrally and peripherally*) lasts for a long period and mitochondrial activity is disturbed throughout the intestine, with colonic expression of CRF_1 increased [50].

The mechanisms of CRH in colitis are complicated. Firstly, CRH/CRF_1 signal pathway is observed to play a role in GI motility directly or by influencing the enteric nervous system [51, 52] or directly taking part in brain-gut sensitization [35], contributing to the symptoms as chronic abdominal pain or discomfort due to altered gut movement and visceral sensation in patients with colitis [4, 51, 53, 54]. This observation is supported by the fact that CRH antagonist, α-helical-CRH, blocks the colorectal distention-induced sensitization of the visceral perception in rats [35, 54, 55]. Moreover, peripheral CRH also functions in colitis via interacting with immune/inflammatory processes [2] (also see Sect. 2). UCN1 is also observed to cause rats' GI hyperpermeability via both microvessels and macrophages [56] and CRH induces human colonic mucosal hyperpermeability by stimulating subepithelial mast cells [57]. In addition, in our laboratory, we find that expressions of UCN1 and CRH are enhanced in the colon of wild type ($Crhr_1^{+/+}$) mice under the treatment of azoxymethane (AOM) and DSS [45]. The extent and severity of colon inflammation are drastically reduced in $Crhr_1^{-/-}$ mice with a decrease in inflammatory cytokines (IL-1, IL-6, and TNF-α), grade of dysplasia, and ulcer numbers in the colon mucosa. In contrast, the anti-inflammatory factor, IL-10, is increased in $Crhr_1^{-/-}$ mice. These results are consistent with the reported research observation that activation of CRF_1 promotes inflammation [2, 58, 59]. On the other hand, CRF_2 is found to have a counter-regulatory action against CRF_1, maintaining a balance between CRF_1 and CRF_2 during the process of inflammation [59, 60]. Differently, activation of CRF_2 is reported to take opposite effects in acute and chronic colitis, promoting inflammation during the former process but inhibiting inflammation during the latter one, partly backed up by the result that mucosal repair is delayed after administration of a CRF_2 antagonist in DSS-induced colitis [61]. In isoflurane-anesthetized rats, it is also found that contrary to CRH, peripheral use of UCN2 decreases colonic vascular resistance (CVR) inducing hyperemia, which is inhibited by L-NAME or Astressin 2B, suggesting that peripheral CRF_2 activation induces colonic hyperemia through NO synthesis [62]. Moreover, CRF_2 is downregulated in distal/sigmoid biopsies of ulcerative colitis (UC) patients. The colonic mucosal biopsies from patients with UC show no CRF_2 expression while those from healthy controls display CRF_2 expression in the epithelial cells [63]. In a word, a balance between CRF_1 and CRF_2 may decide the process of inflammation, which may well interpret that both CRF_1 and CRF_2 are found to participate in acute inflammation while CRF_2 is the main type for repair [59]. Thirdly, CRFp may influence the tight junctions (TJ) leading to permeability impairment. Intestinal tissue samples' analysis shows that both transcriptional and post-transcriptional mechanisms are involved in the modulation of intestinal epithelial barrier function in inflammatory bowel disease (IBS) patients, which includes miRNAs as master regulators in controlling the expression of TJ proteins, being associated with major clinical symptoms [64]. Consistently, in HT29 cells, CRH is found to increase the permeability using a transwell assay and the structural changes of TJ are observed under transmission electron microscopy, accompanied by reduced TJ protein expression [65].

Using a rat model of Crohn's colitis, it is observed that UCN3 decreases with the inflammation processing. With the onset of colitis, UCN3 mRNA levels reduce markedly while surprisingly, during colitis UCN3 alters neither histopathological outcomes nor the levels of pro-inflammatory cytokines (IL-6 and TNF-α). At baseline, colon-specific knockdown of CRF_1 markedly decreases UCN3 mRNA, whereas during colitis, opposite results are obtained. No significant change is found with the knockdown of CRF_2. In cultured cells, co-expression of CRF_1 and CRF_2 attenuates UCN3-elicited intracellular calcium concentration ($[Ca^{2+}]_i$) peak significantly as compared to the results in cells expressing CRF_2 alone. Phosphorylation of p38 kinase shows a drastic increase during colitis, which is significantly attenuated by UCN3 treatment. The results suggest a requirement of balanced and coordinated expression of CRFr, properly regulating the expression and function of UCN3 during inflammation [42]. In SD rats and colon carcinoma cell lines (HT-29 and Caco-2 cell lines), UCN3 is found to induce colon epithelial hyperpermeability and enterocyte cell differentiation via CRF_2. CRF_2 is preferentially expressed in undifferentiated epithelial cells in the colon crypts and human colon carcinoma cell lines. With differentiation, CRF_2 expression is downregulated in HT-29 cells. UCN3-induced CRF_2 signaling causes changes in both para- and trans-cellular permeability of differentiated HT-29 and Caco-2 cells [66]. Taken together, the above results suggest that UCN3 participates in colonic inflammatory processes and may play a role in IBS.

Role of CRFp in CAC

Up to date, limited reports about the peripheral direct effects of CRFp on CAC are presented. We first report the influences of CRF_1 signaling on CAC development by using CRF_1 deficient mice in AOM- and DSS-induced CAC model [45]. Our investigation reveals that CRF_1, UCN1, and CRH are significantly enhanced and tumors develop severely in the colon during AOM and DSS treatment in WT ($Crhr_1^{+/+}$) mice. Interestingly, in $Crhr_1^{-/-}$ mice, tumorigenesis is dramatically reduced (Fig. 4.1). Meanwhile, inflammatory responses are much lower and the pro-inflammatory factors, IL-1β, IL-6, and TNF-α, are remarkably reduced, accompanied by significantly alleviated macrophage infiltration. Moreover, inhibition of NF-κB activation and STAT3 phosphorylation and decreased proliferating and enhanced apoptotic cells are observed in the colon [45]. Our in vitro experiments

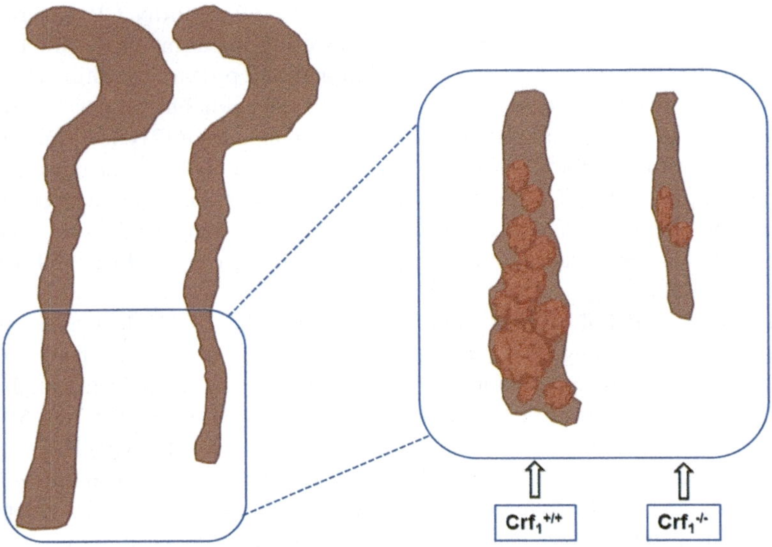

Fig. 4.1 Role of CRF_1 signaling in colitis-associated colon cancer. Tumor numbers are remarkably less in *Crh1*$^{-/-}$ colon

further support the pro-tumorigenesis effect of CRF_1 [67]. CRH is observed to enhance colon cancer cell proliferation, promoting colony formation. Also, CRH significantly promotes angiogenesis of HUVECs in tube formation assay. In the further mechanism-exploring experiments, CRH/CRF_1 is shown to significantly activate NF-κB, upregulating the levels of IL-6 and VEGF. The CRH-induced tube formation is abolished by silencing VEGF [67]. These data are in line with a newly reported research outcome demonstrating that CRF_1 deficiency inhibits CRC in AOM/DSS mouse model [46]. On the other hand, CRF_2 expression is not detected in the human colorectal adenocarcinoma cell line Caco2 [63]. Consistently, Baritaki group report that human colon tissues from CRC patients and CRC cell lines show decreased CRF_2 expression [68]. Contrary to CRH/CRF_1 functions, UCN2/CRF_2 signaling exerts an inhibitory effect on cancer cell proliferation, migration, invasion, and colony formation. The CRF_2-mediated tumor-inhibiting results are supported by the reductions in IL-1β, IL-6, and IL-6R mRNA in CRC-CRF_2^+ cells and the fact that in CRC patients' colon samples, CRF_2 mRNA expression is inversely correlated with IL-6R [68]. Furthermore, CRF_2 deficiency exacerbates CRC in AOM/DSS model [46]. These results indicate that CRF_2 has a protective effect from colon inflammation and cancer. However, opposite effect (tumor-promoting) of CRF_2 is also reported, i.e., CRF_2 exerts a harmful colonic effect, CRF_2 activation stimulating CRC development [69]. In addition, a blood sample analysis demonstrates that CRF_2 is a risk factor for CRC development in Mexican patients [70], increasing the controversial dispute over CRF_2 functions. Recently, the methylation status of both CRF_1 and CRF_2 has been reported, which is being considered a promising screening approach for CAC diagnosis [71, 72].

1.3 CRFp in the Pancreas

CRFp and the receptors (CRFr) are also found in the human and rodent pancreas [73–77] and may change with the body status, for instance, CRF_2 and UCN2 increase in pancreatic β cells of mice in pregnancy [73]. CRH stimulates dog pancreatic bicarbonate and protein secretion both under basal conditions and in response to secretin or cholecystokinin (CCK), accompanied by an increase in plasma levels of pancreatic polypeptide [78]. Moreover, in rat pancreatic β-cells, CRH modulates Ca^{2+} influx via CRF_1 [79]. Microfluorimetric experiments show that both CRH and UCN1 elevate $[Ca^{2+}]_i$ levels, which is attenuated by the unselective CRFr antagonist, astressin, whereas the CRF_2 selective antagonist, anti-sauvagine-30 (aSvg30), appears to enhance the UCN1 effect on the elevation of $[Ca^{2+}]_i$ [79]. These results suggest that CRF_1 has an antagonizing action on CRF_2 in influencing $[Ca^{2+}]_i$ and hence in insulin secretion. Consistently, expression of CRF_1 and its activation potentiating glucose-stimulated insulin secretion has been showed on mouse and human primary pancreatic β cells, being inhibited by the selective CRF_1 antagonist, antalarmin, and the mechanisms involving cAMP/MAPK pathway [80]. In isolated single β cells of the rat islet, immunohistochemical staining reveals the presence of both CRF_1 and CRF_2. And CRH increases cytosolic Ca^{2+} concentration, dependent upon extracellular Ca^{2+} causing depolarization of the cell membrane [81]. In mice lacking CRF_1 ($Crhr_1^{-/-}$ mice), the glucose profile in response to a glucose tolerance test is similar to that of wild-type mice, while serum insulin levels are significantly lower, reflecting high insulin sensitivity. Meanwhile, histology examination reveals islet hypoplasia in $Crhr_1^{-/-}$ mice, suggesting a role of CRF_1 in maintaining the β cell mass. Furthermore, in response to a high-fat diet, $Crhr_1^{-/-}$ mice shows insulin resistance while serum insulin levels during glucose challenge remains at a low level [82]. In rat and mouse insulin-secreting cell lines (INS-1 and MIN6), CRF_1 agonists upregulate insulin receptor substrate 2 expression, increase AKT activation, and inhibit apoptosis [75]. Moreover, UCNs are found to regulate fuel utilization in the periphery by acting locally within key metabolic tissues including skeletal muscle and pancreas, with UCN2 (and UCN3) modulating glucose homeostasis and metabolic functions via CRF_2 [74]. In accordance, in vivo experiments show that UCN2 gene transfer alters the metabolites' signaling pathways in mice. UCN2 gene transfer increases amino acids and peptides, associated with reduced protein synthesis. In insulin-resistant mice, many metabolites are altered, some of which can be reversed by UCN2 gene transfer, likely explaining UCN2 effects on increasing glucose disposal and reducing insulin assistance [83], which is consistent with the finding that UCN1 is a key mediator in mouse acute pancreatic inflammation via CRF_2 [84]. These results are in line with the reported beneficial effects of UCN2/CRF_2 in diabetic mice, increasing glucose proposal and insulin sensitivity [85], improving the retinopathy reducing ocular manifestations such as vascular leak [86], being an insulin sensitizer in the skeletal muscle of obese mice [87]. UCN3 (CRF_2-selective ligand as UCN2) is found to express in pancreatic β cells and in a mouse beta-cell line, MIN6, stimulation of which by high potassium, forskolin, or high glucose induces UCN3 secretion. In vivo studies in rats show that UCN3 administration causes a significant elevation of plasma glucagon, plasma glucose, and plasma insulin levels, which is blocked by the CRF_2 antagonist, astressin2B [76]. Interestingly, UCN3 is observed to be stored and co-released with insulin [88] and regulate insulin secretion, particularly in the presence of nutrient excess [76, 89]. UCN3 secretion from cultured β cells is stimulated by high glucose and insulin secretagogs, and mouse pancreatic UCN3 mRNA levels in vivo are increased during the positive energy balance caused by high-fat diet. Immunoneutralization of UCN3 or CRF_2 blockade attenuates high glucose-induced insulin secretion from isolated islets in vitro, supported by the finding that cultured islets of UCN3-null mice secrete less insulin in high glucose, which is consistent with the result that pretreatment with a selective CRF_2 antagonist significantly attenuates glucose-induced insulin secretion in vivo [89]. Taken together, these results demonstrate that pancreatic UCN3 is induced under excessive caloric conditions and acts locally to augment insulin production, likely leading to reduced insulin sensitivity. Moreover, UCN3 induces increases in cAMP formation in human BON cells, which are pancreatic carcinoid-derived and endocrine-like cells sharing functional similarities with intestinal enterochromaffin cells, where CRFr mRNA is detected, with CRF_2 mRNA levels much higher than those of CRF_1 mRNA [90], supporting the participation of CRF_2 in insulin release.

1.4 CRFp in the Liver

The expression of CRFp and CRFr in the liver has been demonstrated in human and other species [91, 92]. In rat liver cells, upregulation of p53 mRNA induced by hypoxia, which is involved in tumorigenesis, is blocked by pretreatment with the specific CRF_1 antagonist, CP-154,526. And CRH stimulates p53 mRNA via the ERK1/2 pathway in the BRL-3A cell line, confirmed by the result that the effect is blocked by the ERK1/2 antagonist U0126 [93]. In addition, in the human hepatoma NPLC-KC cell line, CRH is detected and stimulated to secret by IL-1 [94, 95].

Simopoulos et al. report that in normal human liver tissue, UCN1 is localized in hepatocytes. CRF_1 and $CRF_{2\alpha}$ gene expression are also found, with the receptor protein of a similar distribution to UCN1, while CRF_{2B} is not detected. Moreover, in hepatic biopsies from patients with liver carcinoma and cirrhosis, UCN1 and the CRFr expression is demonstrated while CRH, UCN2, and UCN3 are not observed [92]. These results suggest that UCN1 may be the major ligand acting in an autocrine or paracrine manner via the local receptors. Consistently, the nonselective CRFr antagonist astressin, but not the selective CRF_2 antagonist astressin2B, reverses the induced liver cell apoptosis in a rat experimental model, suggesting that antagonism of CRF_1 blocks the apoptotic process [96]. Moreover, in our laboratory, UCN1 is observed to inhibit the growth of hepatocellular carcinoma (HCC) and reduce tumor micro-vessel density in nude mice. CRFr expression, mainly CRF_2, is detected in vessels but not in hepatoma cells. In vitro three-dimensional culture assay shows that UCN1 inhibits angiogenesis, which is abolished by aSvg30, demonstrating involvement of CRF_2. Furthermore, UCN1 inhibits the proliferation and promotes the apoptosis of vascular endothelial cells and downregulates VEGF expression in vivo via CRF_2 [97]. These results are in line with the report that CRF_2 gene may influence the risk of developing HCC in patients with HBV infection in Chinese population [98]. In addition, inconsistently, in hepatoma carcinoma cell lines, HepG2 and SMMC-7721, we also find that UCN1 stimulates $cPLA_2$ expression inducing cell migration via CRF_1 [99].

The expression of UCN1 and CRFr is also detected in liver Kupffer cells, the resident macrophages that play a crucial role in the antigen-specific immune response [100] (see Sect. 2).

2 CRFp Action on Immune/Inflammatory Cells in Digestive System

CRFp have important effects on immune/inflammatory cells influencing activities of digestive organs. Especially, CRH is found to communicate with immune/inflammatory system at multilevels [2]. Besides its central effects on the systemic immunity via hypothalamic-pituitary-adrenal (HPA) axis (see Chap. 1), CRH has direct peripheral effects on the immune/inflammatory cells [2].

CRH is identified in mouse intestinal mucosal *eosinophils* related to psychological stress and gut dysfunction, and eosinophils express CRH in the jejunum in response to psychological stress while eosinophil-derived CRH activates mast cells to induce the jejunum epithelial barrier dysfunction [101]. Moreover, substance P (SP) induces CRH expression/release in eosinophils. And by co-culturing SP-primed eosinophils with the mast cells (HMC-1), it is found that cells are activated by eosinophil-derived CRH inducing cell monolayer barrier dysfunction, which is further confirmed by a mouse model investigation [102]. As well known, IBS is characterized by altered intestinal motility, immune activation, and increased gut barrier permeability. It is observed that in cases of GI disorders such as functional dyspepsia (FD), IBS, and colon cancer, increased eosinophils and their degranulation are observed [103–106]. In IBS patients, the jejunal mucosal eosinophils display higher degranulation, with increased content of CRH in the cytoplasmic granules, which is significantly correlated with IBS clinical severity in particular [102]. Collectively, these results suggest that intestinal mucosal eosinophils are potential contributors to gut dysfunction through peripheral CRH production and release.

By utilizing a porcine ex vivo intestinal model, it is found that CRH causes intestinal epithelial barrier disturbances by increasing intestinal paracellular permeability related to *mast cells* [107]. Pigs' ileum exposed to CRH displays higher FITC dextran flux, which is inhibited by the non-selective CRFr antagonist astressin and the mast cell stabilizer sodium cromolyn, demonstrating that CRH functions via mast cell activation. Consistently, in a rat model of FD induced by iodoacetamide, which displays mucosal inflammation and immune activation related to gastric mast cell infiltration [108, 109], RNA interference of gastric CRH expression significantly decreases gastric mast cell infiltration, suggesting that CRH contributes to inflammation via modulating mast cell infiltration [110]. Also in rats, chronic CRH administration is found to mediate the colonic permeability and ion transport functions involving the role of mast cells. CRH used subcutaneously for 12d results in colonic mucosal dysfunction with increased colonic permeability in wild-type but not in mast cell-deficient rats. Moreover, stimulation of CRF_1 or CRF_2 induces the elevated secretory state of mast cells and colonic permeability dysfunction, respectively [111]. Pigs weaning early are also demonstrated to display deleterious effects on mucosal barrier function in jejunum and colon mediated through peripheral CRFr signaling pathways [112]. It is observed that the mast cell stabilizer drug sodium cromoglycate ameliorates barrier dysfunction and hypersecretion in early-weaned pigs' jejunum while activation of mast cells ex vivo with c48/80 and CRH induces barrier dysfunction of the jejunum. By administration of CRF_1 antagonists to early-weaned pigs, it is demonstrated that CRF_1 activation induces barrier dysfunction and hypersecretion [113]. Moreover, early weaning results in reductions in transepithelial electrical resistance and increases in mucosal permeability in the jejunum and colon. Interestingly, early-weaned piglet intestinal mucosa exhibits increased expression of CRF_1 protein, increased mucosal mast cell tryptase levels, and enhanced mast cell degranulation compared with late-weaned intestinal mucosa, which is abolished by pretreatment of piglets with the mast cell stabilizer cromolyn [114]. Also, it is reported that neonatal maternal deprivation (NMD) causes visceral hypersensitivity, promoting gut paracellular permeability (GPP) through mast cells and nerve growth factor (NGF) [115, 116]. Peripheral CRH is observed to be involved in the elevated GPP observed in NMD adult rats through a mast cell-mediated mechanism, since the increase of GPP induced by exogenous CRH is abolished by the mast cell stabilizer, doxantrazole. Moreover, anti-NGF antibody treatment also reduces the elevated GPP induced by CRH or BRX-537A (mast cell activator), suggesting that CRH acts through CRF_1 to stimulate NGF release from mast cells, which participates in the elevated GPP observed in NMD adult rats [115]. Consistently, rats' acute stress is reported to increase histamine content in colonic mucosa mast cells, which is blocked by intravenous pretreatment with IL-1α or α-helical-CRH(9–41), the CRFr antagonist. However, both IL-1ß and CRH injections reproduce the stress-linked changes [117]. However, there is also report that mast cell activation and subsequent visceral hypersensitivity are not targeted by α-helical-CRH(9–41) [118].

It is observed that peripheral use of CRH significantly increases water flux, permeability, and tryptase release in the jejunal segments of IBS patients, whose abdominal pain is worsened after CRH administration, correlated with jejunal tryptase release, water flux, and albumin output. And IBS patients are found to display jejunal upregulation of CRF_2 and downregulation of CRF_1 compared with healthy controls [119]. Altered intestinal barrier is associated with immune activation and clinical symptoms in IBS patients with increased mucosal antigen load and local antibody production. IBS patients display enhanced small bowel humoral immunity, mucosal Ig production contributing to local inflammation and clinical manifestations [120]. Moreover, patients with IBS show a higher number and activation of mucosal *B lymphocytes* and *plasma cells*. Glycocalyx thickness is lower in IBS, correlating with plasma cell activation, proximity to nerves, and clinical symptoms [121]. These results support humoral activity and epithelial integrity loss as important contributors to gut dysfunction and clinical manifestations in IBS. In addition, B lymphocytes contain CRH and CRH is found to be able to stimulate B lymphocytes' proliferation [122, 123], suggesting that CRH may affect the barrier integrity via humoral immune activity. Interestingly, *mast cell* density is also increased in IBS patients in close proximity to plasma cells. IBS patients show ultrastructural alteration in the intestinal epithelial cells and intercellular apical junctional complexes (AJC) [124], and the genes related to mast cells and AJC are expressed differently compared to those of healthy subjects [125]. IBS patients have increased mast cell counts and activation and changed AJC, i.e., increased claudin-2 expression, reduced occludin phosphorylation and enhanced redistribution (from membrane to cytoplasm), increased myosin kinase expression, reduced myosin phosphatase, and hence enhanced myosin phosphorylation, which is associated with ultrastructural abnormalities at the AJC. And the AJC structural alterations are positively related to mast cell activation and clinical symptoms [125]. Based on that mast cells are highly associated with CRH/CRF_1 as described above, these results imply that CRH may influence AJC participating in intestinal barrier function. Moreover, increased TLR4 mRNA expression is observed in the small bowel mucosa from IBS patients [126], which suggests the involvement of bacteria or abnormal immune response to commensal flora in small bowel mucosa. However, rare evidence is presented for a direct peripheral effect of CRF-system on gut flora.

Macrophages are also found to contribute to GI inflammation [127, 128] and macrophage migration inhibitory factor, expressing in enterocytes, participates in maintaining the intestinal barrier [129]. It is observed that in the human colonic mucosa, CRF_1 expression is different between healthy subjects and UC patients. In sigmoid colonic biopsies, both immunohistochemically double-labeled cells with CRF_1 and CD163 (a marker for macrophages) and CRF_1-IR cells are increased in UC patients compared to those in healthy subjects [41]. The results indicate that CRF_1 is significantly enhanced in macrophages in UC patients, providing anatomical support for a CRF_1 signaling role in the modulation of the immune-inflammatory process of UC. UCN1, which appears in human colon only after birth, is detected in human colonic mucosa, in lamina propria mononuclear cells. Interestingly, UCN1 distribution is detected together with CRF_1 much higher than CRF_2. UCN1 is found to be locally synthesized in lamina propria macrophages, exerting an effect on the local inflammatory cells in an autocrine/paracrine way regulating the mucosal immune functions [33]. Moreover, in rat GI system, Bhargava group also observe an inflammation-promoting effect of endogenous UCN1, synergistically augmenting

LPS-induced vascular permeability, with which macrophages are increased, suggesting macrophages' involvement in this UCN1 effect [56]. In addition, locally released CRH from immune cells or enterochromaffin cells in the GI mucosa is likely to be involved in the regulation of rectal afferent nerve function [130].

Kupffer cells (KCs) are resident macrophages in the liver, being the first line fighting invading agents via the portal circulation, but KCs' overactivity contributes to liver pathology [131]. It is observed that in highly purified rat KCs, transcripts of UCN1 and the two receptors, CRF_1 and CRF_2, are present while that of CRH is not detectable. Also, immunoreactive UCN1 and CRF_1 and CRF_2 are easily detectable by immunohistochemistry and immunofluorescence in both the whole rat liver (localized in KCs) and purified KCs while CRH is absent. Exposure of purified KCs to CRH or UCN1 suppresses LPS-induced TNF-α production, which is completely prevented by CRFr antagonist astressin [100]. These data demonstrate that UCN1 is the main functioning type of CRFp affecting local inflammatory phenomena in the liver acting in an auto−/paracrine manner via KCs. Consistently, Ghezzi group show that in mice, exogenous UCN1 significantly reduces LPS-induced serum TNF and IL-1β levels in vivo, paralleled by a rise in corticosterone levels, blockade of which by cyanoketone does not prevent the TNF inhibition by UCN1, suggesting that UCN1 has anti-inflammatory mechanisms independent of HPA axis. Furthermore, UCN1 has a direct inhibitory effect on LPS-induced TNF in rat KCs, related to increased cAMP levels. On the other hand, the in vivo inhibition of LPS-induced IL-1β by UCN1 can be reversed by cyanoketone, which remains to be studied [132].

3 The Influence of Peripheral CRFp on GI Tract via Enteric Nervous System

Increasing evidence demonstrates that CRFp also function through regulating ENS influencing GI activities. In rats' GI and related cells, the presence of CRH and UCN1 in ENS is observed contributing to their roles in GI functions [40, 133–135].

As precedingly described, the mapping of UCN1 distribution in the rat GI is presented using an immunofluorescence histochemical technique. Besides its expression in all parietal cells of the stomach, UCN1 is observed in myenteric and submucosal plexuses in small and large intestine [18]. In rat duodenum, CRH is detected within both myenteric plexus perikarya and nerve fibers [23]. Immunoreactivity assay shows that CRH is also expressed in both the myenteric and submucosal plexuses of all regions of the large and small intestine and the myenteric plexus of the stomach in the guinea pig. The proportions of CRH-IR cell bodies in the myenteric plexus, mostly with uni-axonal morphology, increase progressively from the stomach to the distal colon. Interestingly, CRH-IR cell bodies are more abundant in the submucosal plexus, also found being vasoactive-intestinal peptide (VIP) positive [136]. Consistently, in rat small and large intestines,

CRH-IR enteric neurons are detected, showing networks of CRH-containing nerve cell bodies and fibers. Moreover, CRH-IR neurons are also found containing VIP to a high degree. However, in cultured myenteric neurons from rat ileum, a low number of cells contain CRH-IR, with CRH-, UCN1-, or CRFr-antagonist not influencing, but VIP significantly enhancing the neuronal survival [135]. Also, VIP contributes to peripheral CRH-induced CRF_1-mediated stimulation of colonic motor function and diarrhea in rats. It is observed that the VIP antagonist, [4Cl-D-Phe6, Leu17]VIP completely prevents CRH-induced fecal output and diarrhea. In submucosal plexus neurons, CRH induces c-Fos expression most prominently in the terminal ileum (most VIP-positive neurons expressing CRF_1), whereas no c-Fos is observed in the proximal colon. However, in myenteric neurons, CRH induces a more robust expression of c-Fos in the proximal colon neurons than in the ileum neurons. The CRH-induced c-Fos induction is also prevented by the VIP antagonist [137]. These data demonstrate that CRH activates intestinal submucosal VIP neurons most prominently in the ileum and myenteric neurons in the colon, suggesting VIP signaling in ileum and colon as downstream effectors of CRH.

By in situ hybridization, UCN1-containing cells are found to be exclusively localized to the submucosal plexus and myenteric plexus in the duodenum, small intestine and colon of rats, suggesting that UCN1 may play an important role in the regulation of GI *motor function* throughout ENS [134]. Yamato group also report the presence of both CRH and UCN1 in the neurons of the myenteric plexus [133]. By measuring the isometric tension of rat colonic muscle strips, it is found that CRH and UCN1 increase both the phasic contractions and electrical field stimulation (EFS)-induced off-contractions, with UCN1 exerting a more potent effect than CRH. The CRF_1 antagonist, antalarmin, abolishes the contractile effects of UCN1. Interestingly, UCN1 and choline acetyltransferase, as well as UCN1 and 5-HT, are colocalized in some neurons of the myenteric plexus [133]. These results suggest that CRH and UCN1 may act on the ENS increasing colonic contractility by enhancing cholinergic and serotonergic neurotransmission. Consistently, the group report in another work that UCN1 causes a significant increase in phasic contractions, which is completely inhibited by antalarmin, TTX, and atropine, further supporting that UCN1 acts as an excitatory neurotransmitter in the ENS enhancing the cholinergic neurotransmission [138].

Correspondingly, evaluations of CRF_1 and CRF_2 expression in the rat small intestine (duodenum and ileum) show that $CRF_{1,2}$-IR is localized in the fibers and neurons of the myenteric and submucosal ganglia, with a stronger expression of CRF_1 than CRF_2 in the duodenum and whereas, higher CRF_2 expression in the ileum. Functional studies demonstrate that CRFp increase duodenal phasic contractions and reduce ileal contractions. CRF_1 antagonists (CP-154,526 and SSR125543Q) block the CRFp-induced activation of duodenal motility but do not influence CRFp-induced inhibition of ileal motility. In contrast, the CRF_2 inhibitor Astressin 2B blocks the effects of CRFp on ileal muscle contractions but does not influence CRFp-induced activation of duodenal motility [139]. These findings suggest that CRFp stimulate the contractile activity of the duodenum through CRF_1 while inhibiting phasic contractions of the ileum through CRF_2. And in rat colon, CRF_1

expression in the myenteric and submucosal nervous plexus is detected while CRF_2 expression is localized mainly in the luminal surface of the crypts and in blood vessels of the submucosal layer [40].

More works are presented demonstrating different effects of the two distinct CRFr in ENS. By using intracellular recording with microelectrodes, it is found that in guinea pig colonic tissue, UCN1 depolarizes membrane elevating excitability of S-type colonic myenteric neurons, which is suppressed by the CRF_1 antagonist NBI 27914, but unaffected by the CRF_2 antagonist aSvg30. UCN2 or UCN3 evokes depolarizing responses in part of the AH-type myenteric neurons (but has no effect on S-type neurons), which is suppressed by aSvg30, but not NBI 27914. Moreover, in ganglion cell somas, immunohistochemical staining identifies CRF_1 as the predominant CRFr, while CRF_2-IR neuronal somas are sparse [140]. These results clearly demonstrate that UCNs act as neuromodulators to influence ENS excitability, the activating effect of UCN1 being primarily on S-type neurons via CRF_1 while the excitatory action of UCN2 and UCN3 being on AH-type neurons via CRF_2. Inconsistently, it is reported that neither UCN1-antiserum nor α-helical-CRH(9–41) affects gastroduodenal motility, demonstrating that endogenous UCN1 may not be a factor involved in basal GI motility mediation [141]. Additionally, it is observed that both central CRH and peripheral CRH exert an influence on visceral pain, the former being found to enhance colorectal distention-induced visceral pain in rats and the latter to reduce pain threshold to colonic distention in human. Both nonselective CRFr antagonists and selective CRF_1 antagonists are found to inhibit exogenous CRH- and stress-induced stimulation of colonic myenteric neurons, motor function, and visceral hyperalgesia. No effect is observed with selective CRF_2 antagonists [130, 142, 143]. These findings support that CRF_1 may be the main functioning receptor in ENS of colon.

4 Summary

The main content is summarized as shown in Fig. 4.2. More and more researches show that peripheral CRFp and CRFr are important participants in mediating the functions of the digestive system. They exert an influence on digestive organs directly or via local immune/inflammatory cells and ENS, contributing to a lot of digestive activities and abnormality, such as GI motility and insulin secretion and some dysfunctions. Particularly, CRFp are involved in the development of GI inflammation and tumorigenesis, as colitis and CAC. Targeting CRFp and CRFr may be a promising approach for the preventive and therapeutic measures for digestive diseases in the future. As mentioned in the text, nowadays, detection of CRF_2 hypermethylation may become an effective way for cancer screening in UC patients [72]. Moreover, peripherally acting CRFr antagonists might be directly beneficial for improving IBS symptoms and functional GI disorders [144].

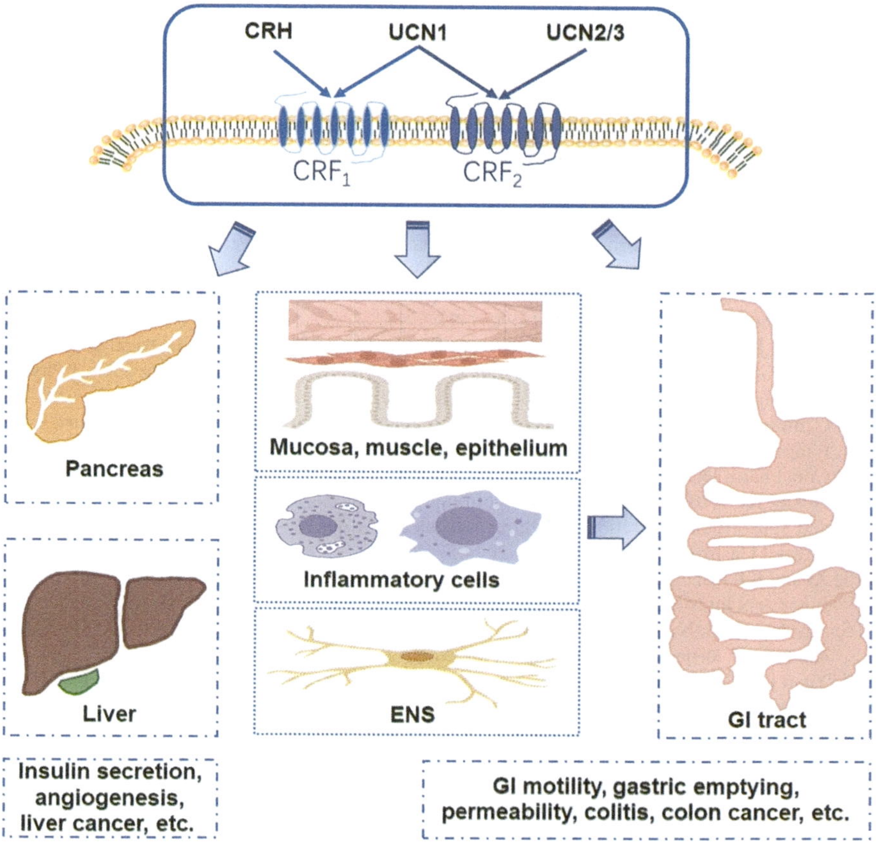

Fig. 4.2 The distribution and role of CRFp in the digestive system

References

1. Vale W, et al. Characterization of a 41-residue ovine hypothalamic peptide that stimulates secretion of corticotropin and beta-endorphin. Science. 1981;213(4514):1394–7.
2. Bamberger CM, Bamberger AM. The peripheral CRH/urocortin system. Ann N Y Acad Sci. 2000;917:290–6.
3. Perrin MH, Vale WW. Corticotropin releasing factor receptors and their ligand family. Ann N Y Acad Sci. 1999;885:312–28.
4. Tache Y, Perdue MH. Role of peripheral CRF signalling pathways in stress-related alterations of gut motility and mucosal function. Neurogastroenterol Motil. 2004;16(Suppl 1):137–42.
5. Hussain Z, Park H. Inflammation and impaired gut physiology in post-operative ileus: mechanisms and the treatment options. J Neurogastroenterol Motil. 2022;28(4):517–30.
6. Fekete EM, et al. Systemic urocortin 2, but not urocortin 1 or stressin 1-A, suppresses feeding via CRF2 receptors without malaise and stress. Br J Pharmacol. 2011;164(8):1959–75.

7. Yin Y, Dong L, Yin D. Peripheral and central administration of exogenous urocortin 1 disrupts the fasted motility pattern of the small intestine in rats via the corticotrophin releasing factor receptor 2 and a cholinergic mechanism. J Gastroenterol Hepatol. 2008;23(7 Pt 2):e79–87.
8. Rodino-Janeiro BK, et al. Role of corticotropin-releasing factor in gastrointestinal permeability. J Neurogastroenterol Motil. 2015;21(1):33–50.
9. Hill LT, Kidson SH, Michell WL. Corticotropin-releasing factor is present in intestinal tissue of patients with gastrointestinal dysfunction following shock and abdominal surgery. Nutrition. 2013;29(4):650–4.
10. Tache Y, Bonaz B. Corticotropin-releasing factor receptors and stress-related alterations of gut motor function. J Clin Invest. 2007;117(1):33–40.
11. Chatzaki E, et al. Urocortin in human gastric mucosa: relationship to inflammatory activity. J Clin Endocrinol Metab. 2003;88(1):478–83.
12. Huang IH, et al. Effects of corticotropin-releasing hormone on gastric electrical activity and sensorimotor function in healthy volunteers: a double-blinded crossover study. Am J Physiol Gastrointest Liver Physiol. 2024;326(5):G622–30.
13. Czimmer J, Tache Y. Peripheral corticotropin releasing factor signaling inhibits gastric emptying: mechanisms of action and role in stress-related gastric alterations of motor function. Curr Pharm Des. 2017;23(27):4042–7.
14. Huang IH, et al. The effects of corticotropin-releasing hormone on gastric electrical activity and sensorimotor function in healthy volunteers: a double-blinded crossover study. Am J Physiol Gastrointest Liver Physiol. 2024;326:G622.
15. Anand KJ, Runeson B, Jacobson B. Gastric suction at birth associated with long-term risk for functional intestinal disorders in later life. J Pediatr. 2004;144(4):449–54.
16. Smith C, et al. Neonatal gastric suctioning results in chronic visceral and somatic hyperalgesia: role of corticotropin releasing factor. Neurogastroenterol Motil. 2007;19(8):692–9.
17. Yuan PQ, Wu SV, Tache Y. Urocortins and CRF type 2 receptor isoforms expression in the rat stomach are regulated by endotoxin: role in the modulation of delayed gastric emptying. Am J Physiol Gastrointest Liver Physiol. 2012;303(1):G20–31.
18. Kozicz T, Arimura A. Distribution of urocortin in the rat's gastrointestinal tract and its colocalization with tyrosine hydroxylase. Peptides. 2002;23(3):515–21.
19. Chatzaki E, et al. Differential profile of CRF receptor distribution in the rat stomach and duodenum assessed by newly developed CRF receptor antibodies. J Neurochem. 2004;88(1):1–11.
20. Nozu T, et al. Water-avoidance stress enhances gastric contractions in freely moving conscious rats: role of peripheral CRF receptors. J Gastroenterol. 2014;49(5):799–805.
21. Lenz HJ, Hester SE, Brown MR, Corticotropin-releasing factor. Mechanisms to inhibit gastric acid secretion in conscious dogs. J Clin Invest. 1985;75(3):889–95.
22. Suda T, et al. Distribution and characterization of immunoreactive corticotropin-releasing factor in human tissues. J Clin Endocrinol Metab. 1984;59(5):861–6.
23. Wolter HJ. Corticotropin-releasing factor is contained within perikarya and nerve fibres of rat duodenum. Biochem Biophys Res Commun. 1984;122(1):381–7.
24. Bulbul M, et al. Peripheral apelin mediates stress-induced alterations in gastrointestinal motor functions depending on the nutritional status. Clin Exp Pharmacol Physiol. 2019;46(1):29–39.
25. Lenz HJ. Regulation of duodenal bicarbonate secretion during stress by corticotropin-releasing factor and beta-endorphin. Proc Natl Acad Sci USA. 1989;86(4):1417–20.
26. Zhu C, et al. Sini San ameliorates duodenal mucosal barrier injury and low-grade inflammation via the CRF pathway in a rat model of functional dyspepsia. Int J Mol Med. 2020;45(1):53–60.
27. Estienne M, et al. Maternal deprivation alters epithelial secretory cell lineages in rat duodenum: role of CRF-related peptides. Gut. 2010;59(6):744–51.
28. Sun Y, et al. Stress-induced corticotropin-releasing hormone-mediated NLRP6 inflammasome inhibition and transmissible enteritis in mice. Gastroenterology. 2013;144(7):1478–87.

29. Bruce JK, et al. Defects in NLRP6, autophagy and goblet cell homeostasis are associated with reduced duodenal CRH receptor 2 expression in patients with functional dyspepsia. Brain Behav Immun. 2022;101:335–45.
30. van Tol EA, et al. Local production of corticotropin releasing hormone is increased in experimental intestinal inflammation in rats. Gut. 1996;39(3):385–92.
31. Duridanova DB, et al. Corticotropin-releasing hormone acts on Guinea pig ileal smooth muscle via protein kinase A. Pflugers Arch. 1999;438(2):205–12.
32. Takeuchi K, et al. Involvement of corticotropin-releasing factor and corticotropin-releasing factor 2 receptors in pathogenesis of ischemia/reperfusion-induced enteritis in rats. J Physiol Pharmacol. 2016;67(5):697–707.
33. Muramatsu Y, et al. Urocortin and corticotropin-releasing factor receptor expression in the human colonic mucosa. Peptides. 2000;21(12):1799–809.
34. O'Malley D, Dinan TG, Cryan JF. Alterations in colonic corticotropin-releasing factor receptors in the maternally separated rat model of irritable bowel syndrome: differential effects of acute psychological and physical stressors. Peptides. 2010;31(4):662–70.
35. Fukudo S. Role of corticotropin-releasing hormone in irritable bowel syndrome and intestinal inflammation. J Gastroenterol. 2007;42(Suppl 17):48–51.
36. Tache Y, Million M. Role of corticotropin-releasing factor signaling in stress-related alterations of colonic motility and hyperalgesia. J Neurogastroenterol Motil. 2015;21(1):8–24.
37. Kawahito Y, et al. Local secretion of corticotropin-releasing hormone by enterochromaffin cells in human colon. Gastroenterology. 1994;106(4):859–65.
38. Goebel M, et al. Lipopolysaccharide increases plasma levels of corticotropin-releasing hormone in rats. Neuroendocrinology. 2011;93(3):165–73.
39. Kawahito Y, et al. Corticotropin releasing hormone in colonic mucosa in patients with ulcerative colitis. Gut. 1995;37(4):544–51.
40. Chatzaki E, et al. CRF receptor type 1 and 2 expression and anatomical distribution in the rat colon. J Neurochem. 2004;90(2):309–16.
41. Yuan PQ, et al. Expression of corticotropin releasing factor receptor type 1 (CRF1) in the human gastrointestinal tract and upregulation in the colonic mucosa in patients with ulcerative colitis. Peptides. 2012;38(1):62–9.
42. Mahajan S, et al. Urocortin 3 expression at baseline and during inflammation in the colon: corticotropin releasing factor receptors cross-talk. Peptides. 2014;54:58–66.
43. Saruta M, et al. Urocortin 3/stresscopin in human colon: possible modulators of gastrointestinal function during stressful conditions. Peptides. 2005;26(7):1196–206.
44. Chatoo M, et al. Involvement of corticotropin-releasing factor and receptors in immune cells in irritable bowel syndrome. Front Endocrinol (Lausanne). 2018;9:21.
45. Liu Y, et al. The role of corticotropin-releasing hormone receptor 1 in the development of colitis-associated cancer in mouse model. Endocr Relat Cancer. 2014;21(4):639–51.
46. Lee Y, et al. Corticotropin-releasing hormone receptor alters the tumor development and growth in Apcmin/+ Mice and in a chemically-induced model of colon cancer. Int J Mol Sci. 2021;22(3)
47. Rogler G. Chronic ulcerative colitis and colorectal cancer. Cancer Lett. 2014;345(2):235–41.
48. Olen O, et al. Colorectal cancer in ulcerative colitis: a Scandinavian population-based cohort study. Lancet. 2020;395(10218):123–31.
49. Zhu C, Li S. Role of CRH in colitis and colitis-associated cancer: a combinative result of central and peripheral effects? Front Endocrinol (Lausanne). 2024;15:1363748.
50. Vicario M, et al. Chronic psychosocial stress induces reversible mitochondrial damage and corticotropin-releasing factor receptor type-1 upregulation in the rat intestine and IBS-like gut dysfunction. Psychoneuroendocrinology. 2012;37(1):65–77.
51. Mancinelli R, et al. In vitro excitatory actions of corticotropin-releasing factor on rat colonic motility. J Auton Pharmacol. 1998;18(6):319–24.
52. Maillot C, et al. Peripheral corticotropin-releasing factor and stress-stimulated colonic motor activity involve type 1 receptor in rats. Gastroenterology. 2000;119(6):1569–79.

53. Ordas I, et al. Ulcerative colitis. Lancet. 2012;380(9853):1606–19.
54. Sagami Y, et al. Effect of a corticotropin releasing hormone receptor antagonist on colonic sensory and motor function in patients with irritable bowel syndrome. Gut. 2004;53(7):958–64.
55. Tanaka Y, et al. Differential activation in amygdala and plasma noradrenaline during colorectal distention by administration of corticotropin-releasing hormone between healthy individuals and patients with irritable bowel syndrome. PLoS One. 2016;11(7):e0157347.
56. Cureton EL, et al. Local secretion of urocortin 1 promotes microvascular permeability during lipopolysaccharide-induced inflammation. Endocrinology. 2009;150(12):5428–37.
57. Wallon C, et al. Corticotropin-releasing hormone (CRH) regulates macromolecular permeability via mast cells in normal human colonic biopsies in vitro. Gut. 2008;57(1):50–8.
58. Wu Y, et al. Enhanced intracellular calcium induced by urocortin is involved in degranulation of rat lung mast cells. Cell Physiol Biochem. 2008;21(1–3):173–82.
59. Nozu T, Okumura T. Corticotropin-releasing factor receptor type 1 and type 2 interaction in irritable bowel syndrome. J Gastroenterol. 2015;50(8):819–30.
60. Li B, et al. Inhibition of corticotropin-releasing hormone receptor 1 and activation of receptor 2 protect against colonic injury and promote epithelium repair. Sci Rep. 2017;7:46616.
61. Hoffman JM, et al. Corticotropin-releasing hormone receptor 2 signaling promotes mucosal repair responses after colitis. Am J Pathol. 2016;186(1):134–44.
62. Akiba Y, Kaunitz JD, Million M. Peripheral corticotropin-releasing factor receptor type 2 activation increases colonic blood flow through nitric oxide pathway in rats. Dig Dis Sci. 2015;60(4):858–67.
63. Chatzaki E, et al. Corticotropin-releasing factor receptor subtype 2 in human colonic mucosa: down-regulation in ulcerative colitis. World J Gastroenterol. 2013;19(9):1416–23.
64. Martinez C, et al. miR-16 and miR-125b are involved in barrier function dysregulation through the modulation of claudin-2 and cingulin expression in the jejunum in IBS with diarrhoea. Gut. 2017;66(9):1537–8.
65. Yue H, et al. Potential regulatory effects of corticotropin-releasing factor on tight junction-related intestinal epithelial permeability are partially mediated by CK8 upregulation. Cell Physiol Biochem. 2017;44(3):1161–73.
66. Ducarouge B, et al. Involvement of CRF2 signaling in enterocyte differentiation. World J Gastroenterol. 2017;23(28):5127–45.
67. Fang X, et al. CRH promotes human colon cancer cell proliferation via IL-6/JAK2/STAT3 signaling pathway and VEGF-induced tumor angiogenesis. Mol Carcinog. 2017;56(11):2434–45.
68. Rodriguez JA, et al. Diminished expression of CRHR2 in human colon cancer promotes tumor growth and EMT via persistent IL-6/Stat3 signaling. Cell Mol Gastroenterol Hepatol. 2015;1(6):610–30.
69. Ducarouge B, et al. CRF2 signaling is a novel regulator of cellular adhesion and migration in colorectal cancer cells. PLoS One. 2013;8(11):e79335.
70. Ramirez-Guerrero AA, et al. Association between genetic variant rs2267716 of CRHR2 gene with colorectal cancer. J Investig Med. 2022;70(4):947–52.
71. Panagopoulou M, et al. Methylation status of corticotropin-releasing factor (CRF) receptor genes in colorectal cancer. J Clin Med. 2021;10(12)
72. Kobayashi M, et al. Hypermethylation of corticotropin releasing hormone receptor-2 gene in ulcerative colitis associated colorectal cancer. In Vivo. 2020;34(1):57–63.
73. Simpson SJS, et al. UCN2: a new candidate influencing pancreatic beta-cell adaptations in pregnancy. J Endocrinol. 2020;245(2):247–57.
74. Kuperman Y, Chen A. Urocortins: emerging metabolic and energy homeostasis perspectives. Trends Endocrinol Metab. 2008;19(4):122–9.
75. Blaabjerg L, et al. CRFR1 activation protects against cytokine-induced beta-cell death. J Mol Endocrinol. 2014;53(3):417–27.
76. Li C, et al. Urocortin III is expressed in pancreatic beta-cells and stimulates insulin and glucagon secretion. Endocrinology. 2003;144(7):3216–24.

77. Huising MO, et al. Glucocorticoids differentially regulate the expression of CRFR1 and CRFR2alpha in MIN6 insulinoma cells and rodent islets. Endocrinology. 2011;152(1):138–50.
78. Konturek SJ, et al. Gastrointestinal secretory, motor and circulatory effects of corticotropin releasing factor (CRF). Life Sci. 1985;37(13):1231–40.
79. Kageyama K, et al. Modulation of Ca2+ influx by corticotropin-releasing factor (CRF) family of peptides via CRF receptors in rat pancreatic beta-cells. Peptides. 2006;27(7):1814–9.
80. Huising MO, et al. CRFR1 is expressed on pancreatic beta cells, promotes beta cell proliferation, and potentiates insulin secretion in a glucose-dependent manner. Proc Natl Acad Sci USA. 2010;107(2):912–7.
81. Kanno T, et al. Corticotropin-releasing factor modulation of Ca2+ influx in rat pancreatic beta-cells. Diabetes. 1999;48(9):1741–6.
82. Sakamoto R, et al. Roles for corticotropin-releasing factor receptor type 1 in energy homeostasis in mice. Metabolism. 2013;62(12):1739–48.
83. Kim YC, et al. Significant alteration of liver metabolites by AAV8.Urocortin 2 gene transfer in mice with insulin resistance. PLoS One. 2019;14(12):e0224428.
84. Kubat E, et al. Corticotropin-releasing factor receptor 2 mediates sex-specific cellular stress responses. Mol Med. 2013;19(1):212–22.
85. Gao MH, et al. One-time injection of AAV8 encoding urocortin 2 provides long-term resolution of insulin resistance. JCI Insight. 2016;1(15):e88322.
86. Gao MH, et al. Urocortin 2 gene transfer improves glycemic control and reduces retinopathy and mortality in murine insulin deficiency. Mol Ther Methods Clin Dev. 2020;17:220–33.
87. Borg ML, et al. Modified UCN2 peptide acts as an insulin sensitizer in skeletal muscle of obese mice. Diabetes. 2019;68(7):1403–14.
88. van der Meulen T, et al. Urocortin3 mediates somatostatin-dependent negative feedback control of insulin secretion. Nat Med. 2015;21(7):769–76.
89. Li C, et al. Urocortin 3 regulates glucose-stimulated insulin secretion and energy homeostasis. Proc Natl Acad Sci USA. 2007;104(10):4206–11.
90. von Mentzer B, et al. Functional CRF receptors in BON cells stimulate serotonin release. Biochem Pharmacol. 2007;73(6):805–13.
91. Paschos KA, et al. The corticotropin releasing factor system in the liver: expression, actions and possible implications in hepatic physiology and pathology. Hormones (Athens). 2013;12(2):236–45.
92. Simopoulos C, et al. Neuropeptide urocortin 1 and its receptors are expressed in the human liver. Neuroendocrinology. 2009;89(3):315–26.
93. Zhao Y, et al. CRHR1 mediates p53 transcription induced by high altitude hypoxia through ERK 1/2 signaling in rat hepatic cells. Peptides. 2013;44:8–14.
94. Parkes DG, et al. Characterization and regulation of corticotropin-releasing factor in the human hepatoma NPLC-KC cell line. Neuroendocrinology. 1993;57(4):663–9.
95. Kasckow JW, et al. Interleukin-1 alpha induces corticotropin-releasing factor secretion and synthesis from NPLC-KC cells through various second messenger pathways. Synapse. 1994;18(4):354–8.
96. Paschos KA, et al. Corticotropin-releasing hormone receptors mediate opposing effects in cholestasis-induced liver cell apoptosis. Endocrinology. 2010;151(4):1704–12.
97. Wang J, et al. Urocortin' inhibition of tumor growth and angiogenesis in hepatocellular carcinoma via corticotrophin-releasing factor receptor 2. Cancer Investig. 2008;26(4):359–68.
98. Gu X, et al. An intronic polymorphism in the corticotropin-releasing hormone receptor 2 gene increases susceptibility to HBV-related hepatocellular carcinoma in Chinese population. Hum Genet. 2010;127(1):75–81.
99. Zhu C, et al. Urocortin affects migration of hepatic cancer cell lines via differential regulation of cPLA2 and iPLA2. Cell Signal. 2014;26(5):1125–34.
100. Charalampopoulos I, et al. Neuropeptide urocortin and its receptors are expressed in rat Kupffer cells. Neuroendocrinology. 2006;84(1):49–57.

101. Zheng PY, et al. Psychological stress induces eosinophils to produce corticotrophin releasing hormone in the intestine. Gut. 2009;58(11):1473–9.
102. Salvo-Romero E, et al. Overexpression of corticotropin-releasing factor in intestinal mucosal eosinophils is associated with clinical severity in Diarrhea-Predominant Irritable Bowel Syndrome. Sci Rep. 2020;10(1):20706.
103. Talley NJ, et al. Beyond eosinophilic esophagitis: eosinophils in gastrointestinal disease-new insights, "new" diseases. J Can Assoc Gastroenterol. 2023;6(6):199–211.
104. Hari S, et al. Eosinophils, hypoxia-inducible factors, and barrier dysfunction in functional dyspepsia. Front Allergy. 2022;3:851482.
105. Casado-Bedmar M, et al. Elevated F-EDN correlates with mucosal eosinophil degranulation in patients with IBS-A possible association with microbiota? J Leukoc Biol. 2022;111(3):655–65.
106. Lopez-Perez D, et al. Eosinophils in colorectal cancer: emerging insights into anti-tumoral mechanisms and clinical implications. Int J Mol Sci. 2024;25(11)
107. Overman EL, Rivier JE, Moeser AJ. CRF induces intestinal epithelial barrier injury via the release of mast cell proteases and TNF-alpha. PLoS One. 2012;7(6):e39935.
108. Wouters MM, Vicario M, Santos J. The role of mast cells in functional GI disorders. Gut. 2016;65(1):155–68.
109. Kindt S, et al. Intestinal immune activation in presumed post-infectious functional dyspepsia. Neurogastroenterol Motil. 2009;21(8):832–e56.
110. Hagiwara SI, et al. Gastric corticotropin-releasing factor influences mast cell infiltration in a rat model of functional dyspepsia. PLoS One. 2018;13(9):e0203704.
111. Teitelbaum AA, et al. Chronic peripheral administration of corticotropin-releasing factor causes colonic barrier dysfunction similar to psychological stress. Am J Physiol Gastrointest Liver Physiol. 2008;295(3):G452–9.
112. Moeser AJ, et al. Stress signaling pathways activated by weaning mediate intestinal dysfunction in the pig. Am J Physiol Gastrointest Liver Physiol. 2007;292(1):G173–81.
113. Smith F, et al. Early weaning stress impairs development of mucosal barrier function in the porcine intestine. Am J Physiol Gastrointest Liver Physiol. 2010;298(3):G352–63.
114. Moeser AJ, et al. Gastrointestinal dysfunction induced by early weaning is attenuated by delayed weaning and mast cell blockade in pigs. Am J Physiol Gastrointest Liver Physiol. 2007;293(2):G413–21.
115. Barreau F, et al. Pathways involved in gut mucosal barrier dysfunction induced in adult rats by maternal deprivation: corticotrophin-releasing factor and nerve growth factor interplay. J Physiol. 2007;580(Pt 1):347–56.
116. Larauche M. Novel insights in the role of peripheral corticotropin-releasing factor and mast cells in stress-induced visceral hypersensitivity. Neurogastroenterol Motil. 2012;24(3):201–5.
117. Eutamene H, et al. Acute stress modulates the histamine content of mast cells in the gastrointestinal tract through interleukin-1 and corticotropin-releasing factor release in rats. J Physiol. 2003;553(Pt 3):959–66.
118. van den Wijngaard RM, et al. Peripheral alpha-helical CRF (9-41) does not reverse stress-induced mast cell dependent visceral hypersensitivity in maternally separated rats. Neurogastroenterol Motil. 2012;24(3):274–82.
119. Guilarte M, et al. Peripheral Corticotropin-Releasing Factor Triggers Jejunal Mast Cell Activation and Abdominal Pain in Patients With Diarrhea-Predominant Irritable Bowel Syndrome. Am J Gastroenterol. 2020;115(12):2047–59.
120. Vicario M, et al. Increased humoral immunity in the jejunum of diarrhoea-predominant irritable bowel syndrome associated with clinical manifestations. Gut. 2015;64(9):1379–88.
121. Pardo-Camacho C, et al. Mucosal plasma cell activation and proximity to nerve fibres are associated with glycocalyx reduction in diarrhoea-predominant irritable bowel syndrome: jejunal barrier alterations underlying clinical manifestations. Cells. 2022;11(13)
122. McGillis JP, et al. Stimulation of rat B-lymphocyte proliferation by corticotropin-releasing factor. J Neurosci Res. 1989;23(3):346–52.

123. Baker C, et al. Corticotropin-releasing hormone immunoreactivity in human T and B cells and macrophages: colocalization with arginine vasopressin. J Neuroendocrinol. 2003;15(11):1070–4.
124. Zhao DY, et al. Ultrastructure of intestinal mucosa in diarrhea-predominant irritable bowel syndrome. Physiol Int. 2019;106(3):225–35.
125. Martinez C, et al. Diarrhoea-predominant irritable bowel syndrome: an organic disorder with structural abnormalities in the jejunal epithelial barrier. Gut. 2013;62(8):1160–8.
126. Dlugosz A, et al. Increased expression of toll-like receptors 4, 5, and 9 in Small Bowel Mucosa from patients with irritable bowel syndrome. Biomed Res Int. 2017;2017:9624702.
127. Wang X, et al. Probiotic bifidobacterium bifidum G9-1 has a preventive effect on the acceleration of colonic permeability and M1 macrophage population in maternally separated rats. Biomedicines. 2021;9(6)
128. Nylund CM, et al. Granulocyte macrophage-colony-stimulating factor autoantibodies and increased intestinal permeability in Crohn disease. J Pediatr Gastroenterol Nutr. 2011;52(5):542–8.
129. Vujicic M, et al. The effect of macrophage migration inhibitory factor on intestinal permeability: FITC-dextran serum measurement and transmission electron microscopy. Methods Mol Biol. 2020;2080:193–201.
130. Lembo T, et al. Effects of the corticotropin-releasing factor (CRF) on rectal afferent nerves in humans. Neurogastroenterol Motil. 1996;8(1):9–18.
131. Baffy G. Kupffer cells in non-alcoholic fatty liver disease: the emerging view. J Hepatol. 2009;51(1):212–23.
132. Agnello D, et al. Corticosteroid-independent inhibition of tumor necrosis factor production by the neuropeptide urocortin. Am J Phys. 1998;275(5):E757–62.
133. Kimura T, et al. Urocortin I is present in the enteric nervous system and exerts an excitatory effect via cholinergic and serotonergic pathways in the rat colon. Am J Physiol Gastrointest Liver Physiol. 2007;293(4):G903–10.
134. Harada S, et al. Urocortin mRNA is expressed in the enteric nervous system of the rat. Neurosci Lett. 1999;267(2):125–8.
135. Sand E, Themner-Persson A, Ekblad E. Corticotropin releasing factor-distribution in rat intestine and role in neuroprotection. Regul Pept. 2011;166(1–3):68–75.
136. Liu S, et al. Distribution and chemical coding of corticotropin-releasing factor-immunoreactive neurons in the Guinea pig enteric nervous system. J Comp Neurol. 2006;494(1):63–74.
137. Yakabi S, et al. VIP is involved in peripheral CRF-induced stimulation of propulsive colonic motor function and diarrhea in male rats. Am J Physiol Gastrointest Liver Physiol. 2018;314(5):G610–22.
138. Yamato S, et al. Urocortin 1: a putative excitatory neurotransmitter in the enteric nervous system. Neurogastroenterol Motil. 2020;32(10):e13842.
139. Porcher C, et al. Expression and effects of metabotropic CRF1 and CRF2 receptors in rat small intestine. Am J Physiol Gastrointest Liver Physiol. 2005;288(5):G1091–103.
140. Liu S, et al. Differential actions of urocortins on neurons of the myenteric division of the enteric nervous system in Guinea pig distal colon. Br J Pharmacol. 2010;159(1):222–36.
141. Kihara N, et al. Effects of central and peripheral urocortin on fed and fasted gastroduodenal motor activity in conscious rats. Am J Physiol Gastrointest Liver Physiol. 2001;280(3):G406–19.
142. Tache Y, et al. Role of corticotropin releasing factor receptor subtype 1 in stress-related functional colonic alterations: implications in irritable bowel syndrome. Eur J Surg Suppl. 2002;587:16–22.
143. Tache Y, et al. CRF1 receptor signaling pathways are involved in stress-related alterations of colonic function and viscerosensitivity: implications for irritable bowel syndrome. Br J Pharmacol. 2004;141(8):1321–30.
144. Martinez V, Tache Y. CRF1 receptors as a therapeutic target for irritable bowel syndrome. Curr Pharm Des. 2006;12(31):4071–88.

Chapter 5
CRF Peptides in the Cardiovascular System

Chao Zhu and Rong Wan

The corticotropin-releasing hormone (factor) family peptides (CRFp), including corticotropin-releasing hormone (CRH) and urocortins (UCNs, UCN1–3), function through their two distinct receptors (CRFr), CRF_1 and CRF_2 (*See* Chaps. 2 and 3). Since the discovery of CRFp in modulating cardiovascular function, more and more researches have been done to elucidate their existence and roles in vascular and cardiac tissues, and clinical trials have been carried out making some of CRFp as novel promising cardiovascular markers in various cardiovascular diseases (CVD). This chapter will focus on the roles of CRFp-CRFr signaling in maintaining normal physiological function of endothelial cells and cardiac myocytes and thus in protecting the health of vasculatures and hearts. Additionally, the possible harmful effects of CRF system on cardiovascular system are also discussed.

1 CRFp in the Endothelial Function and Health of Vasculatures

Vascular endothelium is a barrier between the blood and the surrounding tissue of the body, which functions as a regulated permeability filter for solutes and cells to leave or to enter the bloodstream to maintain homeostasis [1]. Endothelial cells (ECs) are essential for the maintenance of blood vessel function and are involved in

C. Zhu (✉)
Department of Pharmacology, School of Basic Medical Sciences,
Nanjing Medical University, Nanjing, Jiangsu, China
e-mail: czhu@njmu.edu.cn

R. Wan
Jiangxi Key Laboratory of Molecular Medicine, The Second Affiliated Hospital of Nanchang University, Nanchang, China

© The Author(s), under exclusive license to Springer Nature Singapore Pte Ltd. 2025
C. Zhu et al. (eds.), *The Peripheral Existence and Effects of Corticotropin-releasing Factor Family*, https://doi.org/10.1007/978-981-96-5322-5_5

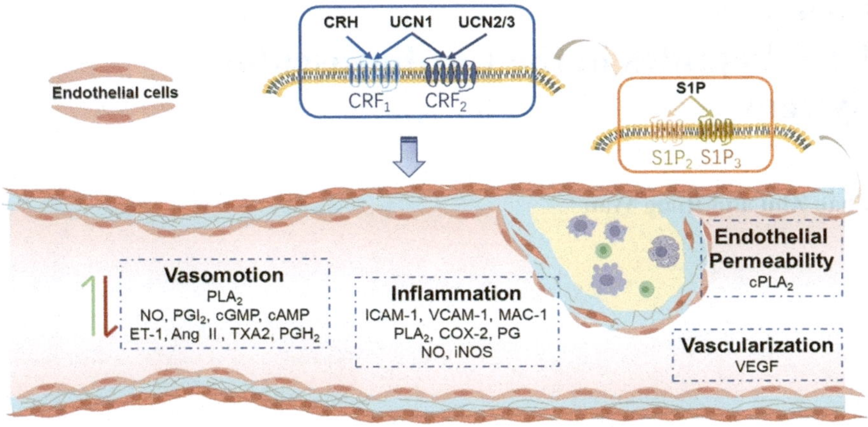

Fig. 5.1 Roles of peripheral CRFp in the endothelial cells and vasculatures

the pathogenesis of almost all cardiovascular diseases [2, 3]. Endothelial dysfunction involves several events, including impaired vasodilation, endothelial nitric oxide synthase (eNOS) uncoupling, leukocyte adhesion, endothelial senescence, and endothelial mesenchymal transition [4]. Since the end of last century, growing evidence has demonstrated the important role of CRFp and CRFr in regulating vascular endothelial function and maintaining the health of vasculatures (as depicted in Fig. 5.1).

1.1 Expression of CRFp in Vascular Endothelium

CRH staining in immunohistochemistry assay is found in vascular endothelium cells of human placenta [5]. Besides, cultured human umbilical vein endothelial cells (HUVECs) are tested to be a source and a target for CRH, as evidenced by the expression and secretion of CRH and the expression of CRFr in these cells [6]. Such findings indicate that CRH can function on vascular endothelial cells in an autocrine/paracrine manner. Moreover, the release of CRH from cultured HUVECs is decreased by dexamethasone while increased by several distinct molecules, including progesterone, 17β-estradiol, forskolin, $PGF_{2\alpha}$, interleukin (IL)-1β, and endothelin [6].

Similar to CRH, high expression of UCN1 is found to be localized in the endothelial layer of coronary arteries and microvessels in rats and humans [7, 8]. A study shows that pitavastatin increases serum UCN1 levels in healthy volunteers, and the in vitro experiments verify that UCN1 is released from human endothelial cells by pitavastatin stimulation [7]. In maternal and fetal vessels of gestational tissues, UCN2 but not UCN3 is present [9]. In another study reported by Kazunori Kageyama et al., all three UCNs, but not CRH, are found to be expressed in HUVECs, and these UCNs can be differentially regulated by the same stimulators [10].

As for the CRFr expressed in vasculatures, CRF_1 is found in human mammary artery [11]. However, the cardiovascular actions of CRFp are thought to be mediated by CRF_2 [12]. By using radioligand binding techniques, highly expressed CRF_2 in human cardiovascular system, including ventricle, intramyocardial blood vessels, and internal mammary arteries, is revealed [13]. Many researchers also examine tissue expression levels of CRFr and find that CRF_2 is mainly expressed in vascular endothelium [14, 15]. CRF_2 mRNA is also expressed in HUVECs [6]. One group further identifies the subtypes of CRF_2 expressing in vasculatures. They report that all the CRF_1, $CRF_{2\alpha}$, and $CRF_{2\beta}$ mRNA are present in human mammary artery [11]. Another group only detects $CRF_{2\beta}$ but not $CRF_{2\alpha}$ in the aorta and uterine vascular bed using RT-PCR and Western blot [16]. Higher expression of $CRF_{2\beta}$ on the aortic endothelial surface than that in the smooth muscle layer is observed by immunohistochemistry [16]. The presence of CRF_2 in vascular endothelium lays a positive foundation for the regulation of endothelial function by CRFp [14, 15].

1.2 Dual Roles of CRFp in Regulating Vasomotor Function

There is a proposal that CRFp play distinct roles in the vessel tissues though targeting brain and periphery: CRH stimulates noradrenergic sympathetic nervous outflow to activate peripheral vessels, whereas activation of CRF_2 directly in peripheral vessels causes strong and sustained vasodilatory response [17–20]. In different species and various vascular beds, CRH and UCNs show endothelial vasodilatory effects. On the other hand, regardless of endothelial function, all the four peptides (CRH and UCN1–3) are tested to produce a potent vasodilator response in endothelium-denuded human internal mammary artery [13].

CRH causes both endothelial-independent and endothelial-dependent vasodilation in rat mesenteric, cerebral, femoral, and uterine vascular beds [21–23]. In rat aorta, CRH induces endothelium-dependent relaxation [24]. Interestingly, CRH-induced relaxation is gestationally regulated, with the unchanged responses during early pregnancy and decreased responses toward the end of gestation [24]. In isolated working rat hearts, CRH increases coronary flow, which can be diminished either by inhibiting nitric oxide (NO) production or prostanoid synthesis [25]. However, CRH is reported to show no effect on colonic blood flow but further increases the vascular resistance [26]. Therefore, whether and how CRH relaxes vessels depends on the various vascular beds studied.

As the mostly investigated one among UCNs in dilating vessels, UCN1 functions via different pathways. UCN1 can relax human internal mammary artery and rat coronary artery dependently or independently of the endothelium [8, 11]. In isolated rat coronary artery, about three times the dose of UCN1 is needed to produce the maximum relaxation in the endothelium-denuded rings compared to that in endothelium-intact rings [8]. Endothelial NO and Ba^{2+}- or tertiapin-Q-sensitive K^+ channel and cyclic guanosine monophosphate (cGMP) seem to be involved in UCN1-induced endothelium-dependent relaxation, whereas cyclic adenosine monophosphate (cAMP)-dependent protein kinase (PKA) and Ca^{2+}-activated K^+ channels appear to mediate its endothelium-independent relaxation [8, 27]. Similar to CRH, UCN1 induces endothelium-dependent relaxation in rat aorta [24, 28]. Because deendothelialization age-dependently reduces UCN1-induced vasodilation and nitric oxide synthase inhibitor significantly decreases UCN1-induced relaxation of aorta with the endothelium in aged rats compared to young rats, aging is seen to increase the role of NO production from the endothelium in UCN1-induced aorta vasodilation [28]. In fact, the underlying mechanism for UCN1-mediated endothelium-dependent vasodilation is always thought to involve NO production and subsequent activation of Ba^{2+}-sensitive K^+ channels [8, 29]. Ba^{2+}, a kind of K^+ channel blocker, reduces the relaxant responses to UCN1 in isolated rat coronary arteries, suggesting that Ba^{2+}-sensitive K^+ channel contributes to UCN1-induced relaxation. Since Ba^{2+} has no effect on UCN1-induced relaxation in the endothelium-denuded arteries but inhibits NO donor-induced relaxation, in addition to that combined treatment with Ba^{2+} and eNOS inhibitor shows no additive inhibition on UCN1's vasodilatory effect, it is speculated that Ba^{2+}-sensitive K^+ channel functions as the downstream of endothelial NO in UCN1-induced endothelium-dependent relaxation in coronary arteries. Likely, Ba^{2+}-sensitive K^+ channel is also involved in UCN1-induced vasodilation in rat pulmonary arteries [30]. Interestingly, UCN1 is also reported to cause endothelium-dependent hyperpolarization and relaxation in rat mesenteric arteries through Ca^{2+}-activated K^+ channels but not through NO or cGMP signaling [31]. Thus, UCN1 can function through multiple potassium channels to induce endothelium-dependent vasodilation. Besides, UCN1 is reported to protect coronary endothelial vasodilatory effect by acetylcholine against ischemia-reperfusion injury [32, 33]. This protective role seems to be mediated by protein kinase C (PKC) but not by Ca^{2+}-dependent potassium channels, K(ATP) channel, endothelial nitric oxide synthase, or cyclooxygenase [32]. As for the endothelium-independent relaxant effect of UCN1 on vasculatures, Na^+-Ca^{2+} exchanger, another ion channel, may contribute to UCN1's role in rat pulmonary arteries [34]. It is found that both the putative Na^+-Ca^{2+} exchanger inhibitor nickel chloride and the Na^+-free solution can reduce UCN1-induced relaxation in endothelium-denuded vascular rings [34]. In addition, PKA activation is also reported to mediate UCN1-exhibited endothelium-independent vasodilatory effect in rat tail artery and rat pulmonary artery [30, 35].

UCN2, the selective CRF_2 agonist, causes coronary artery vasodilation in pigs [36]. For the colonic blood flow in rat, activation of peripheral CRF_2 by UCN2 or sauvagine functions through NO synthesis to induce colonic hyperemia and to decrease colonic vascular resistance [26]. Similar vasodilatory effect of UCN2 via producing endothelial NO is also found in human volunteers [37]. Besides, our recent research also shows that UCN2 protects coronary endothelial vasodilation by acetylcholine against type 2 diabetes [38]. It is found that UCN2 significantly decreases the accumulation of methylglyoxal in diabetic mice and is able to reverse the enrichment of arginase 1 in macrophage extracellular vesicles, both of which are demonstrated to induce diabetes-like coronary microvascular endothelial dysfunction [38]. What's more, the protective effect of UCN2 on diabetic coronary artery seems to be mediated by IL-33 restoring [38]. In addition to UCN2, the other selective CRF_2 agonist UCN3 is also able to induce potent and prolonged arterial vasodilation in healthy volunteers, although it is much less dependent on endothelial NO production [37]. In fact, the different efficiencies on relaxing artery by different CRFp do exist. It is found that UCN1 acts through CRF_2 to induce vasodilation in rat basilar artery, while CRH relaxes the vessel at a 100-fold higher concentration than UCN1, indicating the distinguishing vasodilatory effect of CRF_2 signaling [39]. As for the different sensitivity of CRF_2 signaling-dilated vessels to NO production, the nuances in triggering CRF_2 by UCN2 and UCN3 are worthy of further investigation.

Except for releasing NO for vasodilation, the endothelium also secrets many kinds of contracting factors, like endothelin-1 (ET-1), angiotensin (Ang)II, thromboxane A2 (TXA2), prostaglandin H_2 (PGH_2), and so on, to show vasoconstrictive effects [40]. Therefore, CRFp are speculated to benefit the control of vascular tension either by increasing relaxant factor secretion or decreasing contracting factor secretion from the endothelium. UCN1 and CRF_2 are indeed reported to reduce plasma Ang II and ET-1 in experimental heart failure sheep [41, 42], though other studies show the increased ET-1 release from human coronary artery endothelial cells and human microvascular endothelial cells by CRH [15, 43]. This discrepancy may be caused by differences between in vivo and in vitro experiments, different species of experimental subjects, or different CRFp used.

Among the vasoconstrictors mentioned above, TXA2 and PGH_2 bind to thromboxane receptor to mediate vasoconstriction [44]. Both TXA2 and PGH_2 are the downstream products from the phospholipase A_2 (PLA_2)-arachidonic acid (AA)-cyclooxygenase (COX) pathway [45]. Our recent studies have shown a close relationship between CRF system and various PLA_2 in many types of cells, including endothelial cells [46–50]. Although CRF_1 and CRF_2 seem to regulate PLA_2 activation oppositely, all these findings strongly indicate the involvement of PLA_2 in CRFp-controlled vasomotor function. In addition to TXA2 and PGH_2, prostacyclin (PGI_2), another prostanoid synthesized by COX and released from the endothelium, can increase cAMP in vascular smooth muscle cell to dilate vessels [51]. CRH is shown to abolish IL-1α-induced PGI_2 synthesis through CRFr in bovine aortic endothelial cells [52]. Both IL-1α-induced PLA_2 and prostaglandin H synthase (PGHS) activity can be completely abrogated by CRH, whereas only IL-1β-induced PGHS but not PLA_2 activity is inhibited by CRH [53], suggesting the specific inhibitory effect of CRH on the activation of the arachidonic acid pathway by certain stimulators. In isolated working rat hearts, CRH increases coronary flow, which can be diminished either by inhibiting NO production or prostanoid synthesis [25]. Moreover, UCN1 functions on coronary smooth muscle cells to relax coronary artery endothelium-independently through the inhibition of Ca^{2+}-independent phospholipase A2 ($iPLA_2$) and store-operated Ca^{2+} entry [54]. Therefore, only considering regulating PLA_2 activation and its downstream prostanoid production, CRFp are able to show dual roles in regulating vascular tone. Taken together, most studies have shown the vasodilatory effects of CRFp in diverse vascular beds; it is important to bear in mind that in some certain conditions, CRFp may also show vasoconstrictive activity.

1.3 Dual Roles of CRFp in Maintaining Endothelial Permeability

Enhanced endothelial permeability is a sign of vascular inflammation. CRH is reported to decrease blood–brain barrier (BBB) permeability by directly affecting the endothelium of the cerebral vessels in rats [55]. Likewise, CRH decreases BBB permeability in an experimental model of vasogenic peritumoral brain edema, which is not mediated by the release of corticosteroids [56]. Additionally, peripheral subcutaneous CRH treatment to rat is shown to inhibit tumor vascular permeability, which is speculated to be a consequence of decreased neo-angiogenesis probably [57]. Except for tumor, CRH treatment reduces limb weight gain to about half of control treatment in a pedicled rat hindlimb model [58], suggesting its benefit in controlling vascular permeability. In contrast, it is concluded by another group that CRH is involved in increased rat BBB permeability by acute stress [59]. Our group also reports the activation of CRF_1 in promoting endothelial monolayer hyperpermeability in vitro and mice cortical vascular hyperpermeability in vivo, while CRF_1 interference significantly alleviates hippocampal BBB leakage [48]. What's more and interestingly, CRH/CRF_1 seems to show a crucial role in maintaining cerebrovascular endothelial permeability homeostasis. Our study shows that CRH can reverse both the opposite effects of blocking sphingosine-1-phosphate receptor 2 ($S1P_2$) and sphingosine-1-phosphate receptor 3 ($S1P_3$) on oxidative stress-induced cerebrovascular endothelial cell permeability via regulating the activation of $cPLA_2$ [50].

UCN1 is found to cause an elevation of lung vascular permeability when given by inhalation aerosol to rats, which is markedly reduced by nonselective CRFr antagonist [60]. Mast cells and histamine are considered as the downstream effectors of the peripheral UCN1 in the lung. In triggering skin vascular permeability, one study also points out that mast cell is the target of UCN1, resulting in cell degranulation and thus the skin vasodilation [61]. Compared to that in normal nasal mucosa, the enhanced expression of UCN1 and CRFr in allergic nasal mucosa also indicates their roles in increasing mucosal swelling and vascular permeability [62]. Furthermore, in one of our series studies, UCN1 is found to increase endothelial permeability via CRF_2 in vitro [63]. Oppositely, there are also rare evidence showing the reducing effect of UCN1 on BBB permeability [64, 65].

Whether CRFp promote or inhibit endothelial permeability in both normal conditions and tumor circumstances still need further investigations.

1.4 Dual Roles of CRFp in Vascular Inflammation

Endothelial dysfunction may initiate vascular inflammation. In addition to the effects on endothelial cells, CRFp can also affect vascular inflammation via targeting other cell types.

It is known that the hypothalamic-pituitary-adrenal axis (HPA axis), with CRH involved in the secretion of adrenocorticotropin (ACTH), accounts for the generation of glucocorticoids and thus triggers the anti-inflammatory effects [66]. Direct cerebral CRH injection is also shown to blunt enhanced endothelial expression of intercellular adhesion molecule 1 (ICAM-1) and leukocyte recruitment during endotoxemia in mesenteric venules of rats [67]. Apart from the function through cerebral center, CRF_1 blockade increases tumor necrosis factor (TNF)-α-induced vascular adhesion molecule-1 (VCAM-1) and E-selectin in human aortic endothelial cells, indicating a protective role of peripheral CRF_1 signaling against vascular inflammation [68]. Moreover, IL-1α-enhanced PLA_2 activity and prostaglandin synthesis are significantly suppressed by CRH in bovine aortic endothelial cells, further suggesting the effect of CRH/CRF_1 on inhibiting inflammation at peripheral sites [66]. IL-1α-induced prostacyclin synthesis in endothelial cells is also abolished by simultaneous treatment with CRH, which effect can be further antagonized by CRFr antagonist α-helical CRH(9–41) [52]. In addition to CRH, UCN1 is reported to inhibit the isolated HUVECs to secrete activin-A as a member of the transforming growth factor (TGF)-β superfamily, which indicates the anti-inflammatory action of UCN1 [69].

In contrast to the anti-inflammatory effects, CRFp are also reported to promote inflammatory responses. For example, by targeting monocytes, CRH time- and concentration-dependently increases cell adhesion to human microvascular endothelial cells as well as monocytic MAC-1 expression [70]. Additionally, an ex vivo synovial tissue culture system is established to study the effect of CRH at peripheral sites of inflammation. CRH can time- and dose-dependently increase PGE_2 production from fresh rheumatoid arthritis synovial tissue explants, which is prevented by selective COX-2 inhibitors [71]. CRF_1 might be involved in such joint inflammation, as only CRF_1 but not CRF_2 mRNA is detected in the studied samples of inflamed synovial tissue [72]. It is also found that immunoreactive CRF_1 expresses abundantly on vascular endothelial cells and discrete perivascular cells, which are identified as mast cells [72]. As summarized in our latest review [73], mast cell is another important target for CRH/CRF_1 signaling to play a pro-inflammatory role. CRH can activate mast cell to release histamine and numerous pro-inflammatory mediators and thus increase vascular permeability [74–76]. Likewise, UCN1 significantly induces the activation and degranulation of rat lung mast cells [77]. It can also stimulate the secretion of inflammatory cytokines such as IL-1β and IL-6 from human peripheral blood mononuclear cells, indicating the pro-inflammatory effects of UCN1 [78]. Our previous in vivo work demonstrates that UCN1 promotes vasculitis in a rat model of thromboangitis obliterans via CRF_1 [79]. Unexpectedly, the in vitro study shows the involvement of CRF_2, but not CRF_1, in UCN1-augmented LPS-induced COX-2 and ICAM-1 in rat aortic endothelial cells [80], indicating the pro-inflammatory effect of UCN1/CRF_2 signaling. Moreover, our later research further indicates that UCN1 is a contributory factor to the gender disparity in sodium laurate-induced rat vasculitis, with dihydrotestosterone-promoted UCN1 secretion exacerbating the development of vasculitis [81].

As mentioned above, most vasodilatory roles of CRFp in the endothelium are mediated by gaseous mediator NO. The CRFp-triggered endothelial NO release is thought to be the product catalyzed by eNOS [82]. Actually, in addition to eNOS, inducible NO synthase (iNOS) is also expressed in activated endothelial cells and can synthesize inflammatory NO, showing cytotoxic phenomena during inflammation [83, 84]. Interestingly, CRH is shown to inhibit and potentiate iNOS expression in H5V murine endothelioma cells and HUVECs, respectively [85]. These divergent effects of CRH are associated with different CRFr expressed on these two kinds of endothelial cells with H5V expressing both CRF_1 and CRF_2 and HUVECs expressing only the CRF_2 [85]. In the case of this report, it reminds us of the pro-inflammatory effect of CRF_2 with increasing inflammatory NO from iNOS when we want to take advantage of its anti-ischemic and anti-inflammatory effects with increasing vasodilatory NO from eNOS. Therefore, both CRF_1 and CRF_2 seem to have dual functions in vascular inflammation, at least in regard to the activation of iNOS or eNOS by CRFr.

Despite the possible opposite signaling by CRF_1 and CRF_2, CRH shows a biphasic effect on inflammation which is thought to be dose-dependent [86]. The data show that CRH at low dose is anti-inflammatory while at large dose is pro-inflammatory in a rat model of hind paw edema [86]. Of course, the exact mechanism, for example, whether this phenomenon is caused by the different affinity of CRH to CRF_1 and CRF_2, still needs to be established by additional experiments. Similar to CRH, as we summarize in a latest review [73], UCNs also show both potent protective and harmful effects on the vasculitis, the detailed mechanisms of which also need further investigation.

1.5 *Opposite Roles of CRF_1 and CRF_2 Pathways in Vascularization*

CRF_1 and CRF_2 may oppositely regulate vascularization through different pathways. CRH, a CRF_1-selective agonist having ten-fold lower affinity for CRF_2, is shown to enhance angiogenesis in epithelial cell tumors [87]. In contrast, UCN1 is observed to suppress capillary formation of endothelial cells via CRF_2, supported by the fact that mice lacking CRF_2 develop postnatal hypervascularization [88]. In addition, UCN1 also inhibits smooth muscle cell proliferation and its production of vascular endothelial growth factor (VEGF), which is known as the key factor in vascularity [88]. CRF_2-mutant mice not only have increased tissue capillaries but also have increased larger conductance vessels [88], indicating that blocking CRF_2 may also be a therapeutic strategy in some ischemic diseases; in accompany with that, CRF_2 activation can dilate vessels to increase blood flow to ischemic area. Such similar effects like limiting tumor vascularization by CRF_2 activation even make UCN2 show potential to inhibit tumor growth [89]. Like UCN1, UCN2 also inhibits vascular smooth muscle cell proliferation, which can be reversed by CRF_2 antagonist astressin-2B [90].

1.6 Opposite Roles of CRF_1 and CRF_2 Pathways in Inducing Oxidative Stress

Oxidative stress is one of the main contributors to endothelial damage [91]. CRH induces a significant increase of reactive oxygen species (ROS) levels and a simultaneous significant decrease of eNOS activity and NO levels in endothelial EAhy926 cells [92]. It is found that CRF_1 blockade but not CRF_2 blockade reverses the increased ROS by CRH, indicating the regulatory role of CRH/CRF_1 in elevating ROS levels [92]. On the contrary, UCN1 is reported to suppress angiotensin II-induced ROS in isolated endothelial cells [7]. As known, diabetic nephropathy is one of the major microvascular complications in diabetes. Our early work demonstrates that UCN1 ameliorates diabetic nephropathy in db/db mice, accompanied by a markedly increased superoxide dismutase and a significantly decreased malonaldehyde [93]. Such findings indicate the antioxidative effect of UCN1 as well. In conclusion, it is possible that CRFp function through different CRFr to show biphasic effects on the production of ROS, just like its roles in regulating PLA_2, iNOS, or inflammation mentioned above.

1.7 Other Potential Effects of CRFp on Endothelial Physiological Function and Pathological Processes

1.7.1 Glucose Transport

Glucose transporters (GLUT) are found to be expressed in syncytiotrophoblasts and the endothelium of vessels in human placenta [94]. In cultured placenta syncytiotrophoblasts, CRH dose-dependently increases GLUT1 but decreases GLUT3 through CRFr [94]. Further experiments demonstrate that CRF_1 mediates the upregulation of GLUT1 and downregulation of GLUT3, while CRF_2 mediates the downregulation of both GLUT1 and GLUT3 [94]. Although the effect of CRH on GLUT expression is only detected in syncytiotrophoblasts but not in vascular endothelial cells, these results indicate the similar regulatory mechanism underlying the CRFp-CRFr signaling in regulating glucose transport across the vascular endothelium. It may be reasonable to consider CRH effects on the endothelial GLUT. However, rare reports are presented.

1.7.2 Endothelial-to-Mesenchymal Transition and Endothelial Senescence

Endothelial cells have overlapping behaviors and gene expression between initiating endothelial-to-mesenchymal transition and being in inflammatory and angiogenic settings [95]. Considering the existing evidence about CRFp's pro-inflammatory and anti-inflammatory effects, CRFp might play a role in endothelial-to-mesenchymal transition. In addition, endothelial senescence and its associated vascular dysfunction such as dysregulated vascular tone, increased endothelium permeability, arterial stiffness, impaired angiogenesis, and EC mitochondrial biogenesis lead to increased cardiovascular disease in aging [96]. Whether CRFp participate in the above progress of endothelial alteration needs future investigations. The comprehensive understanding of CRFp's roles in regulating endothelial physiological function and pathological processes will help to design new drugs targeting CRFp to treat aging-related vascular diseases.

1.8 Supplement of CRFp's Detrimental Effects on the Endothelium

In the tissue of rats receiving UCN1 intravenous treatment and in aortic endothelial cells treated with UCN1, angiotensin-converting enzyme (ACE), which converts Ang I to Ang II to increase vascular tone and many other cardiovascular responses associated with CVD such as hypertension and heart failure, is found to be more activated [40, 97]. Such effects indicate the possible detrimental effects of CRFp on the endothelium. Combined with the abovementioned pro-inflammatory, pro-oxidative, and rare vasoconstrictive effects of CRFp, it's important not to forget such potential detrimental effects and choose CRFp properly to handle with vascular diseases in the future.

2 CRFp in the Cardiomyocytes and Health of Hearts

The cardiomyocytes in the heart contract rhythmically to deliver oxygenated blood throughout the body, making the heart the crucial and center organ in maintaining normal life. Although there is a considerable progress in developing new strategies for heart disease, ischemic heart diseases and consequent heart failure remain the leading cause of death worldwide [98, 99]. Up to now, most pharmacological interventions have tried to improve hemodynamics or protect cardiomyocytes, with CRFp and especially UCNs as emerging targets in clinical trials [100, 101]. Growing evidence shows the cardioprotective properties and cardiovascular actions of these peptides and their corresponding CRFr (as depicted in Fig. 5.2). Understanding both the seemingly contradictory effects of CRF system on the health of hearts is beneficial for exploring more precise therapeutic regimen of CRFp relevance in heart diseases.

2.1 Expression of CRF System in Cardiac Tissues

All members of the CRF system, including CRH, UCN1–3, CRF_1, CRF_2, and CRF binding protein (CRF-BP), are tested their presence in the human normal or pathological fetal hearts by immunoreactivity [102]. It is found that all other CRF system

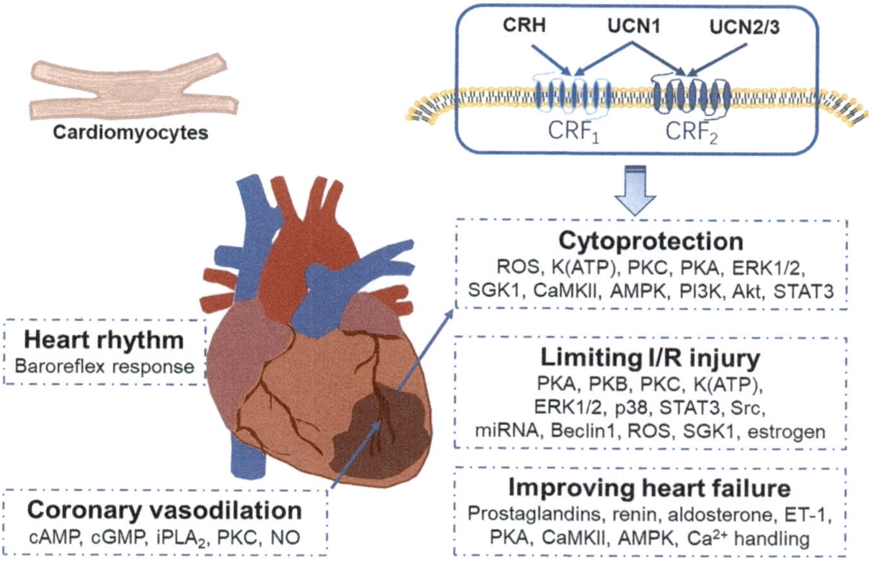

Fig. 5.2 Roles of peripheral CRFp in the cardiomyocytes and hearts

members, but not UCN3, are positive in each group, while UCN3 is only present in almost half of the fetuses with chromosomal abnormalities or congenital disorders but not in normal samples, suggesting the involvement of UCN3 in impaired fetal growth [102]. Another study points out that all UCNs have been detected in the heart and been found to cause increased cardiac output and decreased peripheral resistance [100, 103]. In the absence of intact autonomic nervous system, UCN1 is able to increase cardiac output, heart rate, and cardiac contractility, indicating that CRF receptors present in the heart mediate such response [14]. Some researchers think that only CRF_2 is expressed in the heart, while both CRF_1 and CRF_2 are detected in the brain [104]. In one study, although CRF_1 mRNA is detected in some samples of all tested heart tissues, the signal is much weaker than that of CRF_2 [105]. CRF_2 is thought to mediate CRFp's benefit in therapy of heart failure by improving cardiac output, as evidenced by application of UCN2 and CRF_2-deficient mice [106]. Thus, UCN2 and UCN3, due to their selectivity for CRF_2, exert therapeutic potential for cardiac diseases with few effects on the central nervous system [104].

It is found that UCN1 and UCN2 in cardiomyocytes can be upregulated by two major forms of cardiac stresses, with UCN1 being increased by oxidative stress and UCN2 being increased by inflammation stress-related activation of nuclear factor-κB [107]. This finding may help explain the elevated levels of UCNs in heart diseases, and such regulation can be seen as a cardiac stress adaptation. Among UCNs, UCN1 is found to have a longer half-life (with 2.9 h for alpha phase and 8.3 h for beta phase) than UCN2 (with 15.7 min), while UCN3 has the shortest half-life (with 4.4 min) in healthy sheep [103]. On the other hand, the effects exerted by UCN2 and

UCN3 are more rapid and less prolonged than that by UCN1 [103]. Differently in human volunteers with or without heart failure, the plasma UCN1 half-life is about 50 min [108, 109]. Such comparative information among UCNs and between study species is useful to the design of future studies.

2.2 Beneficial Roles of UCNs/CRF$_2$ in Protecting Cardiomyocytes

CRFp are widely investigated for their protective role in cardiomyocytes. Although some studies have shown that CRH protects cardiomyocytes from lethal ischemic injury or increases cardiac contractility, the more potent effects of UCN1 are usually indicated by these reports [110, 111].

UCN1 and CRFr are found to be expressed in cardiomyocytes [105]. It is reported that UCN1 protects cardiomyocytes from hypoxia-induced cell death [112]. Kir 6.1 cardiac potassium channel subunit, inhibition of which can enhance cell death after ischemia, is found to be induced by UCN1 [113]. Similarly, our previous study also shows that UCN1 dose-dependently activates K(ATP) channel in rat cardiac myocytes [114].The generalized and mitochondrial-specific K(ATP) channel blocker can suppress the cardioprotective effect of UCN1 both in isolated cardiac cells and in intact hearts, indicating the importance of K(ATP) channel in UCN1's cardioprotective roles [113]. What's more, UCN1 can induce another cardioprotective factor cardiotrophin-1 in cardiomyocytes [115]. Additionally, activation of PKCε is also reported to account for the cardioprotective effect of UCN1 on rat cardiomyocytes [116]. While the inhibition of PKCε aggravates cell apoptosis after ischemia and reperfusion, treatment with UCN1 significantly increases the mRNA and protein levels of PKCε in primary rat cardiomyocytes and in ex vivo heart. Moreover, UCN1 can cause a specific translocation/activation of PKCε both in vitro and ex vivo with the incubation time as short as 10 min. With the application of PKCε inhibitor or gene knockout, UCN1's cardioprotective effect loses. Apart from cell apoptosis of cardiomyocytes, non-apoptotic cell death in ischemic heart disease is also considered to be an important therapeutic target. It is also found that UCN1 suppresses anoxia-augmented nuclear shrinkage and caspase-independent cell death in cultured neonatal rat cardiomyocytes, which is abrogated by the nonselective CRFr antagonist astressin [117].

The action of UCN1 on cultured neonatal rat ventricular myocytes in the process of pre- and postconditioning is investigated. UCN1 is reported to prevent cell death and reduce damage, in primary cardiomyocytes in vitro and in isolated rat hearts ex vivo, respectively, when given both prior to simulated hypoxia/ischemia and at the point of reoxygenation [118]. The rapid phosphorylation of extracellular signal-regulated kinase 1/2 (ERK1/2) mediates the survival-promoting effect of UCN1 [118, 119]. Consistently, both preconditioning and postconditioning with UCN1 are reported to induce a powerful cell protective effect, and postconditioning with UCN1 even shows more cardioprotective effect than ischemic postconditioning

[120]. As mentioned above, among CRFp, UCN1 is more potent than CRH in protecting cardiomyocytes from lethal ischemic injury [110], indicating CRF_2 as the dominate receptor for cardioprotection by CRFp. While investigating the effect of serum- and glucocorticoid-responsive kinase-1 (SGK1), a serine-threonine kinase shown to play an important role in cardiomyocyte survival, on UCN1's cardioprotection against hypoxia/reoxygenation injury, CRF_2 antagonist is found to completely reverse UCN1-induced SGK1 activation. This study relatively clearly points out the beneficial role of CRF_2 in cardioprotection [121].

As selective CRF_2 agonists, UCN2 and UCN3 are found to increase cardiac contractility with increased fractional shortening and peak Ca^{2+} transient amplitude and decreased Ca^{2+} decay rate (Tau) in adult feline left ventricular myocytes [122]. Additionally, UCN2 can prolong action potential duration via PKA and Na^+/Ca^{2+} exchange in isolated guinea pig ventricular myocytes both time- and concentration-dependently, showing its potential to participate in cardiac contractility and arrhythmogenesis [123]. By activating CRF_2 and stimulating PKA, UCN2 increases contractility of isolated rabbit cardiomyocytes and exerts positive inotropic effect [124, 125]. The activation of Ca^{2+}/calmodulin-dependent protein kinase II (CaMKII) and AMP-activated protein kinase (AMPK) is reported to take part in the inotropic effect of UCN2 [125, 126]. In addition to PKA, CaMKII, and AMPK, other kinases like ERK, phosphatidylinositol 3-kinase (PI3K), and Akt can also be activated by UCN2 in cardiomyocytes [127]. PI3K/Akt and ERK1/2 mitogen-activated protein kinases (MAPK) are seen as the "reperfusion injury salvage kinase (RISK)" that underlay the cardioprotective mechanism by UCNs in ischemia and reperfusion injury [104, 128]. It is found that UCN2 activates cAMP-PKA, PI3K-Akt, and MEK1/2-ERK1/2 signaling, with cAMP-PKA and PI3K-Akt involved in the phosphorylation of eNOS at Ser1177 and the subsequent cellular NO production [127].

2.3 *UCN1 Protects Cardiomyocytes via Suppressing ROS Production*

In rat cardiac myocytes, pretreatment with UCN1 decreases the level of oxidative stress, the opening of mitochondrial permeability transition pore (MPTP), and cell death following simulated ischemia and reperfusion [129]. In addition to cardiomyocytes, UCN1 also strongly suppresses angiotensin II-induced ROS in human umbilical vein endothelial cells [7], indicating its antioxidative property. Interestingly, pitavastatin, a kind of statin used to treat ischemic heart disease via lowering cholesterol and low-density lipoprotein and stabilizing plaque, is found to increase UCN1 expression and its release from HUVECs and serum UCN1 level in healthy volunteers [7]. Actually, pitavastain is also found to upregulate UCN1 mRNA in human aortic endothelial cells [68]. Taken together, these results indicate that UCN1 released from endothelial cells might protect cardiomyocytes from oxidative stress challenge in a paracrine way.

2.4 Beneficial Roles of UCNs in Coronary Artery Circulation

Coronary artery circulation is crucial to the health of heart. As mentioned above, CRFp can dilate various vascular beds, including coronary artery. UCN1 induces both endothelium-dependent and endothelium-independent relaxation of rat coronary artery [8, 27]. In addition to triggering cGMP- and cAMP-mediated endothelium-dependent coronary vasodilation, UCN1 also functions on coronary smooth muscle cells to relax coronary artery through CRF_2-mediated inhibition of vasoconstriction [54]. Such a new mechanism of vasodilation in coronary artery by UCN1 involves the cAMP/PKA-dependent inhibition of $iPLA_2$ and store-operated Ca^{2+} entry [54]. Beyond its direct vasodilatory effect on coronary artery, which is actually impaired by ischemia/reperfusion (I/R) injury, UCN1 also protects acetylcholine-induced endothelial vasodilation of coronary artery from I/R injury [33]. The dual protective roles of UCN1 in maintaining coronary artery circulation make it a promising drug in preventing ischemic heart disease. To further understand the mechanisms of UCN1's coronary vasoprotective effect, various blockers targeting different enzymes, channels, and kinase are applied. It is found that only PKC inhibitor, but not blockers of Ca^{2+}-dependent potassium channels, K(ATP) channels, nitric oxide synthetase, or cyclooxygenase, is responsible for UCN1-induced improvement of the relaxation to acetylcholine in coronary artery from ischemia-reperfused hearts [32]. These results indicate that UCN1 preserves PKC-dependent endothelial function of coronary artery after the I/R injury.

As for the role of UCN2 in coronary artery circulation, it is found to increase coronary blood flow and cardiac output in anaesthetized pigs, which is mediated by releasing NO and CRF_2 [36]. UCN2 is even verified to induce vasorelaxation of coronary arteries isolated from patients with heart failure, which effect is independent of endothelial integrity and involving adenylyl cyclase activation and PKA stimulation [130]. Similar to the preserved acetylcholine-induced vasodilation of coronary artery by UCN1, UCN2 is also shown by our group to improve the relaxation of coronary artery to acetylcholine in diabetic mice [38]. All these findings further demonstrate the protective role of CRF_2 signaling in coronary artery circulation, thus in cardiac function by preventing ischemic injury.

2.5 Beneficial Role of CRFp in Limiting I/R Injury and Myocardial Infarction

CRFp can limit I/R injury by different mechanisms, including mitochondrial protection, autophagy suppression, miRNA modulation, $iPLA_2$ inhibition, multiple kinase activation, and so on.

As already mentioned, CRH, though less potent than UCN1, exerts a protective effect on rat cardiac cells from ischemia-induced necrotic and apoptotic death [110]. In ex vivo experiments, CRH reduces infarct size when given prior to ischemic insult, though this beneficial effect is not observed when CRH is added during reperfusion [131]. Unexpectedly but reasonably, such a CRH-induced infarction-limiting effect is abolished by selective CRF_2 antagonist astressin-2B [131]. Furthermore, both a selective PKA inhibitor and a selective PKC inhibitor can eliminate CRH's infarct-reducing effect [131]. On the other hand, it is known that the release of coronary constrictive and pro-inflammatory molecules from cardiac mast cells contributes to myocardial ischemia [132]. In this regard, rat cardiac mast cell degranulation is found to be induced by stress, and this effect can be blocked by antiserum against CRH or CRF_1 antagonist, indicating the involvement of CRH in triggering myocardial pathophysiology [132].

In both pre- and postconditioning, UCN1 significantly reduces myocardial cell injury caused by I/R [120]. Beyond the in vitro experiments, UCN1 is shown to decrease damage in isolated rat heart ex vivo subjected to regional I/R [118]. Similarly, administration of UCN1 significantly restores rat cardiac function during myocardial I/R injury as evidenced in ex vivo and in vivo study [133]. Activation of PKB/Akt is required to mediate UCN1's protection on cardiac cells from hypoxia/reoxygenation-induced cell death [134]. UCN1 also protects cardiomyocytes from I/R-induced cell death by preventing mitochondrial damage, with K(ATP), $iPLA_2$, and PKCε involved [135]. PKC activation is reported to account for UCN1-mediated cardioprotection against I/R injury [116]. Besides, in spite of the abovementioned study showing that PKA and PKC, but not ERK1/2, take responsibility for CRH's protection against lethal simulated ischemic stress-induced apoptotic and necrotic cell death in cardiac myocytes [131], more researches demonstrate the involvement of ERK1/2 phosphorylation in UCN1-induced survival-promoting effect on cardiac myocyte [118, 119]. Moreover, through activating ERK1/2, UCN1 can further induce the phosphorylation of signal transducer and activator of transcription 3 (STAT3), a pro-survival and anti-apoptotic transcription, to show cardioprotective potential [136]. Src, a non-receptor tyrosine kinase, is also involved in STAT3 phosphorylation by UCN1 [136]. UCN1 induces STAT3 phosphorylation at Y705 through ERK1/2 and at S727 through Src [136]. In addition, one research group find that Src serves as an upstream modulator of ERK1/2 activation and thus the cardioprotection by UCN1 in immortalized mouse atrial HL-1 cardiomyocytes [137]. Incubation with UCN1 for as short as 5 min triggers the maximal phosphorylation/activation of Src and ERK1/2. Both PP2, the selective Src family kinase inhibitor, and the transfection of dominant-negative mutant of Src can inhibit UCN1-induced phosphorylation of ERK1/2. What's more and unexpected, CRF_1 but not CRF_2 seems to largely mediate these effects [137]. Whether this difference is caused by the specific cell source used here needs to be further clarified.

Our previous data repeatedly demonstrate the regulatory effects of CRFp on the expression and activation of various PLA_2 (as shown above). Among those PLA_2, $iPLA_2$ is found to play an important role in acute myocardial infarction. The activity of $iPLA_2$ is rapidly increased during I/R [138]. When $iPLA_2$-specific inhibitor is used, the infarct size of the rabbit heart in response to I/R is reduced [138]. Furthermore, the attenuated mitochondrial phospholipid loss by $iPLA_2$ inhibition is proposed to be cardioprotective [138]. In caspase-independent myocyte death, high level of $iPLA_2$ is induced by ischemia and is supposed to promote cell death [117]. It is found that UCN1 significantly inhibits $iPLA_2$ expression and thus avoids the ischemic myocyte death [117]. Similarly, K M Lawrence et al. report that UCN1 protects cardiomyocytes from I/R injury by attenuating $iPLA_2$ gene expression [139].

Besides, CRF_2 activation-regulated several miRNAs are seen as novel targets for UCN1 in myocardial protection [133]. UCN1 can enhance or decrease the expression of miR-324-3p or miR-139-3p, the overexpression of which promotes dysregulation of multiple genes related to cell death and apoptosis, cAMP & Ca^{2+} signaling, cell stress, and metabolism [133]. Intracellular calcium handling indeed plays an essential role in the cardioprotective action of postconditioning with UCN1 [140]. In addition to the regulation of multiple miRNA expression, there are many well-established mechanisms underlying the UCN1's effect on preventing cardiomyocytes or heart from I/R injury. Through inhibiting Beclin1, UCN1 inhibits autophagic cell death in cardiomyocytes exposed to I/R injury [141]. Our early study shows that UCN1 dose-dependently prevents the occurrence and incidence of reperfusion ventricular tachycardia and fibrillation, associated with increased NO production and decreased ROS formation [142]. The reduced free radical damage following myocardial infarction is observed by UCN1 treatment [143]. A significant overlap between UCN1-regulated genes and that of anti-oxidant tempol is also revealed [143]. Interestingly, estrogen signaling is demonstrated to play a role in UCN1's effects on female rat heart. Ovariectomy is found to significantly downregulate CRF_2 expression and abrogate the reduced infarct size by UCN1 in simulated myocardial I/R, which can be restored by 17β-estradiol replacement [144]. Therefore, estrogens are thought to maintain CRF_2 expression in myocardium and thus mediate UCN1-induced cardioprotective effects against I/R injury. It is further demonstrated that estrogen increases CRF_2 expression via demethylation of its gene promoter in cardiomyocytes [145]. Moreover, they find that estrogen can enhance UCN1-induced SGK1 expression, which is related to its cardioprotection against I/R injury [146].

As same as UCN1, UCN2 also restores cardiac function during myocardial ischemia-reperfusion injury in both ex vivo and in vivo study [133]. In a model of experimental myocardial infarction, chronic long-term UCN2 treatment is shown to improve cardiovascular function and attenuate cardiac remodeling [147]. Compared with model mice without UCN2 treatment, UCN2-treated mice exhibit reduced infarct size, heart weight-to-body weight ratio, left ventricular mass and end-systolic volumes, and improved ejection fraction and fractional shortening [147]. Decreased expression of collagen 1 and β-myosin heavy chain is also detected by UCN2 treatment [147]. Like UCN1, UCN2 can also regulate the expression of miR-324-3p and miR-139-3p as the targets for its cardioprotection purpose [133]. In addition, UCN2 reduces free radical damage following myocardial infarction [143]. Unsurprisingly, a group points out that UCN2 acts through CRF_2 to mitigate against I/R injury in mice, which is mediated by the activation of the PKC-AMPK pathway [148]. They show that selective CRF_2 antagonist anti-sauvagine-30 increases infarct and exacerbates reperfusion contractile dysfunction in isolated perfused mouse hearts, whereas selective CRF_2 agonist UCN2 decreases the infarct size/area at risk ratio in mice and improves contractility of the isolated perfused heart during reperfusion. The protective effect of UCN2 can be abolished by the selective PKCε inhibitor [148]. UCN2, as well as UCN3, can also bind to CRF_2 to activate ERK1/2 and protect cardiomyocytes from I/R injury [149]. As another member of MAPK kinases other than ERK1/2, p38 MAPK activation is seen as detrimental, but not beneficial, in cardiac I/R injury, and this activation can be reduced by UCN2 treatment [150]. Thus, UCN2 protects ischemic heart through suppressing p38 MAPK as an additional mechanism.

All the abovementioned data strongly indicate the beneficial role of CRFp, especially UCNs which act through CRF_2 mainly, in the treatment of myocardial ischemia and its related bad consequences whether or not followed by prompt reperfusion.

2.6 Roles of CRFp in Regulating Blood Pressure and Hence Cardiac Afterload

Although peripheral CRFp always show lowering blood pressure effect via dilating vessels, central CRH may exert an opposite effect on regulating blood pressure. It is found that CRH administration attenuates NOS inhibition-induced increase in mean arterial pressure [151]. For patients during sepsis, CRH injection is also found to immediately decrease mean arterial pressure and increase heart rate, cardiac index, and stoke index, whereas ACTH released after CRH injection might have an opposite effect on blood pressure [152]. As reported, intracerebroventricular administration of CRH increases arterial pressure and mesenteric vascular resistance, while intravenous administration of CRH does the opposite [153]. These two distinct effects can be reversed by ganglionic blockade and peripheral CRFr blockade, respectively [153]. These results indicate the divergent actions and mechanisms of action of central and peripheral CRH. In another study, human CRH and ovine analogue oCRH show similar opposite results centrally and peripherally, and these effects are inhibited by the CRH antagonist analogue α-helical CRH(9–41) [154]. The number of CRH-positive neurons in the amygdala is significantly greater in spontaneously hypertensive rats [155]. CRH-producing neurons in hypothalamic paraventricular nucleus (PVN) are also found to be elevated in hypertensive patients [156]. A recent study reports the requirement of CRH neurons for chronic stress-induced hypertension [157]. CRH/CRF_1 in PVN is considered to mediate sympathetic responses [158]. Thus, intracerebroventricular injection of CRH increases arterial pressure, HR, and cardiac output [159]. The activation of PVN-solitary tract nucleus CRH-containing projections does increase blood pressure [160]. Moreover, preinjection of CRH antagonist α-helical CRH(9–41) into different nuclei, such as ventromedial nucleus (VMN), dorsomedial nucleus (DMN), and PVN, can reduce their pressor response to glutamate [161], again suggesting the upregulating effect of central CRH on BP. However, microinjection of CRH into the rat nucleus tractus solitarii is reported to decrease arterial blood pressure [162]. In addition, CRH neurotransmission, through activating local CRF_1 in the lateral hypothalamus, only facilitates the tachycardiac response caused by an acute session of restraint stress in rats, without affecting the arterial pressure [163]. In summary, in spite of such just mentioned minority findings showing lowering or no affecting blood pressure effect by central CRH, most researches demonstrate the role of central CRH in elevating BP, while peripheral CRH decreases BP.

As largely described in the first part of this chapter, UCN1 can dilate multiple vascular beds, which probably results in the lowering of BP. Due to the vasodilatory effect on renal arteries, UCN1 can participate in regulating blood pressure at kidney hypertension [100]. In addition to relaxing vessels, UCN1 is also reported to dose-dependently decrease plasma vasopressin, renin activity, aldosterone, and endothelin-1 in sheep with heart failure, which might be other reasons for its lowering BP effect [41]. Central UCN1 by means of microinjection into the rat nucleus tractus solitarii is also reported to decrease arterial blood pressure [162]. Similarly, the inhibitory effect of UCN1 injected into the hypothalamic arcuate nucleus on mean arterial pressure is reported [164]. Additionally, UCN1 decreases mean arterial pressure in thiobutabarbital-anesthetized rats, which is independent of NO synthase, guanylyl cyclase, cyclooxygenase, or K^+ channel including the ATP-sensitive K^+ channel [165]. What's interesting, UCN1 decreases mean blood pressure in heart failure sheep while increases it in healthy sheep [41]. Therefore, the effect of UCN1 on blood pressure differs among the investigated species and morbid state.

While exogenous UCN2 dose-dependently reduces blood pressure, which is blocked by selective CRF_2 antagonist antisauvagine-30, the treatment with antisauvagine-30 itself alone fails to affect blood pressure, indicating the ineffectiveness for endogenous CRF_2 in mediating tone [166]. However, blockade of CRF_2 by CRH(9–41) is reported to increase mean arterial pressure and peripheral resistance and the levels of plasma renin/aldosterone/endothelin-1, indicating the role of endogenous UCNs in reducing vascular tone and renin-aldosterone/endothelin activity [42]. When lowering blood pressure via CRF_2, UCN2 can also reduce plasma catecholamine levels in mice with hyperadrenergic activity, suggesting the regulatory role of UCN2 in exaggerated sympathoadrenal function and thus in the blood pressure [167]. Similar to UCN1, UCN2 also shows central lowering BP effect when given into the rat solitary tract nucleus or hypothalamic arcuate nucleus [162, 164]. Furthermore, UCN2 is shown to improve cardiac function of spontaneously hypertensive rats, with the inhibition of L-type calcium channel in cardiomyocytes as one important mechanism [168]. In human and experimental rat pulmonary arterial hypertension, UCN2 levels in the right ventricular are increased and UCN2 treatment can decrease morbidity, attenuate remodeling, and improve pulmonary vascular function [169]. All these results indicate that UCN2 not only decreases BP via CRF_2 but also shows potential to limit hypertension-related detrimental consequences.

Rare studies show the effects of UCN3 on regulating BP, which are only centrally. On one hand, microinjection of UCN3 into the PVN significantly increases systolic blood pressure, HR, and renal sympathetic nerve activity via activating CRF_2 [170]. On the other hand, the inhibitory effect of UCN3 injected into the hypothalamic arcuate nucleus on mean arterial pressure is also shown [164].

Chronic stress is shown to decrease expression of both CRF_1 and CRF_2 within the bed nucleus of stria terminalis and then increase arterial pressure and impair the baroreflex function [171]. In addition to the possible beneficial effect of CRF_2 on controlling high blood pressure, CRF_1 blockade further augmented plasma noradrenaline and adrenaline and mean blood pressure under surgical stress [172], indicating a pathway to attenuate sympathetic nervous response via CRF_1 signaling. Based on such findings, both CRF_1 and CRF_2 seem to mediate BP lowering effect. However, by bilateral microinjection of selective CRF_1/CRF_2 antagonists, CRF_1 and CRF_2 in the lateral hypothalamus are found to modulate the baroreflex function differently [173]. Thus, not only CRFr expressed in center or periphery but also different CRFr expressed in the same center might show totally distinct effects on regulating blood pression.

2.7 *Protective Roles of CRFp in Heart Failure*

Rare evidence shows the central or local roles of CRH in heart failure. PVN CRH contributes to sympathoexcitation in rats with ischemia-induced heart failure [174]. However, intracerebroventricular injection of CRH can increase cardiac output [159]. On the other hand, positive inotropic effect of peripheral CRH on isolated heart is also observed [175]. Furthermore, CRH injection rapidly increases the release of atrial natriuretic peptide [175], which can be inhibited by indomethacin [176], suggesting the protective role of CRH in heart failure and the possible mechanism with prostaglandins involved.

In patients with heart failure, plasma/serum UCN1 are increased [177, 178]. UCN1 can increase cardiac output and decrease mean blood pressure in sheep with heart failure [41, 179]. In addition, UCN1 administration reduces cardiac preload and peripheral resistance and inhibits a range of vasoconstrictor/volume-retaining factors, including renin, aldosterone, endothelin-1, vasopressin, and atrial/brain natriuretic peptides [180]. Combined with the beneficial effects of UCN1 on vasodilation, especially for coronary artery, and on cardiomyocytes under I/R injury mentioned above, UCN1 shows potent protective roles against heart failure.

As a selective CRF_2 agonist, a large number of studies attempt to elucidate UCN2 as an important agent to treat heart failure. Like UCN1, serum UCN2 levels are also increased in patients with heart failure [181]. UCN2 shows marked and beneficial hemodynamic effects in pacing-induced heart failure in sheep [182]. Similarly, in an ovine model of acute decompensated heart failure, UCN2 has favorable effects on hemodynamics and decreases tissue mediators of inflammation, fibrosis, apoptosis, and hypertrophy in heart tissues [183]. Importantly, UCN2 infusion in human with heart failure also shows great outcomes, with increasing cardiac output and left ventricular ejection fraction and decreasing systemic vascular resistance and cardiac work [184]. Additionally, UCN2 shows positive inotropic effect and is able to stimulate contractility of isolated cardiomyocytes by activating CRF_2 and PKA [124–126]. The activation of CaMKII and AMPK might be the underlying mechanism [125, 126]. In transverse aortic constriction-induced heart failure mice, UCN2 gene transfer significantly improves systolic and diastolic function with higher left ventricular (LV) ejection fraction and more rapid Tau, accompanied with the increased Ser-16 phosphorylation of phospholamban [185]. UCN2 gene transfer in mice is also reported to restore normal cardiac function, shown as increased ejection fraction, reduced LV volume, and reduced global longitudinal strain, in age-related left ventricular dysfunction [186]. Furthermore, the role of intravenous delivery of AAV8 encoding UCN2 in increasing function of failing mice heart is tested. It is found that UCN2 gene transfer increases LV ejection fraction and LV systolic and diastolic function and increases peak systolic Ca^{2+} transient amplitude and rate of Ca^{2+} decline and SERCA2a expression [187]. Moreover, Thr286 phosphorylation of Cam kinase II is reduced, and cardiac myosin light chain kinase expression is increased by UCN2 gene transfer, which would participate in improving failing heart function [187]. As diabetes mellitus is always related to high morbidity of heart failure, whether UCN2 is beneficial for diabetes-related left ventricular dysfunction is investigated. It is found that UCN2 gene transfer not only increases left ventricular systolic and diastolic function but also reduces blood glucose in experimental mice [188]. Moreover, due to the application of mineralocorticoid receptor antagonist (MRAs) as established therapy in heart failure, the interaction of UCN2, as a novel peptide with potential in treating this disease, and an MRA in experimental heart failure is investigated. A favorable profile of effects with the combination therapy of UCN2 and MRA is demonstrated. UCN2 cotreatment with canrenoic acid, an MRA, not only improves hemodynamics and renal function while reducing plasma renin activity, angiotensin II, aldosterone, and vasopressin levels but also prevents the canrenoic acid-induced rises in plasma potassium [189]. Similarly, the adjunct UCN2 therapy with diuretics in heart failure is also demonstrated to be beneficial. Its cotreatment with furosemide significantly enhances hemodynamics, renal function, and diuretic responsiveness without additional potassium elimination in experimental sheep heart failure. UCN2 can also reverse furosemide-induced plasma renin activity and decrease plasma aldosterone and vasopressin [190].

As another selective CRF_2 agonist, UCN3 also shows protective effects on heart failure. UCN3 gene transfer can improve Ca^{2+} handling and left ventricular function in mice with heart failure and reduced ejection fractions [191]. In both patients with heart failure and age- and gender-matched healthy subjects, UCN3, as well as UCN2, causes dose-dependent forearm arterial vasodilation, reduces peripheral vascular resistance, and increases cardiac output, indicating their potential to treat heart failure [192].

2.8 CRFp in Heart Rhythm and Cardiac Baroreflex Responses

Both peripheral and central CRH are shown to regulate heart rate, and those effects seem to be mediated through different CRFr. Peripheral injection of CRH yields a sustained tachycardia, which is blocked by preinjection of CRF_2 antagonist, and such tachycardia effect is absent in CRH-treated CRF_2-deficient mice [193]. Differently, centrally injection of exogenous CRH causes bradycardia via CRF_1 in mice [194]. Unexpectedly, the blockade of central CRF_1 also produces robust bradycardia and prolonged PR interval during stress [195], which is blocked by cholinergic antagonist. This result indicates that stress-induced CRH release may protect heart from elevated cardiac vagal activity. In addition, the involvement of central CRH in producing tachycardia in rats is demonstrated [196]. J M Overton et al. and C L Grosskreutz et al. report that central CRH treatment increases heart rate and arterial pressure [159, 197], which might result from an activation of the sympathetic nervous system. Whether and how central CRH affects the efferent nervous system and hence heart rhythm needs further definition.

As for central UCNs' effect on heart rate, it is found that all three UCNs can decrease HR [162, 164]. CRF_1 or $CRF_{1/2}$ antagonist pretreatment can attenuate the HR response by UCN1, at least suggesting the mediatory effect of CRF_1 here [162]. The bradycardic response to UCN1 is significantly attenuated by bilateral vagotomy [164], further involving the activation of vagus nerves in central UCN1-triggered bradycardia. However, rare evidence shows microinjection of UCN3 into PVN significantly increases HR and renal sympathetic nerve activity via activating CRF_2 [170]. Thus, central UCNs may cause bradycardia via CRF_1 and tachycardia via CRF_2, respectively, which involves the activity of the autonomic nervous system. On the other hand, peripheral UCN1 and UCN2 are reported to cause tachycardia in rat, which is due to autonomic nervous activation mainly through baroreflex mechanisms [198]. Similar results show that UCN2 increases HR and reduces blood pressure dose-dependently, which also seems to be a baroreflex response [166].

Central CRF_1 and CRF_2 are speculated to modulate the cardiac baroreflex activities. CRF_1 antagonist administration in ventral medial prefrontal cortex regions of male Wistar rats is able to increase the slope of the baroreflex tachycardiac activity, while CRF_2 antagonist administration fails to affect bradycardic or tachycardic baroreflex responses [199]. Meanwhile, CRF_1 antagonist, but not CRF_2 antagonist, prevents UCN1-decreased tachycardia slope of the baroreflex, suggesting the inhibitory role of CRF_1 in the baroreflex tachycardic activity. On the opposite, as mentioned above, the activation of local CRF_1 in the lateral hypothalamus is indicated to facilitate the tachycardiac response caused by an acute session of restraint stress in rats [163]. Additionally, both CRF_1 and CRF_2 antagonism within the lateral hypothalamus decrease the tachycardia by both acute and repeated restraint stress, among which CRF_1 antagonism shows more pronounced inhibitory effect during the chronic exposure [200].

2.9 Beneficial Effects of UCN1 on Cardiac Arrest

In addition to the cardioprotective effects mentioned above, UCN1 exerts potential to benefit cardiomyocytes or myocardium after cardiac arrest. Cardiomyocyte apoptosis is increased in patients with long periods of cardioplegic arrest [201]. UCN1 expression can be increased in nonapoptotic myocytes, and K(ATP) channel expression is also increased in these cells [201]. Furthermore, in hearts after cardioplegic arrest and subsequent reperfusion, UCN1 expression is increased, and its presence in viable cells colocalizes with enhanced PKCε phosphorylation and mitochondrial relocation, suggesting the beneficial effect of endogenous UCN1 in the heart and the possible mechanisms [202]. UCN1 can ameliorate acute hemodynamic instability and myocardial damage with increasing Akt, ERK, and STAT3 activation in the myocardium in post-cardiac arrest myocardial dysfunction [203].

2.10 Detrimental Effects of CRFp on Cardiac Function

Besides the various beneficial effects of CRFp on the heart, which includes protecting cardiomyocytes from ischemic condition, maintaining normal coronary artery circulation, alleviating cardiac preload and afterload, and so on, some detrimental effects of CRFp are pointed out to arise our attention.

As one system that can cause increased blood pressure when activated, the sympathetic nervous system seems to be activated when plasma noradrenaline is elevated by CRH administration [204]. In spontaneously hypertensive rats (SHR), CRH expression in PVN is significantly upregulated compared with normotensive Wistar Kyoto rats (WKY) [205]. Exogenous CRH administration into PVN increases renal sympathetic nerve activity, heart rate, and arterial blood pressure in WKY rats. Moreover, blocking CRF_1, but not CRF_2, can inhibit the current-evoked firing of PVN presympathetic neurons in SHRs. All these data indicate the enhanced excitability of presympathetic neurons in SHRs by increased endogenous CRH from PVN via CRF_1 [205]. Cyclooxygenases in spinally projecting neuros seem to be involved in CRH-induced sympathetic activation [206]. During naloxone-precipitated morphine withdrawal, HPA activation and enhanced adrenaline/noradrenaline turnover can be inhibited in CRF_1-knockout mice, indicating the involvement of CRF_1 activation in contributing stress-induced cardiovascular dysfunction [207, 208]. Additionally, the cardiac autonomic imbalance is also implicated with the high CRH level and $CRF_{1/2}$ expression in rostral ventrolateral medulla and/or the nucleus of the solitary tract of immobilization stress rats [209].

UCN1 can be secreted by both cardiomyocytes and cardiac non-myocytes (NMCs) [210]. As UCN1 has cell proliferative effects on NMCs, it is reasonable to believe that UCN1 can proliferate cardiomyocytes as well and thus be involved in cardiac hypertrophy and fibrosis, i.e., cardiac remodeling [210]. While UCN1 protects cardiac myocytes by the ERK-dependent pathway, ERK is tested not to participate in UCN1-induced hypertrophy in rat cardiac myocytes [211]. It is reported that

UCN1 stimulates hypertrophy of adult cardiomyocytes with increasing the expression of a negative regulator of cardiac growth, myostatin [212]. It is also found that UCN1 induces cardiomyocyte hypertrophy associated with GSK-3β phosphorylation in a PI3K-dependent manner [213].

Due to speculation that CRF_2 always mediate beneficial cardioprotective roles of CRFp, the selective CRF_2 agonist is widely used to verify its potential to treat cardiac dysfunction. In the meantime, many negative effects of UCN2 are proposed. Beyond increasing cardiac output and left ventricular ejection fraction while decreasing systemic vascular resistance, intravenous UCN2 injection is found to elevate angiotensin II levels in healthy humans [214]. This phenomenon might be a reflective response due to the decreased peripheral resistance, but it still needs to be paid attention to whether UCN2 would exacerbate some heart diseases through overactivation of renin-angiotensin-aldosterone system (RAAS). RAAS activation may cause hypertension. It is found that serum UCN2 levels, along with left ventricle mass index, are significantly increased in hypertension patients compared to non-hypertension patients, suggesting a relationship between high UCN2 concentrations and hypertension [215]. The logistic regression analysis even shows serum UCN2 values as an independent predictor of hypertension [215]. What's more, on the contrary to the above mostly mentioned, UCN2 and CRF_2 are reported to exacerbate chronic cardiac dysfunction [216]. The plasma UCN2 levels are much higher in patients with heart failure than those in healthy controls. UCN2 can decrease left ventricular ejection fraction, while cardiomyocyte-specific deletion of CRF_2 prevents pressure overload-induced cardiac dysfunction in mice, suggesting the detrimental effect of UCN2/CRF_2 on cardiac function. A novel, oral, small molecule CRF_2 antagonist, RD-00490721, is even developed to protect cardiac function from pressure overload, which is not found to affect basal heart function [217]. Like UCN1, UCN2 also stimulates hypertrophy of adult cardiomyocytes with increasing the expression of myostatin [212]. To identify the different mechanisms underlying the contradictory roles of UCN2 in hearts, both cardioprotective and prohypertrophic, its regulation on different isoforms of nuclear factor of activated T cells (NFAT) transcription factors is postulated. UCN2 is found to regulate the distinct subcellular distribution patterns of isoforms NFATc1 and NFATc3 in cardiac myocytes through PI3K/Akt/eNOS/NO pathways to activate NFAT kinases and/or inactivate NFAT [218]. Collectively, UCNs exert both protective effect and hypertrophic effect on cardiomyocytes, and it would be a promising direction to develop a UCN therapeutic strategy that can dissociate the hypertrophic signal pathway from enhancing cardiomyocyte survival after ischemic injury.

3 Summary

As the two sites of action by CRFp, vascular endothelial cells and cardiomyocytes play crucial roles in maintaining vascular and cardiac health. Compiling evidence from cell, organ, animal, and human studies points to a role of CRFp and CRFr, especially UCNs and CRF_2, in protecting endothelial function and cardiomyocyte viability and thus in treating various cardiovascular diseases. Meanwhile, there are reports showing the detrimental effects of CRFp on cardiovascular system, like pro-inflammatory, pro-oxidative, pro-hypertrophic, and rare vasoconstrictive effects. However, much more data have demonstrated their therapeutic potential to all most all the cardiovascular diseases via dilating vessels to treat hypertension and prevent tissue ischemia, protecting endothelial cells to treat vascular inflammatory diseases, protecting cardiomyocytes against myocardial ischemia, improving cardiac function to treat heart failure, and so on. Generally, CRF_1 or CRF_2 activation and their activation in central or peripheral sites usually exert opposite effects on cardiovascular system. Other more deeper mechanisms of CRFp's roles in either protecting or harming cardiovascular functions are revealed, helping maximize the positive impact of CRFp on cardiovascular health. In conclusion, precise regulation on CRF system may become a promising approach for treating multiple cardiovascular diseases.

References

1. Wettschureck N, Strilic B, Offermanns S. Passing the vascular barrier: endothelial signaling processes controlling extravasation. Physiol Rev. 2019;99(3):1467–525.
2. Monteiro JP, et al. Endothelial function and dysfunction in the cardiovascular system: the long non-coding road. Cardiovasc Res. 2019;115(12):1692–704.
3. Rajendran P, et al. The vascular endothelium and human diseases. Int J Biol Sci. 2013;9(10):1057–69.
4. Parsamanesh N, et al. Resveratrol and endothelial function: a literature review. Pharmacol Res. 2021;170:105725.
5. Zhou F, et al. Expression of corticotrophin-releasing hormone and its receptor in patients with intrahepatic cholestasis of pregnancy. Placenta. 2013;34(5):401–6.
6. Simoncini T, et al. Human umbilical vein endothelial cells: a new source and potential target for corticotropin-releasing factor. J Clin Endocrinol Metab. 1999;84(8):2802–6.
7. Honjo T, et al. Endothelial urocortin has potent antioxidative properties and is upregulated by inflammatory cytokines and pitavastatin. J Vasc Res. 2006;43(2):131–8.
8. Huang Y, et al. Urocortin-induced endothelium-dependent relaxation of rat coronary artery: role of nitric oxide and K+ channels. Br J Pharmacol. 2002;135(6):1467–76.
9. Imperatore A, et al. Urocortin 2 and urocortin 3 are expressed by the human placenta, deciduas, and fetal membranes. Am J Obstet Gynecol. 2006;195(1):288–95.
10. Kageyama K, Hanada K, Suda T. Differential regulation of urocortins1-3 mRNA in human umbilical vein endothelial cells. Regul Pept. 2009;155(1–3):131–8.
11. Chen ZW, et al. Urocortin-induced relaxation in the human internal mammary artery. Cardiovasc Res. 2005;65(4):913–20.
12. Waser B, et al. CRF receptors in the rodent and human cardiovascular systems: species differences. Peptides. 2006;27(12):3029–38.
13. Wiley KE, Davenport AP. CRF2 receptors are highly expressed in the human cardiovascular system and their cognate ligands urocortins 2 and 3 are potent vasodilators. Br J Pharmacol. 2004;143(4):508–14.
14. Parkes DG, Weisinger RS, May CN. Cardiovascular actions of CRH and urocortin: an update. Peptides. 2001;22(5):821–7.

15. Wilbert-Lampen U, et al. Effects of corticotropin-releasing hormone (CRH) on endothelin-1 and NO release, mediated by CRH receptor subtype R2: a potential link between stress and endothelial dysfunction? J Psychosom Res. 2006;61(4):453–60.
16. Jain V, et al. Expression of receptors for corticotropin-releasing factor in the vasculature of pregnant rats. J Soc Gynecol Investig. 2000;7(3):153–60.
17. Abdelrahman AM, Lin Lim S, Pang CC. Influence of urocortin and corticotropin releasing factor on venous tone in conscious rats. Eur J Pharmacol. 2005;510(1–2):107–11.
18. Fisher LA, Jessen G, Brown MR. Corticotropin-releasing factor (CRF): mechanism to elevate mean arterial pressure and heart rate. Regul Pept. 1983;5(2):153–61.
19. Coste SC, et al. Abnormal adaptations to stress and impaired cardiovascular function in mice lacking corticotropin-releasing hormone receptor-2. Nat Genet. 2000;24(4):403–9.
20. Huang Y, et al. Urocortin and cardiovascular protection. Acta Pharmacol Sin. 2004;25(3):257–65.
21. Lei S, et al. Relaxing actions of corticotropin-releasing factor on rat resistance arteries. Br J Pharmacol. 1993;108(4):941–7.
22. Barker DM, Corder R. Studies of the role of endothelium-dependent nitric oxide release in the sustained vasodilator effects of corticotrophin releasing factor and sauvagine. Br J Pharmacol. 1999;126(1):317–25.
23. Jain V, et al. Endothelium-dependent and -independent mechanisms of vasorelaxation by corticotropin-releasing factor in pregnant rat uterine artery. J Pharmacol Exp Ther. 1999;288(2):407–13.
24. Jain V, et al. The relaxation responses to corticotropin-releasing factor in rat aorta are endothelium dependent and gestationally regulated. Am J Obstet Gynecol. 1997;176(1 Pt 1):234–40.
25. Grunt M, et al. Effects of corticotropin-releasing factor on isolated rat heart activity. Am J Phys. 1993;264(4 Pt 2):H1124–9.
26. Akiba Y, Kaunitz JD, Million M. Peripheral corticotropin-releasing factor receptor type 2 activation increases colonic blood flow through nitric oxide pathway in rats. Dig Dis Sci. 2015;60(4):858–67.
27. Huang Y, et al. Roles of cyclic AMP and Ca2+-activated K+ channels in endothelium-independent relaxation by urocortin in the rat coronary artery. Cardiovasc Res. 2003;57(3):824–33.
28. Miki I, et al. Role of corticotropin-releasing factor receptor type 2 beta in urocortin-induced vasodilation of rat aortas. J Pharmacol Sci. 2004;96(2):170–6.
29. Yao X, et al. Endothelium-dependent and -independent coronary relaxation induced by urocortin. J Card Surg. 2002;17(4):347–9.
30. Chan YC, et al. The relaxant effect of urocortin in rat pulmonary arteries. Regul Pept. 2004;121(1–3):11–8.
31. Secilmis MA, et al. Urocortin induces endothelium-dependent vasodilatation and hyperpolarization of rat mesenteric arteries by activating Ca2+-activated K+ channels. Tohoku J Exp Med. 2007;213(1):89–98.
32. Garcia-Villalon AL, et al. Mechanisms of the protective effects of urocortin on coronary endothelial function during ischemia-reperfusion in rat isolated hearts. Br J Pharmacol. 2005;145(4):490–4.
33. Garcia-Villalon AL, et al. Urocortin protects coronary endothelial function during ischemia-reperfusion: a brief communication. Exp Biol Med (Maywood). 2004;229(1):118–20.
34. Lau CW, et al. Nickel inhibits urocortin-induced relaxation in the rat pulmonary artery. Eur J Pharmacol. 2004;488(1–3):169–72.
35. Lubomirov L, et al. Urocortin relaxes rat tail arteries by a PKA-mediated reduction of the sensitivity of the contractile apparatus for calcium. Br J Pharmacol. 2001;134(7):1564–70.
36. Grossini E, et al. The effect of urocortin II administration on the coronary circulation and cardiac function in the anaesthetized pig is nitric-oxide-dependent. Eur J Pharmacol. 2008;578(2–3):242–8.

37. Venkatasubramanian S, et al. Vascular effects of urocortins 2 and 3 in healthy volunteers. J Am Heart Assoc. 2013;2(1):e004267.
38. Zhu C, et al. Urocortin2 attenuates diabetic coronary microvascular dysfunction by regulating macrophage extracellular vesicles. Biochem Pharmacol. 2024;219:115976.
39. Schilling L, et al. Characterization of the relaxant action of urocortin, a new peptide related to corticotropin-releasing factor in the rat isolated basilar artery. Br J Pharmacol. 1998;125(6):1164–71.
40. Yang C, Xu Y, Li S. Urocortin: a beneficial or detrimental agent to endothelium? Biochem Biophys Res Commun. 2008;371(3):345–9.
41. Rademaker MT, et al. Beneficial hemodynamic, endocrine, and renal effects of urocortin in experimental heart failure: comparison with normal sheep. J Am Coll Cardiol. 2002;40(8):1495–505.
42. Rademaker MT, et al. Endogenous urocortins reduce vascular tone and renin-aldosterone/endothelin activity in experimental heart failure. Eur Heart J. 2005;26(19):2046–54.
43. Nickel T, et al. Modification of endothelial biology by acute and chronic stress hormones. Microvasc Res. 2009;78(3):364–9.
44. Luscher TF, Noll G. The pathogenesis of cardiovascular disease: role of the endothelium as a target and mediator. Atherosclerosis. 1995;118(Suppl):S81–90.
45. Badimon L, et al. The key contribution of platelet and vascular arachidonic acid metabolism to the pathophysiology of atherothrombosis. Cardiovasc Res. 2021;117(9):2001–15.
46. Zhu C, et al. Urocortin participates in LPS-induced apoptosis of THP-1 macrophages via S1P-cPLA2 signaling pathway. Eur J Pharmacol. 2020;887:173559.
47. Zhu C, et al. Urocortin affects migration of hepatic cancer cell lines via differential regulation of cPLA2 and iPLA2. Cell Signal. 2014;26(5):1125–34.
48. Cao C, et al. Activation of CRHR1 contributes to cerebral endothelial barrier impairment via cPLA(2) phosphorylation in experimental ischemic stroke. Cell Signal. 2020;66:109467.
49. Zhu C, et al. Corticotrophin-releasing factor participates in S1PR3-dependent cPLA2 expression and cell motility in vascular smooth muscle cells. Vasc Pharmacol. 2015;71:116–26.
50. Mu J, et al. CRH/CRHR1 modulates cerebrovascular endothelial cell permeability in association with S1PR2 and S1PR3 under oxidative stress. Vasc Pharmacol. 2022;142:106941.
51. Bryan RM Jr, et al. Endothelium-derived hyperpolarizing factor: a cousin to nitric oxide and prostacyclin. Anesthesiology. 2005;102(6):1261–77.
52. Fleisher-Berkovich S, Rimon G, Danon A. Modulation of endothelial prostaglandin synthesis by corticotropin releasing factor and antagonists. Eur J Pharmacol. 1998;353(2–3):297–302.
53. Fleisher-Berkovich S, Danon A. IL-1alpha but not IL-1beta-induced prostaglandin synthesis is inhibited by corticotropin-releasing factor. Cytokine. 1999;11(3):239–43.
54. Smani T, et al. Role of Ca2+-independent phospholipase A2 and store-operated pathway in urocortin-induced vasodilatation of rat coronary artery. Circ Res. 2007;101(11):1194–203.
55. Hendryk S, et al. Influence of the corticotropin releasing hormone (CRH) on the brain-blood barrier permeability in cerebral ischemia in rats. J Physiol Pharmacol. 2002;53(1):85–94.
56. Tjuvajev J, et al. Corticotropin-releasing factor decreases vasogenic brain edema. Cancer Res. 1996;56(6):1352–60.
57. Tjuvajev J, et al. Anti-neoplastic properties of human corticotropin releasing factor: involvement of the nitric oxide pathway. In Vivo. 1998;12(1):1–10.
58. Whitney TM, Bentz ML, Johnson PC. Reduction of reperfusion injury edema with corticotropin-releasing factor (CRF): a pilot study. Microsurgery. 1998;18(2):76–8.
59. Esposito P, et al. Corticotropin-releasing factor (CRF) can directly affect brain microvessel endothelial cells. Brain Res. 2003;968(2):192–8.
60. Wu Y, et al. Expression of urocortin in rat lung and its effect on pulmonary vascular permeability. J Endocrinol. 2006;189(1):167–78.
61. Singh LK, et al. Potent mast cell degranulation and vascular permeability triggered by urocortin through activation of corticotropin-releasing hormone receptors. J Pharmacol Exp Ther. 1999;288(3):1349–56.

62. Kim TH, et al. Over-expression of neuropeptide urocortin and its receptors in human allergic nasal mucosa. Laryngoscope. 2007;117(9):1513–8.
63. Wan R, et al. Urocortin increased LPS-induced endothelial permeability by regulating the cadherin-catenin complex via corticotrophin-releasing hormone receptor 2. J Cell Physiol. 2013;228(6):1295–303.
64. Liew HK, et al. Therapeutic effects of human urocortin-1, −2 and −3 in intracerebral hemorrhage of rats. Neuropeptides. 2015;52:89–96.
65. Liew HK, et al. Therapeutic benefit of urocortin in rats with intracerebral hemorrhage. J Neurosurg. 2012;116(1):193–200.
66. Fleisher-Berkovich S, Danon A. Effect of corticotropin-releasing factor on prostaglandin synthesis in endothelial cells and fibroblasts. Endocrinology. 1995;136(9):4068–72.
67. Casadevall M, et al. Mechanisms underlying the anti-inflammatory actions of central corticotropin-releasing factor. Am J Phys. 1999;276(4):G1016–26.
68. Inada Y, et al. Possible involvement of corticotropin-releasing factor receptor signaling on vascular inflammation. Peptides. 2009;30(2):365–72.
69. Borges LE, et al. Expression, localization and control of activin A release from human umbilical vein endothelial cells. Growth Factors. 2015;33(4):243–9.
70. Wilbert-Lampen U, et al. Effects of corticotropin-releasing hormone (CRH) on monocyte function, mediated by CRH-receptor subtype R1 and R2: a potential link between mood disorders and endothelial dysfunction? J Cardiovasc Pharmacol. 2006;47(1):110–6.
71. McEvoy AN, et al. Cyclooxygenase 2-derived prostaglandin E2 production by corticotropin-releasing hormone contributes to the activated cAMP response element binding protein content in rheumatoid arthritis synovial tissue. Arthritis Rheum. 2004;50(4):1132–45.
72. McEvoy AN, et al. Corticotropin-releasing hormone signaling in synovial tissue from patients with early inflammatory arthritis is mediated by the type 1 alpha corticotropin-releasing hormone receptor. Arthritis Rheum. 2001;44(8):1761–7.
73. Zhu C, Li S. The peripheral corticotropin releasing factor family's role in vasculitis. Vasc Pharmacol. 2024;154:107275.
74. Theoharides TC, et al. Mast cells, brain inflammation and autism. Eur J Pharmacol. 2016;778:96–102.
75. Theoharides TC, et al. Mast cells as targets of corticotropin-releasing factor and related peptides. Trends Pharmacol Sci. 2004;25(11):563–8.
76. Theoharides TC, et al. Corticotropin-releasing hormone induces skin mast cell degranulation and increased vascular permeability, a possible explanation for its proinflammatory effects. Endocrinology. 1998;139(1):403–13.
77. Wu Y, et al. Enhanced intracellular calcium induced by urocortin is involved in degranulation of rat lung mast cells. Cell Physiol Biochem. 2008;21(1–3):173–82.
78. Kohno M, et al. Urocortin expression in synovium of patients with rheumatoid arthritis and osteoarthritis: relation to inflammatory activity. J Clin Endocrinol Metab. 2001;86(9):4344–52.
79. Xu Y, et al. Urocortin promotes the development of vasculitis in a rat model of thromboangiitis obliterans via corticotrophin-releasing factor type 1 receptors. Br J Pharmacol. 2009;157(8):1368–79.
80. Zhang R, et al. Urocortin induced expression of COX-2 and ICAM-1 via corticotrophin-releasing factor type 2 receptor in rat aortic endothelial cells. Br J Pharmacol. 2009;158(3):819–29.
81. Wan R, et al. Sex difference in urocortin production is contributory to the gender disparity in a rat model of vasculitis induced by sodium laurate. Endocrinology. 2013;154(12):4663–74.
82. Grossini E, et al. Urocortin II induces nitric oxide production through cAMP and Ca2+ related pathways in endothelial cells. Cell Physiol Biochem. 2009;23(1–3):87–96.
83. Rao KM. Molecular mechanisms regulating iNOS expression in various cell types. J Toxicol Environ Health B Crit Rev. 2000;3(1):27–58.
84. Thiemermann C. The role of the L-arginine: nitric oxide pathway in circulatory shock. Adv Pharmacol. 1994;28:45–79.

85. Cantarella G, et al. Divergent effects of corticotropin releasing hormone on endothelial cell nitric oxide synthase are associated with different expression of CRH type 1 and 2 receptors. Br J Pharmacol. 2001;134(4):837–44.
86. Correa SG, et al. Modulation of the inflammatory response by corticotropin-releasing factor. Eur J Pharmacol. 1997;319(1):85–90.
87. Arbiser JL, et al. Corticotropin-releasing hormone stimulates angiogenesis and epithelial tumor growth in the skin. J Invest Dermatol. 1999;113(5):838–42.
88. Bale TL, et al. Corticotropin-releasing factor receptor 2 is a tonic suppressor of vascularization. Proc Natl Acad Sci USA. 2002;99(11):7734–9.
89. Hao Z, et al. Urocortin2 inhibits tumor growth via effects on vascularization and cell proliferation. Proc Natl Acad Sci USA. 2008;105(10):3939–44.
90. Emeto TI, et al. Urocortin 2 is associated with abdominal aortic aneurysm and mediates anti-proliferative effects on vascular smooth muscle cells via corticotrophin releasing factor receptor 2. Clin Sci (Lond). 2014;126(7):517–27.
91. Yamada T, et al. Role of oxidative stress in vinorelbine-induced vascular endothelial cell injury. Free Radic Biol Med. 2010;48(1):120–7.
92. Gougoura S, Liakos P, Koukoulis GN. Effect of CRH on NO bioavailability, ROS production and antioxidant defense systems in endothelial EAhy926 cells. Free Radic Res. 2010;44(7):803–12.
93. Li X, et al. Urocortin ameliorates diabetic nephropathy in obese db/db mice. Br J Pharmacol. 2008;154(5):1025–34.
94. Gao L, et al. Differential regulation of glucose transporters mediated by CRH receptor type 1 and type 2 in human placental trophoblasts. Endocrinology. 2012;153(3):1464–71.
95. Alvandi Z, Bischoff J. Endothelial-mesenchymal transition in cardiovascular disease. Arterioscler Thromb Vasc Biol. 2021;41(9):2357–69.
96. Jia G, et al. Endothelial cell senescence in aging-related vascular dysfunction. Biochim Biophys Acta Mol basis Dis. 2019;1865(7):1802–9.
97. Yang C, et al. Effects of intravenous urocortin on angiotensin-converting enzyme in rats. Vasc Pharmacol. 2006;44(4):238–46.
98. Berry C, Duncker DJ. Coronary microvascular disease: the next frontier for Cardiovascular research. Cardiovasc Res. 2020;116(4):737–40.
99. Calderon-Sanchez EM, et al. Urocortin role in ischemia cardioprotection and the adverse cardiac remodeling. Int J Mol Sci. 2021;22(22)
100. Chatzaki E, et al. Do urocortins have a role in treating cardiovascular disease? Drug Discov Today. 2019;24(1):279–84.
101. Adao R, et al. Urocortin 2 in cardiovascular health and disease. Drug Discov Today. 2015;20(7):906–14.
102. Chouridou E, et al. Corticotropin-releasing factor (CRF) system localization in human fetal heart. Hormones (Athens). 2016;15(1):55–64.
103. Patel K, et al. Comparative pharmacokinetics and pharmacodynamics of urocortins 1, 2 and 3 in healthy sheep. Br J Pharmacol. 2012;166(6):1916–25.
104. Davidson SM, Yellon DM. Urocortin: a protective peptide that targets both the myocardium and vasculature. Pharmacol Rep. 2009;61(1):172–82.
105. Kimura Y, et al. Expression of urocortin and corticotropin-releasing factor receptor subtypes in the human heart. J Clin Endocrinol Metab. 2002;87(1):340–6.
106. Bale TL, et al. The cardiovascular physiologic actions of urocortin II: acute effects in murine heart failure. Proc Natl Acad Sci USA. 2004;101(10):3697–702.
107. Ikeda K, et al. Regulation of urocortin I and its related peptide urocortin II by inflammatory and oxidative stresses in HL-1 cardiomyocytes. J Mol Endocrinol. 2009;42(6):479–89.
108. Davis ME, et al. Urocortin-1 infusion in normal humans. J Clin Endocrinol Metab. 2004;89(3):1402–9.
109. Davis ME, et al. Effect of urocortin 1 infusion in humans with stable congestive cardiac failure. Clin Sci (Lond). 2005;109(4):381–8.

110. Brar BK, et al. CRH-like peptides protect cardiac myocytes from lethal ischaemic injury. Mol Cell Endocrinol. 1999;158(1–2):55–63.
111. Parkes DG, et al. Cardiac inotropic actions of urocortin in conscious sheep. Am J Phys. 1997;272(5 Pt 2):H2115–22.
112. Okosi A, et al. Expression and protective effects of urocortin in cardiac myocytes. Neuropeptides. 1998;32(2):167–71.
113. Lawrence KM, et al. K(ATP) channel gene expression is induced by urocortin and mediates its cardioprotective effect. Circulation. 2002;106(12):1556–62.
114. Xu H, et al. The cardioprotective peptide, urocortin, activates cardiac KATP channels in adult rat. Protein Pept Lett. 2006;13(1):21–7.
115. Janjua S, et al. The cardioprotective agent urocortin induces expression of CT-1. Cardiovasc Toxicol. 2003;3(3):255–62.
116. Lawrence KM, et al. Cardioprotection mediated by urocortin is dependent on PKCepsilon activation. FASEB J. 2005;19(7):831–3.
117. Takatani-Nakase T, Takahashi K. Cardioprotective activity of urocortin by preventing caspase-independent, non-apoptotic death in cultured neonatal rat cardiomyocytes exposed to ischemia. Biochem Biophys Res Commun. 2010;402(2):216–21.
118. Brar BK, et al. Urocortin protects against ischemic and reperfusion injury via a MAPK-dependent pathway. J Biol Chem. 2000;275(12):8508–14.
119. Schulman D, Latchman DS, Yellon DM. Urocortin protects the heart from reperfusion injury via upregulation of p42/p44 MAPK signaling pathway. Am J Physiol Heart Circ Physiol. 2002;283(4):H1481–8.
120. Cserepes B, et al. Cardioprotective action of urocortin in early pre- and postconditioning. Ann N Y Acad Sci. 2007;1095:228–39.
121. Cong B, et al. SGK1 is involved in cardioprotection of urocortin-1 against hypoxia/reoxygenation in cardiomyocytes. Can J Cardiol. 2014;30(6):687–95.
122. Makarewich CA, et al. Comparative effects of urocortins and stresscopin on cardiac myocyte contractility. J Mol Cell Cardiol. 2015;86:179–86.
123. Yang LZ, Zhu YC. Urocortin2 prolongs action potential duration and modulates potassium currents in Guinea pig myocytes and HEK293 cells. Eur J Pharmacol. 2015;758:97–106.
124. Yang LZ, et al. Urocortin II enhances contractility in rabbit ventricular myocytes via CRF(2) receptor-mediated stimulation of protein kinase A. Cardiovasc Res. 2006;69(2):402–11.
125. Yang LZ, et al. cAMP- and Ca(2)(+) /calmodulin-dependent protein kinases mediate inotropic, lusitropic and arrhythmogenic effects of urocortin 2 in mouse ventricular myocytes. Br J Pharmacol. 2011;162(2):544–56.
126. Chen S, et al. The Modulation of Cardiac Contractile Function by the Pharmacological and Toxicological Effects of Urocortin2. Toxicol Sci. 2015;148(2):581–93.
127. Walther S, et al. Urocortin 2 stimulates nitric oxide production in ventricular myocytes via Akt- and PKA-mediated phosphorylation of eNOS at serine 1177. Am J Physiol Heart Circ Physiol. 2014;307(5):H689–700.
128. Hausenloy DJ, Yellon DM. Survival kinases in ischemic preconditioning and postconditioning. Cardiovasc Res. 2006;70(2):240–53.
129. Townsend PA, et al. Urocortin prevents mitochondrial permeability transition in response to reperfusion injury indirectly by reducing oxidative stress. Am J Physiol Heart Circ Physiol. 2007;293(2):H928–38.
130. Smani T, et al. Urocortin-2 induces vasorelaxation of coronary arteries isolated from patients with heart failure. Clin Exp Pharmacol Physiol. 2011;38(1):71–6.
131. Jonassen AK, et al. Activation of corticotropin releasing factor receptor type 2 in the heart by corticotropin releasing factor offers cytoprotection against ischemic injury via PKA and PKC dependent signaling. Regul Pept. 2012;174(1–3):90–7.
132. Pang X, et al. A neurotensin receptor antagonist inhibits acute immobilization stress-induced cardiac mast cell degranulation, a corticotropin-releasing hormone-dependent process. J Pharmacol Exp Ther. 1998;287(1):307–14.

133. Diaz I, et al. miR-125a, miR-139 and miR-324 contribute to Urocortin protection against myocardial ischemia-reperfusion injury. Sci Rep. 2017;7(1):8898.
134. Brar BK, et al. Activation of protein kinase B/Akt by urocortin is essential for its ability to protect cardiac cells against hypoxia/reoxygenation-induced cell death. J Mol Cell Cardiol. 2002;34(4):483–92.
135. Lawrence KM, et al. The cardioprotective effect of urocortin during ischaemia/reperfusion involves the prevention of mitochondrial damage. Biochem Biophys Res Commun. 2004;321(2):479–86.
136. Corsetti G, et al. Urocortin induces phosphorylation of distinct residues of signal transducer and activator of transcription 3 (STAT3) via different signaling pathways. Med Sci Monit Basic Res. 2019;25:139–52.
137. Yuan Z, et al. Activation of Src protein tyrosine kinase plays an essential role in urocortin-mediated cardioprotection. Mol Cell Endocrinol. 2010;325(1–2):1–7.
138. Williams SD, Gottlieb RA. Inhibition of mitochondrial calcium-independent phospholipase A2 (iPLA2) attenuates mitochondrial phospholipid loss and is cardioprotective. Biochem J. 2002;362(Pt 1):23–32.
139. Lawrence KM, et al. Urocortin protects cardiac myocytes from ischemia/reperfusion injury by attenuating calcium-insensitive phospholipase A2 gene expression. FASEB J. 2003;17(15):2313–5.
140. Calderon-Sanchez EM, et al. Cardioprotective action of urocortin in postconditioning involves recovery of intracellular calcium handling. Cell Calcium. 2011;50(1):84–90.
141. Valentim L, et al. Urocortin inhibits Beclin1-mediated autophagic cell death in cardiac myocytes exposed to ischaemia/reperfusion injury. J Mol Cell Cardiol. 2006;40(6):846–52.
142. Liu CN, et al. In vivo protective effects of urocortin on ischemia-reperfusion injury in rat heart via free radical mechanisms. Can J Physiol Pharmacol. 2005;83(6):459–65.
143. Barry SP, et al. New targets of urocortin-mediated cardioprotection. J Mol Endocrinol. 2010;45(2):69–85.
144. Cong B, et al. Estrogens protect myocardium against ischemia/reperfusion insult by up-regulation of CRH receptor type 2 in female rats. Int J Cardiol. 2013;168(5):4755–60.
145. Cong B, Ni X. Estrogen up-regulates CRHR2 expression via demethylation of CRHR2 gene promoter in cardiomyocytes. Int J Cardiol. 2014;172(2):496–7.
146. Cong B, et al. Estrogen enhancement of SGK1 expression induced by urocortin contributes to its cardioprotection against ischemia/reperfusion insult. Int J Cardiol. 2015;178:200–2.
147. Ellmers LJ, et al. Chronic urocortin 2 administration improves cardiac function and ameliorates cardiac remodeling after experimental myocardial infarction. J Cardiovasc Pharmacol. 2015;65(3):269–75.
148. Li J, et al. Urocortin 2 autocrine/paracrine and pharmacologic effects to activate AMP-activated protein kinase in the heart. Proc Natl Acad Sci USA. 2013;110(40):16133–8.
149. Brar BK, et al. Urocortin-II and urocortin-III are cardioprotective against ischemia reperfusion injury: an essential endogenous cardioprotective role for corticotropin releasing factor receptor type 2 in the murine heart. Endocrinology. 2004;145(1):24–35.
150. Gao XF, et al. Urocortin-2 suppression of p38-MAPK signaling as an additional mechanism for ischemic cardioprotection. Mol Cell Biochem. 2015;398(1–2):135–46.
151. Corder R, Barker DM. Corticotrophin releasing factor attenuates NG-nitro-L-arginine methyl ester induced increases in blood pressure in the anaesthetised rat. J Hum Hypertens. 1999;13(12):875–6.
152. Matejec R, et al. Hemodynamic actions of corticotropin-releasing hormone and proopiomelanocortin derivatives in septic patients. J Cardiovasc Pharmacol. 2011;57(1):94–102.
153. Overton JM, Fisher LA. Differentiated hemodynamic responses to central versus peripheral administration of corticotropin-releasing factor in conscious rats. J Auton Nerv Syst. 1991;35(1):43–51.
154. Richter RM, Mulvany MJ. Comparison of hCRF and oCRF effects on cardiovascular responses after central, peripheral, and in vitro application. Peptides. 1995;16(5):843–9.

155. Porter K, Hayward LF. Stress-induced changes in c-Fos and corticotropin releasing hormone immunoreactivity in the amygdala of the spontaneously hypertensive rat. Behav Brain Res. 2011;216(2):543–51.
156. Goncharuk VD, et al. Paraventricular nucleus of the human hypothalamus in primary hypertension: activation of corticotropin-releasing hormone neurons. J Comp Neurol. 2002;443(4):321–31.
157. Sheng ZF, et al. Corticotropin-releasing hormone neurons in the central nucleus of amygdala are required for chronic stress-induced hypertension. Cardiovasc Res. 2023;119(8):1751–62.
158. Zhang ZH, Felder RB. Hypothalamic corticotrophin-releasing factor and norepinephrine mediate sympathetic and cardiovascular responses to acute intracarotid injection of tumour necrosis factor-alpha in the rat. J Neuroendocrinol. 2008;20(8):978–87.
159. Overton JM, Davis-Gorman G, Fisher LA. Central nervous effects of CRF and angiotensin II on cardiac output in conscious rats. J Appl Physiol. 1985;69(2):788–91.
160. Wang LA, Nguyen DH, Mifflin SW. Corticotropin-releasing hormone projections from the paraventricular nucleus of the hypothalamus to the nucleus of the solitary tract increase blood pressure. J Neurophysiol. 2019;121(2):602–8.
161. Wu JS, et al. Corticotropin releasing factor and substance P mediate the nucleus amygdaloideus centralis-nucleus ventromedialis-nucleus dorsomedialis pressor system. Brain Res. 1999;842(2):392–8.
162. Yamazaki T, et al. Microinjection of urocortin into the rat nucleus tractus solitarii decreases arterial blood pressure. Auton Neurosci. 2008;142(1–2):51–4.
163. Barretto-de-Souza L, et al. Corticotropin-releasing factor neurotransmission in the lateral hypothalamus modulates the tachycardiac response during acute emotional stress in rats. Brain Res Bull. 2021;166:102–9.
164. Chitravanshi VC, Kawabe K, Sapru HN. Mechanisms of cardiovascular actions of urocortins in the hypothalamic arcuate nucleus of the rat. Am J Physiol Heart Circ Physiol. 2013;305(2):H182–91.
165. Abdelrahman AM, et al. Analysis of the mechanism of the vasodepressor effect of urocortin in anesthetized rats. Pharmacology. 2005;73(4):175–9.
166. Mackay KB, et al. Effects of a selective agonist and antagonist of CRF2 receptors on cardiovascular function in the rat. Eur J Pharmacol. 2003;469(1–3):111–5.
167. Gu Y, et al. Urocortin 2 lowers blood pressure and reduces plasma catecholamine levels in mice with hyperadrenergic activity. Endocrinology. 2010;151(10):4820–9.
168. Liu C, et al. The effects of vasoactive peptide urocortin 2 on hemodynamics in spontaneous hypertensive rat and the role of L-type calcium channel and CRFR2. Pharmacol Rep. 2015;67(2):394–8.
169. Adao R, et al. Urocortin-2 improves right ventricular function and attenuates pulmonary arterial hypertension. Cardiovasc Res. 2018;114(8):1165–77.
170. Li X, et al. Excitatory responses of cardiovascular activities to urocortin3 administration into the PVN of the rat. Auton Neurosci. 2010;154(1–2):108–11.
171. Oliveira LA, et al. Both CRF(1) and CRF(2) receptors in the bed nucleus of stria terminalis are involved in baroreflex impairment evoked by chronic stress in rats. Prog Neuro-Psychopharmacol Biol Psychiatry. 2021;105:110009.
172. Uetsuki N, et al. The role of CRF1 receptors for sympathetic nervous response to laparotomy in anesthetized rats. Brain Res. 2005;1044(1):107–15.
173. Reis-Silva LL, et al. CRF(1) and CRF(2) receptors in the lateral hypothalamus differently modulate the baroreflex function in unanesthetized rats. Brain Res. 2021;1751:147195.
174. Kang YM, et al. Paraventricular nucleus corticotrophin releasing hormone contributes to sympathoexcitation via interaction with neurotransmitters in heart failure. Basic Res Cardiol. 2011;106(3):473–83.
175. Grunt M, et al. Dilatory and inotropic effects of corticotropin-releasing factor (CRF) on the isolated heart. Effects on atrial natriuretic peptide (ANP) release. Horm Metab Res. 1992;24(2):56–9.

176. Haug C, et al. Effect of corticotropin releasing factor on atrial natriuretic peptide release from the isolated perfused rat heart. Arzneimittelforschung. 1994;44(5):579–82.
177. Ng LL, et al. Plasma urocortin in human systolic heart failure. Clin Sci (Lond). 2004;106(4):383–8.
178. Yildirim E, et al. Evaluation of the clinical utility of urocortin 1 in systolic heart failure. Kardiol Pol. 2014;72(5):452–8.
179. Rademaker MT, Charles CJ, Richards AM. Urocortin 1 administration from onset of rapid left ventricular pacing represses progression to overt heart failure. Am J Physiol Heart Circ Physiol. 2007;293(3):H1536–44.
180. Rademaker MT, et al. Four-day urocortin-I administration has sustained beneficial haemodynamic, hormonal, and renal effects in experimental heart failure. Eur Heart J. 2005;26(19):2055–62.
181. Topal E, et al. Relationship of urocortin-2 with systolic and diastolic functions and coronary artery disease: an observational study. Anadolu Kardiyol Derg. 2012;12(2):115–20.
182. Rademaker MT, et al. Integrated hemodynamic, hormonal, and renal actions of urocortin 2 in normal and paced sheep: beneficial effects in heart failure. Circulation. 2005;112(23):3624–32.
183. Rademaker MT, et al. Urocortin 2 protects heart and kidney structure and function in an ovine model of acute decompensated heart failure: comparison with dobutamine. Int J Cardiol. 2015;197:56–65.
184. Davis ME, et al. Urocortin 2 infusion in human heart failure. Eur Heart J. 2007;28(21):2589–97.
185. Lai NC, et al. Urocortin 2 gene transfer for systolic and diastolic dysfunction due to chronically increased left ventricular pressure. Hum Gene Ther. 2022;33(19–20):1091–100.
186. Giamouridis D, et al. Urocortin 2 gene transfer improves heart function in aged mice. Mol Ther. 2020;28(1):180–8.
187. Lai NC, et al. Intravenous AAV8 encoding urocortin-2 increases function of the failing heart in mice. Hum Gene Ther. 2015;26(6):347–56.
188. Kim YC, et al. Urocortin 2 gene transfer reduces the adverse effects of a western diet on cardiac function in mice. Hum Gene Ther. 2019;30(6):693–701.
189. Rademaker MT, et al. Interactions of enhanced urocortin 2 and mineralocorticoid receptor antagonism in experimental heart failure. Circ Heart Fail. 2013;6(4):825–32.
190. Rademaker MT, et al. Urocortin 2 inhibits furosemide-induced activation of renin and enhances renal function and diuretic responsiveness in experimental heart failure. Circ Heart Fail. 2009;2(6):532–40.
191. Giamouridis D, et al. Urocortin 3 gene transfer increases function of the failing murine heart. Hum Gene Ther. 2019;30(1):10–20.
192. Stirrat CG, et al. Cardiovascular effects of urocortin 2 and urocortin 3 in patients with chronic heart failure. Br J Clin Pharmacol. 2016;82(4):974–82.
193. Stiedl O, et al. Stress-mediated heart rate dynamics after deletion of the gene encoding corticotropin-releasing factor receptor 2. Eur J Neurosci. 2003;17(10):2231–5.
194. Stiedl O, et al. Corticotropin-releasing factor receptor 1 and central heart rate regulation in mice during expression of conditioned fear. J Pharmacol Exp Ther. 2005;312(3):905–16.
195. Wood SK, et al. Facilitation of cardiac vagal activity by CRF-R1 antagonists during swim stress in rats. Neuropsychopharmacology. 2006;31(12):2580–90.
196. Gao HR, et al. Corticotropin releasing factor excites neurons of posterior hypothalamic nucleus to produce tachycardia in rats. Sci Rep. 2016;6:20206.
197. Grosskreutz CL, Brody MJ. Regional hemodynamic responses to central administration of corticotropin-releasing factor (CRF). Brain Res. 1988;442(2):363–7.
198. Gardiner SM, et al. A comparison between the cardiovascular actions of urocortin 1 and urocortin 2 (stresscopin-related peptide) in conscious rats. J Pharmacol Exp Ther. 2007;321(1):221–6.
199. Brufatto JPT, et al. Ventromedial prefrontal cortex CRF1 receptors modulate the tachycardic activity of baroreflex. Pflugers Arch. 2021;473(4):697–709.

200. Barretto-de-Souza L, et al. Role of CRF(1) and CRF(2) receptors in the lateral hypothalamus in cardiovascular and anxiogenic responses evoked by restraint stress in rats: evaluation of acute and chronic exposure. Neuropharmacology. 2022;212:109061.
201. Scarabelli TM, et al. Warm blood cardioplegic arrest induces mitochondrial-mediated cardiomyocyte apoptosis associated with increased urocortin expression in viable cells. J Thorac Cardiovasc Surg. 2004;128(3):364–71.
202. Chen-Scarabelli C, et al. Warm-blood cardioplegic arrest induces selective mitochondrial translocation of protein kinase Cepsilon followed by interaction with 6.1 inwardly rectifying potassium channel subunit in viable myocytes overexpressing urocortin. J Thorac Cardiovasc Surg. 2009;138(5):1213–21.
203. Huang CH, et al. Urocortin treatment improves acute hemodynamic instability and reduces myocardial damage in post-cardiac arrest myocardial dysfunction. PLoS One. 2016;11(11):e0166324.
204. Petrakova L, et al. Salivary alpha-amylase and noradrenaline responses to corticotropin-releasing hormone administration in humans. Biol Psychol. 2017;127:34–9.
205. Ma HY, et al. Endogenous corticotropin-releasing factor potentiates the excitability of presympathetic neurons in paraventricular nucleus via activation of its receptor 1 in spontaneously hypertensive rats. Sheng Li Xue Bao. 2023;75(4):487–96.
206. Yamaguchi N, Okada S. Cyclooxygenase-1 and -2 in spinally projecting neurons are involved in CRF-induced sympathetic activation. Auton Neurosci. 2009;151(2):82–9.
207. Martinez-Laorden E, et al. Corticotropin-releasing factor (CRF) receptor-1 is involved in cardiac noradrenergic activity observed during naloxone-precipitated morphine withdrawal. Br J Pharmacol. 2014;171(3):688–700.
208. Garcia-Carmona JA, et al. Sympathetic activity induced by naloxone-precipitated morphine withdrawal is blocked in genetically engineered mice lacking functional CRF1 receptor. Toxicol Appl Pharmacol. 2015;283(1):42–9.
209. Zhu L, et al. Electroacupuncture intervention on stress-induced cardiac autonomic imbalance in rats involves corticotropin-releasing hormone system activity. Neuroreport. 2023;34(7):401–10.
210. Ikeda K, et al. Urocortin has cell-proliferative effects on cardiac non-myocytes. Life Sci. 2002;71(16):1929–38.
211. Railson JE, et al. Cardiotrophin-1 and urocortin cause protection by the same pathway and hypertrophy via distinct pathways in cardiac myocytes. Cytokine. 2002;17(5):243–53.
212. Gruson D, et al. Urotensin II and urocortin trigger the expression of myostatin, a negative regulator of cardiac growth, in cardiomyocytes. Peptides. 2012;33(2):351–3.
213. Gruson D, et al. Urocortin-induced cardiomyocytes hypertrophy is associated with regulation of the GSK-3beta pathway. Heart Vessel. 2012;27(2):202–7.
214. Davis ME, et al. Urocortin 2 infusion in healthy humans: hemodynamic, neurohormonal, and renal responses. J Am Coll Cardiol. 2007;49(4):461–71.
215. Aslan G, Aytekin S. Evaluation of serum urocortin 2 levels in patients with hypertension. High Blood Press Cardiovasc Prev. 2020;27(1):35–42.
216. Tsuda T, et al. Corticotropin releasing hormone receptor 2 exacerbates chronic cardiac dysfunction. J Exp Med. 2017;214(7):1877–88.
217. Mori Y, et al. Corticotropin releasing hormone receptor 2 antagonist, RQ-00490721, for the prevention of pressure overload-induced cardiac dysfunction. Biomed Pharmacother. 2022;146:112566.
218. Walther S, et al. NFAT transcription factor regulation by urocortin II in cardiac myocytes and heart failure. Am J Physiol Heart Circ Physiol. 2014;306(6):H856–66.

Chapter 6
CRF Peptides in the Immune/Inflammatory System

Rong Wan and Chao Zhu

It is well known that stress can elicit hypothalamic-pituitary-adrenal axis (HPA) axis activation and promote the following cortisol release, which finally contributes to oxidative, inflammatory, physiological, and mental stress [1]. As described precedingly, under the stimulation of stress, corticotropin-releasing hormone (CRH) can be released from the paraventricular nucleus (PVN) of the hypothalamus (Chap. 1). Over the past few decades, CRH and other corticotropin-releasing hormone (factor) family peptides (CRF peptides, CRFp) have been shown to play important roles both centrally and peripherally, balancing the interplay of hormonal, behavioral, and immune systems in response to stress [2]. Up to this point, our comprehension of the intricate interactions between CRFp and immune-mediated inflammatory responses has undergone remarkable advancement.

On one hand, the response of the pituitary-adrenal axis to localized inflammation is predominantly orchestrated through mechanisms that are intricately dependent on CRH [3]. CRH is primarily synthesized within the PVN of the hypothalamus and subsequently transported into the portal capillaries that converge upon the anterior lobe of the pituitary gland [4]. Subsequently, CRH binds to its own specific CRF receptors (CRFr) and contributes to the HPA-derived hormone glucocorticoid (GC) synthesis and secretion from the adrenal gland as demonstrated previously [5]. GCs are widely recognized for their profound anti-inflammatory properties and potent immunosuppressive effects [6, 7]. As reported, GCs possess the remarkable ability to attenuate the production of pro-inflammatory cytokines and mitigate cellular inflammatory infiltrates through the downregulation of adhesion molecules [8–10].

R. Wan (✉)
Jiangxi Key Laboratory of Molecular Medicine, The Second Affiliated Hospital of Nanchang University, Nanchang, China

C. Zhu
Department of Pharmacology, School of Basic Medical Sciences, Nanjing Medical University, Nanjing, Jiangsu, China

© The Author(s), under exclusive license to Springer Nature Singapore Pte Ltd. 2025
C. Zhu et al. (eds.), *The Peripheral Existence and Effects of Corticotropin-releasing Factor Family*, https://doi.org/10.1007/978-981-96-5322-5_6

In brief, due to the contribution of GCs, CRH-adrenocorticotropin (ACTH)-cortisol axis, the principal components of the HPA axis, is critical for inflammatory suppression processes [11].

However, recently, different opinions have been raised about the role of central CRFp in inflammation. Firstly, the HPA axis has been shown to exert both anti-inflammatory and pro-inflammatory influences on the immune response [12]. Meanwhile, more and more different ideas have emerged about the role of GCs in inflammation. Further examination of the GC's impact on the kainate-induced inflammatory response reveals that persistently elevated levels of corticosterone significantly enhance the expression of interleukin (IL)-1β [13] and promote an increased accumulation of the pro-inflammatory cytokine monocyte/macrophage chemotactic protein-1 (MCP-1) [14] in the hippocampus. Evidence which support the pro-inflammatory activity of CRH have confirmed that chronic stress can induce CRH release and further engage the microglial 1 phenotype through its receptor interactions on microglia, thereby catalyzing a cascade of inflammatory responses [15]. All the data suggest that central CRFp promote the processes of inflammation, and what's more, it is nonspecific.

On the other hand, numerous studies have elucidated that the CRH gene is extensively expressed in extracranial tissues; however, its expression levels are significantly lower than those observed in the hypothalamus (Fig. 6.1). CRFp are

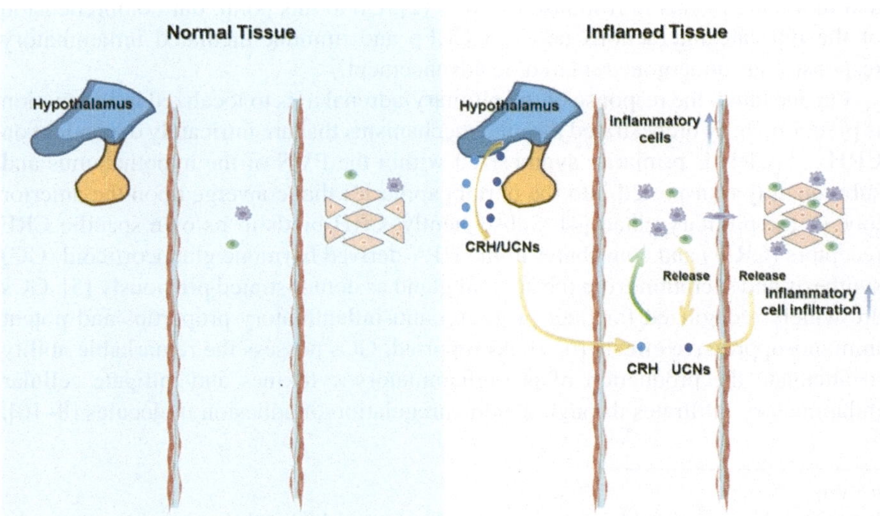

Fig. 6.1 Role of CRFp in inflammation

demonstrated to be produced in peripheral inflammatory sites [16–18]. Moreover, emerging lines of evidence indicate that immune-derived UCNs, encompassing UCN1, UCN2, and UCN3, exert localized and direct modulation over pro-inflammatory responses to perceived environmental adversities. The nature of this influence is contingent upon the specific tissue type or CRFr subtype involved [18]. Indeed, it has been documented that CRH plays a significant role in the subcutaneous inflammation triggered by carrageenan [16]. In peripheral tissue, CRFp can be stimulated by the cytokines IL-1 and IL-6 and tumor necrosis factor (TNF)-α [19]. In addition, prostaglandins, epidermal growth factor, and platelet growth factor can also enhance the production of CRH [20–22]. Immunoreactive CRH is synthesized in peripheral sites of inflammation, where it functions as an autocrine or paracrine inflammatory cytokine. Immunoreactive CRH is produced in peripheral inflammatory sites, where it acts as an autocrine or paracrine inflammatory cytokine [23]. Consistently, CRFp possesses the remarkable ability to either suppress or enhance local immune responses, contingent upon its specific cellular targets [23,24]. On the contrary, CRH may exert a contrasting immunoactivity effect in the periphery by inciting pro-inflammatory responses [16]. Jing Cao and colleagues advocate the notion that CRH possesses the capacity to either instigate or amplify inflammatory processes [25] by promoting vascular endothelial growth factor (VEGF) releasing [26].

The previous section has introduced the effects and functions of UCNs as a member of the CRFp. Without a doubt, UCNs can act as inflammatory regulators. Tsatsanis et al. have elucidated that UCN1 and UCN2 orchestrate anti-inflammatory effects by stimulating the synthesis of IL-6, thereby exerting their immunomodulatory influence in vitro [27]. Similar to CRH, in the gastric and colonic mucosa of humans, UCNs play a pivotal role in modulating inflammatory responses, exhibiting both anti-inflammatory and pro-inflammatory effects [28,29]. Additional evidence indicates that UCNs may serve as powerful pro-inflammatory neuropeptides through the activation of nuclear factor-κ-gene binding (NF-κB) and mitogen-activated protein kinase (MAPK) signaling pathways [30].

It should be noted that the interaction between CRFp and immune cells has been emerged and clear. CRH is found to be produced by immune cells, including mast cells (MCs) and macrophages [2, 31, 32]. Additionally, the distribution of CRFr (CRF_1 and CRF_2) in immune cells has attracted researchers' attention. A sophisticated single-cell RNA sequencing assay has been meticulously conducted on adult zebrafish kidney samples, which are readily accessible to the public at the following link: https://molpath.shinyapps.io/zebrafishblood/#pltly [33]. As reported, CRF_1 is also prominently expressed in neutrophils, macrophages, and T cells, while CRF_2 exhibits its highest expression levels within myeloid cells/macrophages, with lesser quantities found in various other cell types. CRF_1 expression is upregulated by lipopolysaccharide (LPS) stimulation (Table 6.1) [34].

Table 6.1 The distribution of CRH, UCNs, and CRFr in immune cells

	CRH	UCN1	UCN2	UCN3	CRF_1	CRF_2
Mast cells	√ [35]	√ [35]	Unavailable	√ [36]	Unavailable	√ [35]
Monocytes	√ [37]	√ [37]	√ [37]	Unavailable	Unavailable	√ [35]
Macrophages	√ [35]	Unavailable	Unavailable	Unavailable	Unavailable	√ [35]
Neutrophils	√ [35]	Unavailable	Unavailable	Unavailable	Unavailable	√ [35]
B cells	√ [32]	Unavailable	Unavailable	Unavailable	Unavailable	√ [38]
T cell	√ [32]	√ [39]	Unavailable	Unavailable	Unavailable	Unavailable
NK cell	Unavailable	Unavailable	Unavailable	Unavailable	Unavailable	Unavailable

1 Relationships between CRFp and Immune Cells

1.1 CRFp and Monocytes

Peripherally circulating CRH plays an important role in influencing specific homeostatic properties of monocytes [40]. CRH induces the production of IL-1β and IL-6 by peripheral blood mononuclear cells [4, 23, 41]. Additionally, CRH stimulates in vitro migration of human monocytes [4]. Moreover, in the absence of LPS, CRH enhances the expression of IL-1 receptor alpha (IL-1Rα) and IL-1β messenger RNA and promotes protein synthesis in human peripheral monocytes. Moreover, the addition of UCN1 to cultures of human peripheral blood mononuclear cells, similar to CRH, results in an increased production of IL-1β and IL-6 [41, 42].

In contrast, anti-inflammatory activities are demonstrated of CRH in monocytes. In conjunction with high concentrations of LPS (1 mg/ml), CRH induces the suppression of IL-1Rα and IL-1β transcription and secretion. The varying effects of CRH on the modulation of the IL-1 system may be contingent upon the activation state of monocytes. Specifically, CRH exerts an inhibitory influence on activated cells while simultaneously promoting a stimulatory effect on resting monocytes [18]. The effects of CRH on human monocytes are indicated to be mediated by the activation of phosphatidylinositol 3-kinase (PI3K)/protein kinase B (PKB/AKT) [43]. Furthermore, CRH attenuates the production of cytokines induced by endotoxins in human mononuclear cells (MNCs) [24].

1.2 CRFp and Macrophages

The reported inflammatory-mediated effect of CRF appears to involve macrophages and is limited to the early stages of inflammation [44]. Emerging evidence have confirmed the involvement of macrophages in CRH-mediated inflammation process. Bhargava group has discovered that endogenous UCN1 synergistically enhances LPS-induced vascular permeability, a process that is accompanied by an increase in macrophage presence [45]. In contrast, the anti-inflammatory activities of CRH on macrophages exist. For instance, CRH mitigates the influx of macrophages induced by doxorubicin, thereby manifesting a pronounced anti-inflammatory effect [46]. Investigations from Park et al.'s group reveal that CRH diminishes the cholesterol efflux in macrophages and fosters the formation of foam cells within murine peritoneal macrophages as well as human monocyte-derived macrophages via CRF_1-AKT signaling [47]. Most intriguingly, CRFp assumes a pivotal role in modulating macrophage functionality through the engagement of CRF_2, as evidenced by the upregulation of TLR4 and the inhibitory influence exerted by LPS on toll-like receptor 4 (TLR4) expression [48].

However, not CRH, but UCN1, emerges as a detectable entity within rat Kupffer cells (KC)—the resident macrophages of the liver. This peptide plays a pivotal role in modulating local inflammatory phenomena within hepatic tissue, exerting its effects through a paracrine mechanism [49]. Moreover, UCN1 has been elucidated to play a pivotal role in the modulation of macrophage apoptosis induced by LPS through the action of cytoplasmic phospholipase A2 ($cPLA_2$) [50]. In vitro studies conducted by Tsatsanis et al. have elucidated that both UCN1 and UCN2 orchestrate anti-inflammatory responses through the induction of macrophage apoptosis, a process mediated by the activation of CRF_2 receptors [27]. In alternative investigations, UCN2 significantly enhances the secretion of IL-10 while concurrently diminishing the release of TNF-α from murine RAW264.7 macrophages that have been infected with *Listeria* [4, 51].

1.3 CRFp and MCs

MCs are versatile immune cells, widely acknowledged as the vigilant sentinels of the human body. They play a pivotal role in defending against external threats and orchestrating responses to various stressors, including allergic reactions [52]. A principal immunological target of CRH is the MCs [4, 53]. Both CRF_1 and CRF_2 abundantly exist on the surface of MCs, which have tight relationship with MCs [54]. In response to the crosslinking of immunoglobulin E receptors (FcεRI), MCs possess the remarkable ability to both synthesize and secrete CRH as well as UCN1 [55]. Consistently, decreased CRF_1 expression on the surface of MCs is found to be associated with inhibited MC degranulation [54]. Similarly, when macrophage cells are activated by inflammatory stimuli, the expression of CRF_2 is significantly upregulated [56]. The impairment of CRF_2 functionality has been demonstrated to exacerbate MC degranulation, thereby facilitating IgE-mediated anaphylaxis and precipitating dysfunction of the intestinal barrier induced by psychological stress [57, 58].

Furthermore, both the human leukemic mast cell line (HMC-1) and MCs derived from human umbilical cord blood exhibit a notable expression of CRH [26]. Interestingly, research has unveiled that MCs possess the remarkable ability to synthesize and secrete substantial quantities of CRH, thereby playing a pivotal role in the progression of inflammation through an autocrine mechanism [54, 59]. Likewise,

CRH may activate MCs [60] and promote MC maturation [61], which subsequently leads to the release of histamine and various inflammatory mediators, including IL-6 and TNF-α, and culminates in heightened vascular permeability and pronounced vasodilation [62]. As well as CRH, human MCs are demonstrated to synthesize and secrete UCN1 in response to FcεRI crosslinking [63], which can stimulate MCs and incite MC-mediated vascular permeability [55, 64].

Besides immune cells, other cells are also found to express CRFp during inflammation. As evidenced, adipose tissue exerts profound systemic effects primarily implicated in the regulation of energy and immune homeostasis through a diverse array of protein signals and factors [65]. A comprehensive CRF system is also prominently expressed in adipose tissues and may play an instrumental role in the onset of chronic low-grade inflammation, a hallmark characteristic of obesity [35]. In a similar vein, the activation of CRF_2 induced by UCN2 within aortic smooth muscle cells culminates in an augmented production of IL-6 [66]. In addition, elevated expression levels of CRH, UCN1, and their respective receptors, CRF_1 and CRF_2, have been observed in the spleen and thymus of rats subjected to an immunological challenge [34, 67].

In conclusion, inflammation may arise as a consequence of the activation of CRH and the immune system, wherein cytokines such as IL-1 and IL-6 engender a positive feedback loop that enhances CRH stimulation. This process is further compounded by the secretion of CRH beyond the confines of the central nervous system (CNS) (Fig. 6.2). Detailed effects of CRFp on inflammation will be discussed as follows.

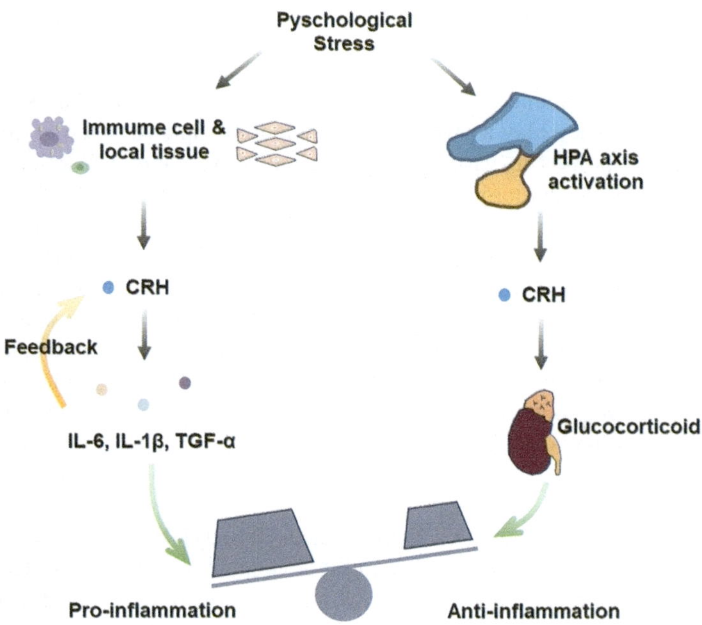

Fig. 6.2 Roles of CRH in inflammation

2 Roles of CRFp in Neuroinflammation

2.1 CRH and Neuroinflammation

In CNS, the physiological response to stress is intricately rooted in the activation of the HPA axis, and further released CRH acts on immune reaction [68]. Acute stress precipitates an increase in blood–brain barrier (BBB) permeability, a phenomenon intricately linked to the signaling pathways of CRH [69]. Reportedly, pro-inflammatory cytokines, including TNF-α, IL-1β, and IL-6, orchestrate the activation of the HPA axis through both CRH-dependent and CRH-independent mechanisms. This intricate interplay culminates in an augmented secretion of ACTH from the pituitary gland and a subsequent release of glucocorticoids from the adrenal cortex [70]. Many studies have explored the involvement of CRFp in linking pathways between the immune system and chronic stress.

Chronic stress-induced release of CRH has the capacity to activate microglial cells, specifically promoting the M1 phenotype through its interaction with receptors located on these immune cells. This activation subsequently fosters a cascade of inflammatory responses [71]. Meanwhile, CRH induces the cell proliferation and release of TNF-α from rat microglia cells [72] and induces neurogenic inflammation [61]. Accordingly, CRH has the potential to markedly enhance the levels of TNF-α and phospho-NF-κB within the ischemic penumbra. Furthermore, CRH conspicuously elevates the population of CD16/Iba-1-positive cells while simultaneously diminishing the count of CD206/Iba-1-positive cells in this region, thereby providing compelling evidence for the pro-inflammatory role of CRH in an ischemic stroke model [73].

2.2 UCN1 and Neuroinflammation

The role of UCN1 in the context of stress has been elucidated through studies conducted on mouse models [74, 75], rat [76–79] and nonhuman primate [80] depression models. Exogenous administration of UCN1 exerts palliative effects in experimental models of autoimmune encephalomyelitis [81]. Systemic treatment with UCN1 following intracerebral hemorrhage (ICH) significantly mitigates striatal injury and neurological deficits, likely through the suppression of microglial activation and the production of inflammatory cytokines [82]. Human UCN1 significantly disrupts BBB after ICH insult [83]. In vitro studies have demonstrated that UCN1 exhibits anti-inflammatory properties, which contribute to the reduction of neurotoxicity induced by endotoxin-activated microglia [84].

2.3 UCN2 and Neuroinflammation

UCN2 is located in the motor neurons of the brainstem, including the supraoptic nucleus and paraventricular nucleus of the hypothalamus, as well as in the arcuate nucleus and locus coeruleus within both the brainstem and spinal cord [85]. Intraperitoneal administration of LPS leads to a significant upregulation of c-fos and UCN2 gene expression in the PVN. UCN2 may play a crucial role in the regulation of the HPA axis in response to immune challenges [86].

2.4 UCN3 and Neuroinflammation

UCN3 is predominantly found in the amygdala, brainstem, and hypothalamus [87]. Effects of UCN3 on neuroinflammation is largely unknown.

2.5 CRFr and Neuroinflammation

In the CNS, CRH plays a crucial role in regulating the stress response, primarily through its interaction with CRF_1 receptors [88, 89]. During neuroinflammation, CRF_1 is implicated in the production of inflammatory factors and plays a crucial role in the transformation of activated BV2 cells from a neuroprotective phenotype (M2) to a cytotoxic phenotype (M1) [73]. Consistent with previous data, CRF_1 activation plays a significant role in modulating brain plasticity, as well as in neuronal inflammation and injury. Additionally, it is involved in the recovery of function following ischemic brain insults [90]. Eric et al. have demonstrated that CRF_1 plays a crucial role in mediating the antigen-specific antibody response and functions as an immunomodulator, facilitating neuro-immune interactions [91]. CRF_1 in brain regions containing opioid peptides plays a crucial role in the modulation of inflammatory pain [92]. However, raising work demonstrates the contribution of CRF_2 to neuroinflammation. Deng et al. demonstrate that the absence of CRF_2 results in dysregulation of the HPA axis and activates neuroinflammation by disrupting the polarization balance between microglia and astrocytes [93]. Interestingly, the translocator protein (TSPO) and the activation of microglial M1 phenotype (CD11b), both of which are neuroinflammatory markers, have been found to be significantly elevated in *Crfr2*$^{-/-}$ zebrafish [93, 94].

3 Roles of CRFp in Intestinal Inflammation

Intestinal inflammation is one of the most common inflammatory diseases that CRFp are involved in. A growing body of research has shown that CRFp and their receptors play a significant role in the regulation of inflammation within the gastrointestinal tract, both in humans and rodents [28, 95–97]. In addition, there is a growing body of experimental and clinical evidence suggesting that the induction and progression of inflammatory and functional intestinal disorders may be influenced by CRH signaling pathways [98]. Intestinal inflammatory diseases have become the most common inflammation disease which CRFp are involved in.

3.1 CRH and Intestinal Inflammation

Several studies have demonstrated that stress can influence various intestinal functions, including gut motor and mucosal activity, visceral hypersensitivity, as well as the integrity of the epithelial barrier and local immune responses. These effects appear to be mediated through pathways involving peripheral CRH signaling [99]. Peripheral CRH may represent a promising pharmacologic target for the prevention and treatment of necrotizing enterocolitis [100]. For instance, in the digestive tract, CRH has the ability to directly influence the inflammatory and immune responses in the intestine [101, 102]. Moreover, in a rat model of functional dyspepsia, it appears that CRH may play a role in contributing to low-grade inflammation. This could be achieved through the modulation of MC infiltration, cytokine levels, MAPK signaling, and the gut–brain axis [103]. In an experimental model of toxin-induced intestinal inflammation, the inhibition of CRH appears to significantly reduce the inflammatory response. This is evidenced by a decrease in epithelial damage and neutrophil infiltration [104]. Research conducted in both animal models and human subjects suggest that CRH increases intestinal permeability via MC activation [11, 105]. These modifications have been documented as playing a significant role in the onset and pathophysiology of chronic intestinal disorders, including inflammatory bowel disease (IBD) [106–108]. Following attentions will be mainly focused on the participation of CRH in IBD and IBS.

First, the participation of CRH in IBD is discussed. Elevated concentrations of CRH, observed at both the protein and mRNA levels, have been demonstrated in the epithelial cells of the colonic mucosa derived from patients with IBD. Vanuytsel et al. report that the administration of peripheral CRH replicates the effects of psychosocial stress and initiates both the onset and progression of IBD [105]. Macrophages play a crucial role in the exacerbation of IBD mediated by CRH [109]. In LPS-stimulated bone marrow-derived macrophage, CRH significantly enhances M1/M2 polarization, thereby promoting inflammation. In mice with dextran sulfate sodium (DSS)-induced IBD and in LPS-stimulated bone marrow-derived macrophages, the administration of CRH enhances intestinal autophagy. This effect is mediated through the modulation of gut microbiota and inflammation, ultimately exacerbating IBD [110].

Second, IBD, encompassing ulcerative colitis (UC), is intricately linked to a discernible inflammatory response that precipitates damage to the intestinal tissue [111]. CRH is prominently expressed within the intestinal milieu and exhibits a marked upregulation in individuals afflicted with UC [112]. Systemic deficiency of

CRH has been shown to elicit localized inflammatory responses within colonic tissues, as evidenced by an experimental model of colitis in mice [112]. In a murine model of acute experimental colitis induced by trinitrobenzene sulfonic acid, our research team elucidates that, despite the presence of diminished glucocorticoid levels, CRF_1-deficient mice exhibit markedly attenuated local inflammatory responses [112].

3.2 UCN1 and Intestinal Inflammation

Elevated levels of UCN1, in contrast to CRH expression, have been observed to correlate with the presence of active gastritis. Furthermore, patients who exhibit a favorable response to treatment for this condition demonstrate even more pronounced elevations in UCN1 expression. In addition, and in stark contrast to the findings regarding CRH in UC, a remarkably significant yet negative correlation has been observed between UCN1 levels and gastric inflammation. This intriguing relationship suggests that UCN1 may play a pivotal role in exerting an anti-inflammatory effect within the gastric mucosa [28]. Finally, UCN1 modulates immune signaling in a rat model of colitis [113].

UCN1-positive cells have been found to correlate with the severity of inflammation in the colonic mucosa of patients with UC, and treatment with GCs has been shown to reduce the presence of these cells. The mRNA of UCN1 is expressed in plasma cells located within the lamina propria, and both CRF1 and CRF2 mRNAs are also partially co-expressed in these cells as well as in macrophages [97].

3.3 UCN2 and Intestinal Inflammation

Treatment of HT-29 cells with UCN2, which selectively binds to CRF_2, promotes the expression of IL-8 and MCP-1. In a rat model of chemical colitis induced by trinitrobenzene sulfonic acid (TNBS), which is commonly accepted as a model for Crohn's disease, UCN2 levels are observed to be increased, while the expression levels of its only identified receptor, CRF_2, appear to be decreased. These findings suggest that UCN2 may exert its effects partially through CRF_2 in a rat model of chemically induced colitis [114]. CRF_2 and UCN2 are expressed in MCs located within the gastric mucosa [36]. The central administration of UCN2 can significantly exacerbate the infiltration of CD68- and CC chemokine receptor 2 (CCR2)-positive cells in the intestinal mucosa of rats treated with LPS. In vitro treatment with UCN2 significantly decreases the production of TNF-α and IL-6 in LPS-stimulated NR8383 cells [51]. Chatzaki et al. have reported that treatment with UCN2 exacerbates *Listeria monocytogenes* infection in mice through the upregulation of IL-10 [28]. The protective effects of UCN2, which include anti-inflammatory and anti-necrotic properties, involve the activation of CRF_2, $[Ca2+]_i$ signaling pathways, and the inhibition of NF-κB activity in a caerulein-induced acute pancreatitis

(AP) model in rats [115]. Additionally, UCN2 dose-dependently inhibits prostaglandin E2 (PGE2) and prostaglandin F2α (PGF2α) secretion induced by inflammatory stimuli [116].

3.4 *UCN3 and Intestinal Inflammation*

UCN3 appears to play various physiological or pathological roles in modulating gastrointestinal functions under stressful conditions, and it does so in ways that differ from UCN1 [96]. Treatment with UCN1 and UCN3 encourages the secretion of PGE2 and PGF2α in a manner that is dependent on the dosage [116].

3.5 *CRFr and Intestinal Inflammation*

CRF_1 antagonists have shown promising effectiveness in alleviating IBD by blocking colonic hypersensitivity that arises from inflammatory reactions in the colon. This offers a novel therapeutic option for treating stress-aggravated IBD, which we believe could be beneficial for many patients [117–119]. Predominantly, the expression of CRF_1 is upregulated in the colonic mucosa in patients with UC [99]. Activation of CRF_1 appears to enhance the disease activity index (DAI) and histological scores in colons affected by dextran sodium sulfate-induced colitis. This effect seems to be linked to the promotion of M1 macrophage polarization, as evidenced by increased NF-κB activation along with elevated levels of TNF-α and IL-6 release [118].

Likewise, it is noteworthy that CRF_2 mRNA is expressed in human colonic epithelial HT-29 cells. CRF_2-deficient mice have been observed to exhibit a decrease in intestinal inflammatory responses as well as a reduction in MCP-1 production [120]. Collectively, these findings offer compelling evidence that CRF_2 plays a significant role in mediating intestinal inflammatory responses through the release of pro-inflammatory mediators at the level of colonocytes [102]. In contrast, CRF_2 activation initiates an anti-inflammatory response in the intestinal mucosa by modulating the migration, proliferation, and apoptosis of intestinal epithelial cells in mice with colitis [121].

4 Roles of CRFp in Vascular Inflammation

CRFp/CRFr have been universally recognized to influence vascular immunity. The pro-vasculitis effects of CRFp encompass several mechanisms, including the enhancement of vascular endothelial permeability, disruption of endothelial adherens or tight junctions resulting in hyperpermeability, stimulation of immune and inflammatory cells to release various inflammatory factors, and promotion of angiogenesis through the release of VEGF [122].

Despite of the pro-inflammatory activities in the development of vasculitis, CRH has been found to counteract vascular inflammation. For instance, CRF_1 signaling has been shown to play a protective role against vascular inflammatory stress in human aortic endothelial cells (HAECs) [123].

4.1 CRH and Vascular Inflammation

CRH has been shown to play a role in vascular inflammation and permeability. Data from our laboratory have indicated that the blockade of CRF_1 may effectively inhibit H_2O_2-induced hyperpermeability in brain endothelial cells. This effect appears to be mediated through the inhibition of $cPLA_2$ phosphorylation [124, 125]. Moreover, CRH peptides play a significant role in vasculitis by influencing inflammatory cells, modulating angiogenesis, and regulating the migration of vascular smooth muscle cells (VSMC) [125].

4.2 UCN1 and Vascular Inflammation

UCN1 is a neuropeptide that plays a crucial role in the regulation of vascular tone and is involved in both vascular responses and immune cell-mediated reactions to inflammation. Consider thromboangiitis obliterans (TAO) as an example; it serves as a rat vasculitis model induced by sodium laurate. The findings derived from our research group suggest that UCN1 exacerbates vasculitis involving cyclooxygenase-2 (COX-2) and intercellular adhesion molecule-1 (ICAM-1) both in vivo and in vitro [4,126]. In depth, UCN1 increases COX-2 and ICAM-1 expressions mainly dependent of $cPLA_2$ [127]. In terms of the mechanism, it appears that the local secretion of UCN1 plays a significant role in promoting microvascular permeability during inflammation induced by LPS [45]. In accordance, our group have found that UCN1 can increase LPS-induced endothelial permeability by regulating the cadherin–catenin complex [128]. Parallelly, UCN1 enhances endothelial ICAM1 expression through $cPLA_2$-dependent NF-κB and protein kinase A (PKA) signaling pathways in human umbilical vein endothelial cells (HUVECs) [127].

However, a protective effect of UCN1 has been observed against diabetic nephropathy in two distinct diabetic mouse models, both of which are associated with endothelial damage [129, 130]. It attracts our attention that UCN1 is responsible for sex difference in vasculitis. Specifically, males TAO rats exhibit higher plasma levels and femoral artery tissue levels of UCN1 compared to females, along with more pronounced symptoms of vasculitis. Orchidectomy appears to significantly improve the symptoms of vasculitis, accompanied by a reduction in plasma

UCN1 levels. Additionally, rabbit antiserum to UCN1 seems to nearly eliminate the differences between sexes in relation to vasculitis [131]. In vitro work by our group also supports the relationship between sex differences and UCN1 [132].

4.3 CRFr and Vascular Inflammation

In the context of vascular inflammation, different CRFr exhibit distinct roles. It is widely acknowledged that the activation of CRF_1 contributes to pro-inflammatory processes, which include stimulating MCs, enhancing endothelial permeability, promoting angiogenesis, and regulating the migration of VSMCs. Conversely, the activation of CRF_2 may exert opposing effects. However, evidence has demonstrated that the pro-inflammatory effects induced by LPS are exacerbated by the CRF_1 blocker NBI-27914, while they are diminished by the CRF_2 blocker astressin 2B [45]. In HAECs, CRF_1 signaling has been confirmed to play against TNF-α-induced inflammation [123]. The activation of CRF_2, which involves the release of VEGF, plays a crucial role in enhancing vascular permeability in the bladder [133]. Consistently, in *Crhr1*$^{-/-}$mice, but not in *Crhr2*$^{-/-}$ or *Crhr1 + 2* $^{-/-}$ mice, increased bladder vascular permeability is observed.

5 Roles of CRFp in Rheumatoid Arthritis (RA)

5.1 CRFp and RA

CRH has been demonstrated to be expressed in carrageenan-induced rat granulomas, streptococcal cell wall-induced rat arthritis, as well as in the synovial fluids and tissues of patients with RA [16]. Immunoreactive CRH has been identified in the synovial tissue of patients with rheumatoid arthritis, which is associated with elevated levels of VEGF. Furthermore, inflammatory arthritis exhibits a significant reduction in CRH knockout mice [134].

Not only is CRH significantly elevated, but UCN1-like immunoreactivity and UCN1 mRNA levels are also markedly increased in the synovium of individuals with RA. Furthermore, the quantity of UCN1-positive cells present in the synovial tissue [135], including leukocytes and macrophages, is elevated and exhibits a significant correlation with the severity of inflammation [29]. This elevation contributes to a reduction in both inflammation and bone erosion in a murine model of the disease [136]. It is noteworthy that the expression levels of UCN1 and its corresponding mRNA within synovial tissues in RA exceed those observed in osteoarthritis (OA). This finding demonstrates a significant correlation of UCN1 expression with the degree of inflammation. While the expression of UCN1 in RA-affected joints is marginally lower than that of CRH, it demonstrates a comparable distribution pattern [29].

5.2 CRFr and RA

CRFr are prominently expressed within the synovial lining cell layer, subsynovial stromal cells, and endothelial cells of blood vessels. Notably, their expression is markedly intensified in infiltrating mononuclear inflammatory cells residing in the synovium of patients afflicted with RA and OA. MCs are notably elevated [137, 138] and exhibit the expression of $CRF_{1\alpha}$ within the joints of patients afflicted with RA [139]. In this context, the presence of mRNAs for both CRF_1 and CRF_2 has been identified [140]. Collagen-induced arthritis is significantly mitigated by the CRF_1 antagonist, antalarmin [134].

6 Roles of CRFp in Skin Inflammation

CRF peptides are expressed in human skin [141], and there is substantial evidence indicating that the cutaneous neuroendocrine system may play a role in skin inflammatory diseases through CRH [142]. Psychological stress has been identified as being associated with elevated levels of CRH in the serum of patients suffering from atopic dermatitis [143]. CRH accumulation in mouse skin is elevated following acute stress or in models of inflammatory skin diseases [144–147]. Stress-increased skin vascular permeability in human [148] and rodent [149] depends on CRH. Rodent skin, specifically that of mice and rats, also expresses UCN2 [150–153]. The effects of CRFp during skin inflammation is mainly attributed to MCs, and the role of CRFp on MCs has been represented previously in this chapter. Mouse UCN3 is found to be expressed peripherally in the small intestine and skin [154].

7 Summary

In summary, it is entirely comprehensible that CRFp, functioning as both a centrally active endocrine hormone and a peripherally active peptide, assumes a pivotal role in the intricate processes of inflammation. In addition, based on the recent data focused on CRFp and inflammation, it is not difficult to conclude that the local effects of the CRFp can act as either pro- or anti-inflammatory factors. The activities of both CRH and UCNs are intricately influenced by the concentration of each neuropeptide variant present, as well as the local expression ratios of their respective receptors, CRF_1 and CRF_2 [35]. It is widely acknowledged that the activation of CRF_1 exerts a pro-inflammatory influence, inciting MC activity, enhancing endothelial permeability, promoting angiogenesis, and orchestrating the migration of VSMCs. In contrast, the activation of CRF_2 may elicit an opposing effect (Table 6.2). Given the pivotal role of CRH in mediating stress and inflammation, coupled with forthcoming evidence that may further illuminate its significance, CRF receptor pathways could emerge as a promising therapeutic target for combating inflammatory diseases.

Table 6.2 CRFp act through CRFr in inflammation

Peptide	Receptor	Effects in inflammation
CRF_1	CRH	Pro-inflammatory activity
	UCN1	
CRF_2	CRH	Anti-inflammatory activity
	UCN1	
	UCN2	
	UCN3	

Primarily, it is acknowledged that CRF_1 functions as a pro-inflammatory agent, whereas, in stark contrast, CRF_2 assumes an opposing role. The local effects of the CRFp can act as either pro- or anti-inflammatory factors. The activities of CRH or UCNs are profoundly shaped by the concentration of each neuropeptide variant present, as well as the local expression ratios of their respective receptors CRF_1 and CRF_2

References

1. Saxena A, et al. A systems biology-based mathematical model demonstrates the potential anti-stress effectiveness of a multi-nutrient botanical formulation. Sci Rep. 2024;14(1):9582.
2. Tache Y, Bonaz B. Corticotropin-releasing factor receptors and stress-related alterations of gut motor function. J Clin Invest. 2007;117(1):33–40.
3. Turnbull AV, et al. CRF type I receptor-deficient mice exhibit a pronounced pituitary-adrenal response to local inflammation. Endocrinology. 1999;140(2):1013–7.
4. Aguilera G. Corticotropin releasing hormone, receptor regulation and the stress response. Trends Endocrinol Metab. 1998;9(8):329–36.
5. Herman JP, et al. Regulation of the hypothalamic-pituitary-adrenocortical stress response. Compr Physiol. 2016;6(2):603–21.
6. Marx J. How the glucocorticoids suppress immunity. Science. 1995;270(5234):232–3.
7. DeRijk R, et al. Exercise and circadian rhythm-induced variations in plasma cortisol differentially regulate interleukin-1 beta (IL-1 beta), IL-6, and tumor necrosis factor-alpha (TNF alpha) production in humans: high sensitivity of TNF alpha and resistance of IL-6. J Clin Endocrinol Metab. 1997;82(7):2182–91.
8. Kern JA, et al. Dexamethasone inhibition of interleukin 1 beta production by human monocytes. Posttranscriptional Mech J Clin Invest. 1988;81(1):237–44.
9. Lew W, Oppenheim JJ, Matsushima K. Analysis of the suppression of IL-1 alpha and IL-1 beta production in human peripheral blood mononuclear adherent cells by a glucocorticoid hormone. J Immunol. 1988;140(6):1895–902.
10. Goulding NJ, et al. Novel pathways for glucocorticoid effects on neutrophils in chronic inflammation. Inflamm Res. 1998;47(Suppl 3):S158–65.
11. Baritaki S, et al. Chronic stress, inflammation, and colon cancer: a CRH system-driven molecular crosstalk. J Clin Med. 2019;8(10)
12. Kritas SK, et al. Neuropeptide NGF mediates neuro-immune response and inflammation through mast cell activation. J Biol Regul Homeost Agents. 2014;28(2):177–81.
13. Sorrells SF, et al. Glucocorticoid signaling in myeloid cells worsens acute CNS injury and inflammation. J Neurosci. 2013;33(18):7877–89.
14. Sorrells SF, et al. Glucocorticoids increase excitotoxic injury and inflammation in the hippocampus of adult male rats. Neuroendocrinology. 2014;100(2–3):129–40.
15. Theoharides TC, Asadi S, Patel AB. Focal brain inflammation and autism. J Neuroinflammation. 2013;10:46.
16. Karalis K, et al. Autocrine or paracrine inflammatory actions of corticotropin-releasing hormone in vivo. Science. 1991;254(5030):421–3.

17. Saperstein A, et al. Interleukin 1 beta mediates stress-induced immunosuppression via corticotropin-releasing factor. Endocrinology. 1992;130(1):152–8.
18. Paez Pereda M, et al. Corticotropin-releasing hormone differentially modulates the interleukin-1 system according to the level of monocyte activation by endotoxin. Endocrinology. 1995;136(12):5504–10.
19. Brunetti L, et al. Involvement of nitric oxide in basal and interleukin-1 beta-induced CRH and ACTH release in vitro. Life Sci. 1993;53(13):PL219.
20. Petraglia F, et al. Peptide signaling in human placenta and membranes: autocrine, paracrine, and endocrine mechanisms. Endocr Rev. 1996;17(2):156–86.
21. Petraglia F, et al. Mechanism of action of interleukin-1 beta in increasing corticotropin-releasing factor and adrenocorticotropin hormone release from cultured human placental cells. Am J Obstet Gynecol. 1990;163(4 Pt 1):1307–12.
22. Roe CM, et al. Nitric oxide regulation of corticotropin-releasing hormone release from the human perfused placenta in vitro. J Clin Endocrinol Metab. 1996;81(2):763–9.
23. Angioni S, et al. Corticotropin-releasing hormone modulates cytokines release in cultured human peripheral blood mononuclear cells. Life Sci. 1993;53(23):1735–42.
24. Hagan P, Poole S, Bristow AF. Immunosuppressive activity of corticotrophin-releasing factor. Inhibition of interleukin-1 and interleukin-6 production by human mononuclear cells. Biochem J. 1992;281(Pt 1):251–4.
25. Theoharides TC, Cochrane DE. Critical role of mast cells in inflammatory diseases and the effect of acute stress. J Neuroimmunol. 2004;146(1–2):1–12.
26. Cao J, et al. Human mast cells express corticotropin-releasing hormone (CRH) receptors and CRH leads to selective secretion of vascular endothelial growth factor. J Immunol. 2005;174(12):7665–75.
27. Tsatsanis C, et al. Urocortin 1 and Urocortin 2 induce macrophage apoptosis via CRFR2. FEBS Lett. 2005;579(20):4259–64.
28. Chatzaki E, et al. Urocortin in human gastric mucosa: relationship to inflammatory activity. J Clin Endocrinol Metab. 2003;88(1):478–83.
29. Kohno M, et al. Urocortin expression in synovium of patients with rheumatoid arthritis and osteoarthritis: relation to inflammatory activity. J Clin Endocrinol Metab. 2001;86(9):4344–52.
30. Novembri R, et al. Corticotropin releasing hormone and Urocortin 2 activate inflammatory pathways in cultured trophoblast cell lines. Eur J Obstet Gynecol Reprod Biol. 2015;195:200–5.
31. McCann SM, et al. Role of the hypothalamic pituitary adrenal axis in the control of the response to stress and infection. Braz J Med Biol Res. 2000;33(10):1121–31.
32. Kravchenco IV, Furalev VA. Secretion of immunoreactive corticotropin releasing factor and adrenocorticotropic hormone by T- and B-lymphocytes in response to cellular stress factors. Biochem Biophys Res Commun. 1994;204(2):828–34.
33. Tang Q, et al. Dissecting hematopoietic and renal cell heterogeneity in adult zebrafish at single-cell resolution using RNA sequencing. J Exp Med. 2017;214(10):2875–87.
34. Radulovic M, et al. Corticotropin-releasing factor receptor 1 in mouse spleen: expression after immune stimulation and identification of receptor-bearing cells. J Immunol. 1999;162(5):3013–21.
35. Dermitzaki E, et al. The multi-faceted profile of corticotropin-releasing factor (CRF) Family of neuropeptides and of their receptors on the paracrine/local regulation of the inflammatory response. Curr Mol Pharmacol. 2018;11(1):39–50.
36. Kozakai Y, et al. The role of peripheral corticotropin-releasing factor signaling in a rat model of stress-induced gastric hyperalgesia. Biochem Biophys Res Commun. 2019;519(4):797–802.
37. Koido S, et al. Production of corticotropin-releasing factor and urocortin from human monocyte-derived dendritic cells is stimulated by commensal bacteria in intestine. World J Gastroenterol. 2014;20(39):14420–9.
38. Harle G, et al. Murine splenic B cells express corticotropin-releasing hormone receptor 2 that affect their viability during a stress response. Sci Rep. 2018;8(1):143.

39. Bamberger CM, et al. Human lymphocytes produce urocortin, but not corticotropin-releasing hormone. J Clin Endocrinol Metab. 1998;83(2):708–11.
40. Wilbert-Lampen U, et al. Effects of corticotropin-releasing hormone (CRH) on monocyte function, mediated by CRH-receptor subtype R1 and R2: a potential link between mood disorders and endothelial dysfunction? J Cardiovasc Pharmacol. 2006;47(1):110–6.
41. Leu SJ, Singh VK. Stimulation of interleukin-6 production by corticotropin-releasing factor. Cell Immunol. 1992;143(1):220–7.
42. Singh VK, Leu SJ. Enhancing effect of corticotropin-releasing neurohormone on the production of interleukin-1 and interleukin-2. Neurosci Lett. 1990;120(2):151–4.
43. Chandras C, et al. Activation of phosphatidylinositol 3-kinase/protein kinase B by corticotropin-releasing factor in human monocytes. Endocrinology. 2009;150(10):4606–14.
44. Tsatsanis C, et al. Corticotropin releasing factor receptor 1 (CRF1) and CRF2 agonists exert an anti-inflammatory effect during the early phase of inflammation suppressing LPS-induced TNF-alpha release from macrophages via induction of COX-2 and PGE2. J Cell Physiol. 2007;210(3):774–83.
45. Cureton EL, et al. Local secretion of urocortin 1 promotes microvascular permeability during lipopolysaccharide-induced inflammation. Endocrinology. 2009;150(12):5428–37.
46. McLoon LK, Wirtschafter J. Local injections of corticotropin releasing factor reduce doxorubicin-induced acute inflammation in the eyelid. Invest Ophthalmol Vis Sci. 1997;38(5):834–41.
47. Cho W, Kang JL, Park YM. Corticotropin-releasing hormone (CRH) promotes macrophage foam cell formation via reduced expression of atp binding cassette transporter-1 (ABCA1). PLoS One. 2015;10(6):e0130587.
48. Tsatsanis C, et al. Corticotropin-releasing factor and the urocortins induce the expression of TLR4 in macrophages via activation of the transcription factors PU.1 and AP-1. J Immunol. 2006;176(3):1869–77.
49. Charalampopoulos I, et al. Neuropeptide urocortin and its receptors are expressed in rat Kupffer cells. Neuroendocrinology. 2006;84(1):49–57.
50. Zhu C, et al. Urocortin participates in LPS-induced apoptosis of THP-1 macrophages via S1P-cPLA2 signaling pathway. Eur J Pharmacol. 2020;887:173559.
51. Yamawaki H, et al. Acotiamide attenuates central urocortin 2-induced intestinal inflammatory responses, and urocortin 2 treatment reduces TNF-alpha productions in LPS-stimulated macrophage cell lines. Neurogastroenterol Motil. 2020;32(8):e13813.
52. Li N, et al. Bidirectional relationship of mast cells-neurovascular unit communication in neuroinflammation and its involvement in POCD. Behav Brain Res. 2017;322(Pt A):60–9.
53. Elenkov IJ, Chrousos GP. Stress hormones, Th1/Th2 patterns, pro/anti-inflammatory cytokines and susceptibility to disease. Trends Endocrinol Metab. 1999;10(9):359–68.
54. Ayyadurai S, et al. Frontline science: corticotropin-releasing factor receptor subtype 1 is a critical modulator of mast cell degranulation and stress-induced pathophysiology. J Leukoc Biol. 2017;102(6):1299–312.
55. Theoharides TC, et al. Mast cells as targets of corticotropin-releasing factor and related peptides. Trends Pharmacol Sci. 2004;25(11):563–8.
56. Papadopoulou NG, et al. Regulation of corticotropin-releasing hormone receptor-2 expression in human cord blood-derived cultured mast cells. J Mol Endocrinol. 2005;35(3):R1–8.
57. Vicario M, et al. Chronological assessment of mast cell-mediated gut dysfunction and mucosal inflammation in a rat model of chronic psychosocial stress. Brain Behav Immun. 2010;24(7):1166–75.
58. D'Costa S, et al. Mast cell corticotropin-releasing factor subtype 2 suppresses mast cell degranulation and limits the severity of anaphylaxis and stress-induced intestinal permeability. J Allergy Clin Immunol. 2019;143(5):1865–1877 e4.
59. Zouboulis CC, et al. Corticotropin-releasing hormone: an autocrine hormone that promotes lipogenesis in human sebocytes. Proc Natl Acad Sci USA. 2002;99(10):7148–53.

60. Theoharides TC, et al. High serum corticotropin-releasing hormone (CRH) and bone marrow mast cell CRH receptor expression in a mastocytosis patient. J Allergy Clin Immunol. 2014;134(5):1197–9.
61. Fukuoka H, et al. The mechanisms underlying autonomous adrenocorticotropic hormone secretion in cushing's disease. Int J Mol Sci. 2020;21(23)
62. Theoharides TC, et al. Mast cells and inflammation. Biochim Biophys Acta. 2012;1822(1):21–33.
63. Kempuraj D, et al. Corticotropin-releasing hormone and its structurally related urocortin are synthesized and secreted by human mast cells. Endocrinology. 2004;145(1):43–8.
64. Singh LK, et al. Potent mast cell degranulation and vascular permeability triggered by urocortin through activation of corticotropin-releasing hormone receptors. J Pharmacol Exp Ther. 1999;288(3):1349–56.
65. Trayhurn P, Wood IS. Signalling role of adipose tissue: adipokines and inflammation in obesity. Biochem Soc Trans. 2005;33(Pt 5):1078–81.
66. Kageyama K, Suda T. Urocortin-related peptides increase interleukin-6 output via cyclic adenosine 5′-monophosphate-dependent pathways in A7r5 aortic smooth muscle cells. Endocrinology. 2003;144(6):2234–41.
67. Baigent SM, Lowry PJ. mRNA expression profiles for corticotrophin-releasing factor (CRF), urocortin, CRF receptors and CRF-binding protein in peripheral rat tissues. J Mol Endocrinol. 2000;25(1):43–52.
68. Armario A. Activation of the hypothalamic-pituitary-adrenal axis by addictive drugs: different pathways, common outcome. Trends Pharmacol Sci. 2010;31(7):318–25.
69. Theoharides TC, Konstantinidou AD. Corticotropin-releasing hormone and the blood-brain-barrier. Front Biosci. 2007;12:1615–28.
70. Chesnokova V, Melmed S. Minireview: Neuro-immuno-endocrine modulation of the hypothalamic-pituitary-adrenal (HPA) axis by gp130 signaling molecules. Endocrinology. 2002;143(5):1571–4.
71. Theoharides TC, et al. Dysregulated brain immunity and neurotrophin signaling in Rett syndrome and autism spectrum disorders. J Neuroimmunol. 2015;279:33–8.
72. Wang W, et al. Corticotropin-releasing hormone potentiates neural injury induced by oxygen-glucose deprivation: a possible involvement of microglia. Neurosci Lett. 2004;371(2–3):133–7.
73. Wu Q, et al. Corticotropin-releasing factor aggravates ischemic stroke injury by the inflammatory activation of microglia. Endocrinology. 2022;163(3)
74. Kormos V, et al. Reduced response to chronic mild stress in PACAP mutant mice is associated with blunted FosB expression in limbic forebrain and brainstem centers. Neuroscience. 2016;330:335–58.
75. Farkas J, et al. Construct and face validity of a new model for the three-hit theory of depression using PACAP mutant mice on CD1 background. Neuroscience. 2017;354:11–29.
76. Gaszner B, Csernus V, Kozicz T. Urocortinergic neurons respond in a differentiated manner to various acute stressors in the Edinger-Westphal nucleus in the rat. J Comp Neurol. 2004;480(2):170–9.
77. Gaszner B, et al. Neuropeptide Y activates urocortin 1 neurons in the nonpreganglionic Edinger-Westphal nucleus. J Comp Neurol. 2007;500(4):708–19.
78. Gaszner B, et al. Effects of maternal separation on dynamics of urocortin 1 and brain-derived neurotrophic factor in the rat non-preganglionic Edinger-Westphal nucleus. Int J Dev Neurosci. 2009;27(5):439–51.
79. Aschrafi A, et al. MicroRNA-326 acts as a molecular switch in the regulation of midbrain urocortin 1 expression. J Psychiatry Neurosci. 2016;41(5):342–53.
80. Kozicz T, et al. Chronic psychosocial stress affects corticotropin-releasing factor in the paraventricular nucleus and central extended amygdala as well as urocortin 1 in the non-preganglionic Edinger-Westphal nucleus of the tree shrew. Psychoneuroendocrinology. 2008;33(6):741–54.

81. Poliak S, et al. Stress and autoimmunity: the neuropeptides corticotropin-releasing factor and urocortin suppress encephalomyelitis via effects on both the hypothalamic-pituitary-adrenal axis and the immune system. J Immunol. 1997;158(12):5751–6.
82. Liew HK, et al. Systemic administration of urocortin after intracerebral hemorrhage reduces neurological deficits and neuroinflammation in rats. J Neuroinflammation. 2012;9:13.
83. Liew HK, et al. Therapeutic effects of human urocortin-1, −2 and −3 in intracerebral hemorrhage of rats. Neuropeptides. 2015;52:89–96.
84. Wang MJ, et al. Urocortin modulates inflammatory response and neurotoxicity induced by microglial activation. J Immunol. 2007;179(9):6204–14.
85. Reyes TM, et al. Urocortin II: a member of the corticotropin-releasing factor (CRF) neuropeptide family that is selectively bound by type 2 CRF receptors. Proc Natl Acad Sci USA. 2001;98(5):2843–8.
86. Tillinger A, Mravec B. Vagotomy affects lipopolysaccharide-induced changes of urocortin 2 gene expression in the brain and on the periphery. Neurochem Res. 2021;46(2):159–64.
87. Choy KW, et al. The role of urocortins in intracerebral hemorrhage. Biomol Ther. 2020;10(1)
88. Hauger RL, et al. Corticotropin releasing factor (CRF) receptor signaling in the central nervous system: new molecular targets. CNS Neurol Disord Drug Targets. 2006;5(4):453–79.
89. Takefuji M, Murohara T. Corticotropin-releasing hormone family and their receptors in the cardiovascular system. Circ J. 2019;83(2):261–6.
90. de la Tremblaye PB, et al. CRHR1 exacerbates the glial inflammatory response and alters BDNF/TrkB/pCREB signaling in a rat model of global cerebral ischemia: implications for neuroprotection and cognitive recovery. Prog Neuro-Psychopharmacol Biol Psychiatry. 2017;79(Pt B):234–48.
91. Smith EM, et al. Corticotropin releasing factor (CRF) activation of NF-kappaB-directed transcription in leukocytes. Cell Mol Neurobiol. 2006;26(4–6):1021–36.
92. Mousa SA, et al. Superior control of inflammatory pain by corticotropin-releasing factor receptor 1 via opioid peptides in distinct pain-relevant brain areas. J Neuroinflammation. 2022;19(1):148.
93. Deng S, et al. The exploration of neuroinflammatory mechanism by which CRHR2 deficiency induced anxiety disorder. Prog Neuro-Psychopharmacol Biol Psychiatry. 2024;128:110844.
94. Liddelow SA, et al. Neurotoxic reactive astrocytes are induced by activated microglia. Nature. 2017;541(7638):481–7.
95. Gonzalez-Rey E, et al. Therapeutic effect of urocortin and adrenomedullin in a murine model of Crohn's disease. Gut. 2006;55(6):824–32.
96. Saruta M, et al. Urocortin 3/stresscopin in human colon: possible modulators of gastrointestinal function during stressful conditions. Peptides. 2005;26(7):1196–206.
97. Saruta M, et al. Urocortin 1 in colonic mucosa in patients with ulcerative colitis. J Clin Endocrinol Metab. 2004;89(11):5352–61.
98. Kiank C, Tache Y, Larauche M. Stress-related modulation of inflammation in experimental models of bowel disease and post-infectious irritable bowel syndrome: role of corticotropin-releasing factor receptors. Brain Behav Immun. 2010;24(1):41–8.
99. Larauche M, Kiank C, Tache Y. Corticotropin releasing factor signaling in colon and ileum: regulation by stress and pathophysiological implications. J Physiol Pharmacol. 2009;60(Suppl 7):33–46.
100. Bell RL, et al. Stress and corticotropin releasing factor (CRF) promote necrotizing enterocolitis in a formula-fed neonatal rat model. PLoS One. 2021;16(6):e0246412.
101. Wallon C, et al. Corticotropin-releasing hormone (CRH) regulates macromolecular permeability via mast cells in normal human colonic biopsies in vitro. Gut. 2008;57(1):50–8.
102. Kokkotou E, et al. Corticotropin-releasing hormone receptor 2-deficient mice have reduced intestinal inflammatory responses. J Immunol. 2006;177(5):3355–61.
103. Hagiwara SI, et al. Gastric corticotropin-releasing factor influences mast cell infiltration in a rat model of functional dyspepsia. PLoS One. 2018;13(9):e0203704.

104. la Fleur SE, et al. Role of peripheral corticotropin-releasing factor and urocortin II in intestinal inflammation and motility in terminal ileum. Proc Natl Acad Sci USA. 2005;102(21):7647–52.
105. Vanuytsel T, et al. Psychological stress and corticotropin-releasing hormone increase intestinal permeability in humans by a mast cell-dependent mechanism. Gut. 2014;63(8):1293–9.
106. Buckinx R, et al. Corticotrophin-releasing factor, related peptides, and receptors in the normal and inflamed gastrointestinal tract. Front Neurosci. 2011;5:54.
107. Collins SM. Stress and the Gastrointestinal Tract IV. Modulation of intestinal inflammation by stress: basic mechanisms and clinical relevance. Am J Physiol Gastrointest Liver Physiol. 2001;280(3):G315–8.
108. Chatoo M, et al. Involvement of corticotropin-releasing factor and receptors in immune cells in irritable bowel syndrome. Front Endocrinol (Lausanne). 2018;9:21.
109. Zhao SB, et al. Corticotropin releasing hormone promotes inflammatory bowel disease via inducing intestinal macrophage autophagy. Cell Death Discov. 2021;7(1):377.
110. Wang SL, et al. Intestinal autophagy links psychosocial stress with gut microbiota to promote inflammatory bowel disease. Cell Death Dis. 2019;10(6):391.
111. Shih DQ, Targan SR. Immunopathogenesis of inflammatory bowel disease. World J Gastroenterol. 2008;14(3):390–400.
112. Gay J, et al. Corticotropin-releasing hormone deficiency is associated with reduced local inflammation in a mouse model of experimental colitis. Endocrinology. 2008;149(7):3403–9.
113. Chang J, et al. Urocortin 1 modulates immunosignaling in a rat model of colitis via corticotropin-releasing factor receptor 2. Am J Physiol Gastrointest Liver Physiol. 2011;300(5):G884–94.
114. Chang J, et al. Urocortin 2 expression in the rat gastrointestinal tract under basal conditions and in chemical colitis. Peptides. 2007;28(7):1453–60.
115. Yuan J, et al. Protective effects of urocortin 2 against caerulein-induced acute pancreatitis. PLoS One. 2019;14(5):e0217065.
116. You X, et al. Urocortins exhibit differential effects on PGE2 and PGF2alpha output via CRHR2 in human myometrium. Reproduction. 2021;162(1):11–20.
117. Gravanis A, Margioris AN. The corticotropin-releasing factor (CRF) family of neuropeptides in inflammation: potential therapeutic applications. Curr Med Chem. 2005;12(13):1503–12.
118. Chen H, et al. Activation of corticotropin-releasing factor receptor 1 aggravates dextran sodium sulphate-induced colitis in mice by promoting M1 macrophage polarization. Mol Med Rep. 2018;17(1):234–42.
119. Saito-Nakaya K, et al. Corticotropin-releasing hormone receptor 1 antagonist blocks colonic hypersensitivity induced by a combination of inflammation and repetitive colorectal distension. Neurogastroenterol Motil. 2008;20(10):1147–56.
120. Pincus-Knackstedt MK, et al. Prenatal stress enhances susceptibility of murine adult offspring toward airway inflammation. J Immunol. 2006;177(12):8484–92.
121. Gong SS, et al. Mucosa repair mechanisms of Tong-Xie-Yao-Fang mediated by CRH-R2 in murine, dextran sulfate sodium-induced colitis. World J Gastroenterol. 2018;24(16):1766–78.
122. Zhu C, Li S. The peripheral corticotropin releasing factor family's role in vasculitis. Vasc Pharmacol. 2024;154:107275.
123. Inada Y, et al. Possible involvement of corticotropin-releasing factor receptor signaling on vascular inflammation. Peptides. 2009;30(2):365–72.
124. Cao C, et al. Activation of CRHR1 contributes to cerebral endothelial barrier impairment via cPLA(2) phosphorylation in experimental ischemic stroke. Cell Signal. 2020;66:109467.
125. Zhu C, et al. Corticotrophin-releasing factor participates in S1PR3-dependent cPLA2 expression and cell motility in vascular smooth muscle cells. Vasc Pharmacol. 2015;71:116–26.
126. Xu Y, et al. Urocortin promotes the development of vasculitis in a rat model of thromboangiitis obliterans via corticotrophin-releasing factor type 1 receptors. Br J Pharmacol. 2009;157(8):1368–79.
127. Wan R, et al. Urocortin increased endothelial ICAM1 by cPLA2-dependent NF-kappaB and PKA pathways in HUVECs. J Mol Endocrinol. 2014;52(1):43–53.

128. Wan R, et al. Urocortin increased LPS-induced endothelial permeability by regulating the cadherin-catenin complex via corticotrophin-releasing hormone receptor 2. J Cell Physiol. 2013;228(6):1295–303.
129. Li X, et al. Urocortin ameliorates diabetic nephropathy in obese db/db mice. Br J Pharmacol. 2008;154(5):1025–34.
130. Li X, et al. Urocortin 1 improves renal function in rats with streptozotocin-induced diabetes by inhibiting overproduction of TGF-beta 1 and VEGF. Br J Pharmacol. 2009;157(6):994–1003.
131. Wan R, et al. Sex difference in urocortin production is contributory to the gender disparity in a rat model of vasculitis induced by sodium laurate. Endocrinology. 2013;154(12):4663–74.
132. Wan R, et al. Dihydrotestosterone alters urocortin levels in human umbilical vein endothelial cells. J Endocrinol. 2013;218(3):321–30.
133. Boucher W, et al. Corticotropin-releasing hormone-receptor 2 is required for acute stress-induced bladder vascular permeability and release of vascular endothelial growth factor. BJU Int. 2010;106(9):1394–9.
134. Webster EL, et al. Corticotropin releasing hormone (CRH) antagonist attenuates adjuvant induced arthritis: role of CRH in peripheral inflammation. J Rheumatol. 2002;29(6):1252–61.
135. Uzuki M, et al. Urocortin in the synovial tissue of patients with rheumatoid arthritis. Clin Sci (Lond). 2001;100(6):577–89.
136. Gonzalez-Rey E, et al. Therapeutic effect of urocortin on collagen-induced arthritis by down-regulation of inflammatory and Th1 responses and induction of regulatory T cells. Arthritis Rheum. 2007;56(2):531–43.
137. Olsson N, Ulfgren AK, Nilsson G. Demonstration of mast cell chemotactic activity in synovial fluid from rheumatoid patients. Ann Rheum Dis. 2001;60(3):187–93.
138. Crofford LJ, et al. Local secretion of corticotropin-releasing hormone in the joints of Lewis rats with inflammatory arthritis. J Clin Invest. 1992;90(6):2555–64.
139. Crofford LJ, et al. Corticotropin-releasing hormone in synovial fluids and tissues of patients with rheumatoid arthritis and osteoarthritis. J Immunol. 1993;151(3):1587–96.
140. Singh LK, et al. Acute immobilization stress triggers skin mast cell degranulation via corticotropin releasing hormone, neurotensin, and substance P: a link to neurogenic skin disorders. Brain Behav Immun. 1999;13(3):225–39.
141. Slominski A, et al. Cutaneous expression of corticotropin-releasing hormone (CRH), urocortin, and CRH receptors. FASEB J. 2001;15(10):1678–93.
142. Slominski AT, et al. Key role of CRF in the skin stress response system. Endocr Rev. 2013;34(6):827–84.
143. Vasiadi M, et al. Increased serum CRH levels with decreased skin CRHR-1 gene expression in psoriasis and atopic dermatitis. J Allergy Clin Immunol. 2012;129(5):1410–3.
144. Theoharides TC, Kalogeromitros D. The critical role of mast cells in allergy and inflammation. Ann N Y Acad Sci. 2006;1088:78–99.
145. Huang M, et al. Mast cell deficient W/W(v) mice lack stress-induced increase in serum IL-6 levels, as well as in peripheral CRH and vascular permeability, a model of rheumatoid arthritis. Int J Immunopathol Pharmacol. 2002;15(3):249–54.
146. Lytinas M, et al. Acute stress results in skin corticotropin-releasing hormone secretion, mast cell activation and vascular permeability, an effect mimicked by intradermal corticotropin-releasing hormone and inhibited by histamine-1 receptor antagonists. Int Arch Allergy Immunol. 2003;130(3):224–31.
147. Zhang X, et al. Development of alopecia areata is associated with higher central and peripheral hypothalamic-pituitary-adrenal tone in the skin graft induced C3H/HeJ mouse model. J Invest Dermatol. 2009;129(6):1527–38.
148. Crompton R, et al. Corticotropin-releasing hormone causes vasodilation in human skin via mast cell-dependent pathways. J Clin Endocrinol Metab. 2003;88(11):5427–32.
149. Theoharides TC, et al. Corticotropin-releasing hormone induces skin mast cell degranulation and increased vascular permeability, a possible explanation for its proinflammatory effects. Endocrinology. 1998;139(1):403–13.

150. Slominski A, et al. Differential expression of a cutaneous corticotropin-releasing hormone system. Endocrinology. 2004;145(2):941–50.
151. Chen A, et al. Urocortin II gene is highly expressed in mouse skin and skeletal muscle tissues: localization, basal expression in corticotropin-releasing factor receptor (CRFR) 1- and CRFR2-null mice, and regulation by glucocorticoids. Endocrinology. 2004;145(5):2445–57.
152. Yamauchi N, et al. Distribution of urocortin 2 in various tissues of the rat. J Neuroendocrinol. 2005;17(10):656–63.
153. Chae JI, et al. cDNA cloning and analysis of tissue-specific gene expression of rat urocortin II. Mol Biol (Mosk). 2009;43(1):91–6.
154. Lewis K, et al. Identification of urocortin III, an additional member of the corticotropin-releasing factor (CRF) family with high affinity for the CRF2 receptor. Proc Natl Acad Sci USA. 2001;98(13):7570–5.

Chapter 7
CRF Peptides in Tumors

Rong Wan and Chao Zhu

Evidence suggests that hypothalamus-pituitary-adrenal (HPA) axis imbalance and inflammation such as increased interleukin-1 (IL-1), IL-6, and tumor necrosis factor alpha (TNF-α) cytokine secretion play a crucial role in the etiology of tumors [1, 2]. Dysregulation of the HPA axis has been observed in patients with cancer [3, 4]. Attributed to the participation of corticotrophin-releasing hormone (CRH) in both HPA and inflammation, there is a strong link between CRH and tumorigenesis development (Chap. 1). As reported, CRH-like immunoreactivity can be found in tumors composed of peptide-hormone-producing endocrine cells [5]. The peripheral biosynthesis of CRH has also been demonstrated in a large variety of human cancer cell lines, such as neuroblastomas, small-cell lung cancers, and melanomas [6, 7]. However, the effects of CRH on tumor are complicated because of the absence of an absolute clear-cut between the central and peripheral effects of CRH on inflammation and cancer. Until now, little is known about the direct relationship between central CRH and tumorigenesis. In addition to CRH, other corticotropin-releasing hormone (factor) family peptides (CRF peptides, CRFp), including CRH, urocortin (UCN1), urocortin 2 (UCN2), urocortin 3 (UCN3), and CRF binding protein (CRF-BP), as well as their corresponding receptors (CRFr, including CRF_1 and CRF_2), are found to be involved in tumors [8, 9].

On the one hand, CRFp are involved in the regulation of tumor biology by influencing cell proliferation, migration, invasion, and apoptosis [10–12]. Although a comprehensive and systematic study of the relationship between CRFp and tumor is still needed, the existing evidence suggests that the molecular regulatory

R. Wan (✉)
Jiangxi Key Laboratory of Molecular Medicine, The Second Affiliated Hospital of Nanchang University, Nanchang, China

C. Zhu
Department of Pharmacology, School of Basic Medical Sciences, Nanjing Medical University, Nanjing, Jiangsu, China

© The Author(s), under exclusive license to Springer Nature Singapore Pte Ltd. 2025
C. Zhu et al. (eds.), *The Peripheral Existence and Effects of Corticotropin-releasing Factor Family*, https://doi.org/10.1007/978-981-96-5322-5_7

mechanism of CRFp in tumor formation is worthy of further exploration. On the other hand, data from a human study on tumors indicate that CRF_1 is expressed in 4 out of 19 (21%) surgical specimens obtained from untreated patients with a diagnosis of primary endometrial cancer. Two out of four cases (50%) expressing CRF_1 mRNA have extrauterine spreading of the disease, whereas cases not expressing CRF_1 mRNA are all in federation international gynecology and obstetrics (FIGO) stage I, 2 ($p = 0.015$) [13], which suggest the indispensable role of CRFr in cancer. Just like CRF_2, studies have demonstrated the important role of CRF_2 in the progression, metastasis, and survival of several types of cancer, mostly prostate, pancreatic ductal, lung, kidney, hepatocellular cancer (HCC), and colorectal cancer (CRC) [4, 8, 14, 15]. Understanding the mechanisms underlying the involvement of CRFp and CRFr in tumorigenesis may open new avenues for targeted therapeutic strategies in malignancies.

1 Role of CRFp in Gastrointestinal Neoplasms

1.1 CRC

CRC, commonly referred to as malignancy originating in the colon or rectal epithelium, is the fourth leading cause of death in the world [16]. Multiple lines of evidences have suggested the role of the CRFp in CRC process. Stress, inflammation, and colon cancer are highly related, forming a CRH system-driven crosstalk [17–19]. Moreover, CRFp has been detected to influence the biological behavior of colon cancer through complex mechanisms, including processes such as cell proliferation, migration, invasion, and angiogenesis.

CRH is reported to be expressed in the intestinal submucosa, the interscalene plexus, and the lamina propria nerve fibers [20]. The central role of CRH in colon cancer is accomplished primarily by mediating the HPA axis during chronic stress indirectly [17, 21, 22]. In regard of the relationship between CRH and HPA axis, it is believable that central CRH acts on CAC is based on that central CRH mediates colitis and the crosstalk between inflammation and cancer [21, 23]. Moreover, CRH has been recognized as one of the key regulators of brain-gut-microbiome link under stress, which can regulate CAC [24, 25]. In addition, due to the close relationship between peripheral CRH and gastrointestinal system [4, 26, 27] and the involvement of peripheral CRH in colitis [28, 29], it is not difficult to prove the effects of CRH in CAC. CRH can enhance colon cancer cell proliferation, promoting colony formation [30] and tumor angiogenesis via nuclear factor-κ-gene binding (NF-κB)/vascular endothelial growth factor A (VEGF-A) signaling pathway [31]. Furthermore, CRH treatment significantly promotes angiogenesis of human umbilical vein endothelial cells (HUVECs), which is indicated by tube formation assay [32].

Similarly, a research indicates that UCN1 promotes colorectal cancer cell migration and proliferation while inhibiting apoptosis by suppressing the p53 signaling pathway [33]. Interestingly, UCN1 has been indicated to be an important factor in the correlation between sex and CRC. Specifically, high UCN1 expression is more frequently observed in males with higher incidence than that in female patients [34].

Another CRFp, UCN2 is confirmed to be expressed in the intestinal submucosa, the interscalene plexus, and the lamina propria nerve fibers [20]. The evidence of the involvement of UCN2 in CRC is rare. Nowadays, UCN2 signaling is a negative regulator of CRC cell resistance to immune-mediated apoptotic stimuli [35].

CRF_1 is mainly localized to macrophages in the lamina propria of the colon [16]. CRH/CRF_1 signaling pathway promotes human colon cancer cell proliferation through the NF-κB/IL-6/signal transducer and activator of transcription 3 (STAT3) signaling pathway and tumor angiogenesis through the NF-κB/VEGF signaling pathway [30]. Correspondingly, the absence of CRF_1 can exhibit tumor-suppressive effects [31]. Likewise, in *Crhr1*$^{-/-}$ mice, tumor incidence is significantly reduced, with a decrease in proliferating cells and an increase in apoptotic cells in the colon [36].

The expression of CRF_2 decreases in colon cancer tissues compared with that in normal tissues [37]. Unlike CRF_1, raising evidence suggest that CRF_2 expression in colonic intestinal cells can regulate migration, proliferation, and apoptosis through the modulation of several pathways [37]. The lack of CRF_2 exacerbates tumorigenicity [31]. Moreover, in colonic samples from CRC patients, mRNA levels of IL-1β, IL-6, and IL-6R are reduced in CRC-CRF_2^+ cells, and CRF_2 mRNA expression is negatively correlated with IL-6R [37]. However, opposing effects of CRF_2 have also been reported. It is suggested that CRF_2 may promote CRC development [38]. Additionally, blood sample analyses indicate that CRF_2 is a risk factor for CRC development in Mexican patients [39]. CRF_2 is a potent angiogenic suppressor through phosphatidylinositol-4,5-bisphosphate 3-kinase (PI3K), phospholipase C gamma (PLCγ), and VEGF-A pathways [40, 41].

Thus, this area remains controversial, and further research is needed. Recently, it has been reported that monitoring $CRF_{1/2}$ methylation-based features in colorectal cancer tissues may have significant diagnostic and prognostic value in CRC [15, 42, 43].

1.2 HCC

HCC is one of the most common malignant tumors of the liver and often arises in patients with chronic liver disease [44, 45]. Notably, it has been reported that UCN1, CRF_1, and CRF_2 are expressed in the cytoplasm and cell membranes of hepatocytes, endothelial cells, and cholangiocytes [46]. The CRFp can influence liver cell proliferation, migration, invasion, and apoptosis.

Specifically, the liver can produce a local immune response against harmful stimuli through the secretion of UCN1 [47]. UCN1 affects the occurrence and development of liver cancer by influencing cell growth factors and immune processes [48]. Under hypoxic conditions, UCN1/CRF_1 inhibits apoptosis by activating the phosphorylation of extracellular signal regulated kinase 1/2 (ERK1/2), which in turn activates CCAAT/enhancer-binding protein β (C/EBP-β) to downregulate the pro-apoptotic gene Bcl-2-associated X protein (Bax) [47]. Additionally, UCN1 has been found to inhibit liver cancer growth in nude mice and reduce tumor microvessel density [49]. UCN1 can inhibit cell proliferation and promote the migration of liver tumor cells by increasing the expression of cytoplasmic phospholipase A2 ($cPLA_2$) through the NF-κB pathway [49] and inhibit tumor cell migration by acting on calcium-dependent cytoplasmic phospholipase A2 ($iPLA_2$) [11]. These findings suggest that UCN1 may mediate anti-tumor effects.

CRF-BP, a molecule that interacts with members of the CRFp, may function by regulating the bioavailability of CRH. CRF-BP can form complexes with CRH, reducing its concentration in the bloodstream, which may affect the activity of the CRH signaling pathway [50]. Studies have found that CRF-BP expression is significantly reduced in liver cancer patients, possibly due to p62-mediated autophagy [51]. Recent research has shown that CRF-BP can slow the progression of HCC by reducing the expression of cyclin B2 and inhibiting the interaction between cyclin B2 and cyclin-dependent kinase 1 (CDK1) [52]. Therefore, enhancing the expression or function of CRF-BP may be a potential therapeutic strategy, which requires further basic and clinical research for validation.

1.3 Gastric Cancer

Gastric cancer, a malignancy originating from the gastric epithelium, is the fifth most common cancer worldwide, with significant variations in incidence and mortality across different regions and populations [53]. Treatment for gastric cancer primarily includes surgical resection, chemotherapy, radiation therapy, and targeted therapy. The prognosis for early-stage gastric cancer is relatively favorable, but advanced gastric cancer, which is prone to metastasis, has a poor prognosis. Tissue biopsies from gastric cancer patients have indicated that high levels of CRH may be associated with the progression of chronic gastritis to gastric cancer [54]. UCN1/CRF_2 is expressed in human gastric mucosa and plays a physiological role in regulating apoptosis, whereas CRF_1 is not expressed [55]. Other studies have shown that UCN1 is expressed in most non-tumor gastric glandular epithelial cells and that in gastric adenocarcinoma. Meanwhile, UCN1 expression is negatively correlated with higher tumor grade and advanced tumor/lymph node/metastasis (TNM) stage [56]. These findings suggest that UCN may play a crucial role in the development and progression of gastric cancer, potentially aiding in the development of new diagnostic and therapeutic strategies for gastric cancer.

1.4 Central Nervous System: Glioma

Gliomas are primary brain tumors that are thought to develop from neural stem or progenitor cells that carry tumor-initiating genetic alterations, whose incidence accounts for a high proportion of all brain tumors [57]. Treatment methods primarily include surgical resection, radiation therapy, and chemotherapy, but the prognosis is generally poor due to the tumor's invasiveness and heterogeneity. CRH and CRF_1 are expressed in brain tissue. In gliomas, CRF_1 expression is increased and positively correlated with tumor grade [58]. It is reported that treating gliomas with CRH enhances the cell ability to suppress abnormal proliferation and promote apoptosis by increasing p53 expression, suggesting that CRH can serve as a potential anti-tumor factor with lower toxicity compared to steroid treatments [58, 59]. However, further basic research is needed to elucidate the precise molecular mechanisms of CRH in glioma treatment, as well as clinical studies to assess its safety, efficacy, and long-term outcomes.

2 Role of CRFp in Genitourinary System Cancers

2.1 Renal Cell Carcinoma (RCC)

The most common type of kidney cancer is RCC, which typically arises from the endothelial cells of the renal tubules, with a higher incidence in men than in women [60]. Treatment options include surgical resection, targeted therapy, immunotherapy, and radiation therapy. The prognosis for early-stage kidney cancer is relatively favorable, but it is poor for advanced or metastatic RCC.

CRH is reported to inhibit RCC cell proliferation and regulate angiogenesis [61]. Hossein et al.'s group show the expression of UCN1 in human kidney and renal cell carcinoma for the first time and demonstrate that the nuclear translocation of UCN1 in epithelial cells and microvasculature of tumoral specimens may be involved in the pathobiology of renal cell carcinoma [62]. Further studies have shown that UCN1 can promote the proliferation and migration of RCC and exert pro-cancer effects through the oxidative stress pathway in RCC [63]. Apart from UCN1, UCN3 is significantly downregulated in RCC compared to normal tissues [8]. UCN3 is expressed in the kidneys and reduces VEGF production by binding to CRF_2, leading to decreased angiogenesis in the kidneys and reduced tumor vascular density.

Moreover, CRF-BP is also expressed in the kidneys and is involved in the development and progression of kidney cancer. The direct activity of CRF-BP in RCC cells is only described recently. In RCC patients, decreased CRF-BP expression in tumor tissues is significantly associated with poorer survival rates. Overexpressed CRF-BP inhibits cell proliferation, migration, invasion, and apoptosis both in vitro and in vivo by upregulating NF-κB- and p53-mediated mitochondrial apoptotic pathways [64]. Compared to normal samples, the CpG island (CGI) methylation level of CRF-BP is elevated in kidney cancer tissues, and DNA methylation is inversely correlated with mRNA expression. Re-expression of CRF-BP is associated with changes in the invasive behavior of kidney cancer cells [65]. These studies suggest that CRF-BP has a suppressive effect on the development and progression of kidney cancer and may be an effective therapeutic target for RCC patients, though its efficacy and safety require further clinical research for validation.

2.2 Bladder Cancer

Bladder cancer is one of the most common malignant tumors in the urinary system, with the primary type being transitional cell carcinoma of the bladder. Its occurrence is associated with factors such as smoking, occupational exposure, and genetics [66]. Treatment options include surgery, chemotherapy, radiation therapy, and immunotherapy. The prognosis for early-stage bladder cancer is relatively favorable, but it is poor for advanced or recurrent bladder cancer. CRH, UCN1, and CRFr have been identified in the bladder of experimental animals [67, 68]. Studies suggest that downregulation of the UCN1 may be associated with bladder cancer, contributing to the prognosis, diagnosis, or treatment of urothelial malignancies [69]. Moreover, a recent study indicates that CRH induces bladder cancer cell migration through the protein kinase B (PKB/AKT) and ERK pathways involving supervillin (SVIL), a membrane-associated and actin-binding protein that actively participates in cancer cell proliferation, dissemination, and migration [70]. Although a relationship between the CRF system and the development of bladder cancer has been proposed, studies focused on this area are limited. More basic research is needed to confirm the association between CRFp and the occurrence and progression of bladder cancer.

2.3 Ovarian Cancer

Ovarian cancer is the third most common gynecological malignancy worldwide, but it has the highest mortality rate among genitourinary system cancers [71]. Treatment primarily includes surgery, chemotherapy, and radiation therapy, but many patients develop resistance to chemotherapy drugs, leading to poor prognosis [72]. CRH has been found in the ovarian cortex, stromal cells, and follicular fluid, while CRF_1 and CRF_2 receptors are expressed in the corpus luteum [73]. Increased staining for CRH and factor-related apoptosis ligand (FasL) is associated with advanced tumor stages [74]. CRH/CRF_1 can act on extravillous trophoblast cells (EVTs), leading to upregulation of FasL expression in ovarian cancer cells. FasL is a molecule released by activated T cells and natural killer cells (NK cells) [74]. It binds to its specific receptor Fas, inducing apoptosis in Fas-bearing cells. Based on this, in ovarian cancers exposed to CRH, Fas/FasL apoptotic compounds may significantly induce apoptosis of activated lymphocytes, thereby helping ovarian cancer cells evade immune responses and promoting the development and progression of ovarian cancer [75]. Exploring CRF_1 antagonists to reduce the immune escape capability of ovarian cancer can lead to the development of new therapeutic strategies for ovarian cancer.

2.4 Endometrial Cancer (EMC)

EMC is a malignancy of the inner epithelial lining of the uterus, with an increasing incidence and disease-associated mortality, worldwide. Perimenopausal and post-menopausal women commonly experience these conditions [76]. Standard treatment methods typically include surgery, radiotherapy, and chemotherapy. Patients diagnosed at an early stage tend to have a better prognosis, whereas those with advanced stage disease generally face a poorer prognosis. Both CRH and UCN1 are expressed in normal uterine tissues as well as in endometrial cancer cells, with their receptors CRF_1 and CRF_2 localized in the cytoplasm of uterine cells, particularly within glandular and stromal cells. Progesterone has been shown to stimulate the expression of CRH, while estradiol inhibits the activity of the CRH promoter [77]. Activation of CRF_1 by CRH can inhibit the proliferation of Ishikawa cells, a well-differentiated human endometrial adenocarcinoma cell line, and promote tumor cell invasiveness and migratory capacity by upregulating the expression of matrix metalloproteinases-2 (MMP-2) and MMP-9 [78, 79]. In contrast, UCN1/CRF_2 system has been found to suppress the migratory ability of tumor cells [80]. Additionally, studies have demonstrated that UCN1 leads to the downregulation of estrogen receptor expression. Researchers hypothesize that the loss of UCN1 activity in endometrial cancer may enhance estrogen-induced malignant cell proliferation and migration [77]. The expression of CRFp and the molecular mechanisms underlying their involvement in the development and progression of endometrial cancer remain incompletely understood, necessitating further research to provide insights for identifying potential therapeutic targets in clinical settings.

2.5 Breast Cancer

Breast cancer is one of the most common malignancies among women, with incidence rates increasing with age, and it is estimated that 90–95% of cases are attributable to environmental factors [81]. Early detection is generally associated with a better prognosis, and treatment options include surgery, radiotherapy, chemotherapy, endocrine therapy, and targeted therapy. CRH expression has been detected in breast cancer biopsies, while CRF_1 has been observed in malignant tissues and breast ductal epithelial cells, and CRF_2 has been identified at sites of perineural invasion [7, 82]. The authors, therefore, hypothesize that the differential localization and biological functions of these two receptors may be involved in the complex interactions between malignant cells and adjacent cells, influencing tumor growth, metastasis, and immune surveillance [82].

Studies have shown that CRH/CRF_1 activation inhibits apoptosis and proliferation in breast cancer cell line MCF-7 cells while simultaneously enhancing their migratory and invasive capabilities [83]. When cells are treated with estradiol, CRF_1 expression increases, whereas CRF_2 expression decreases; however, treatment with

UCN2 promotes tumor cell migration through CRF_2 activation and further enhances estradiol-induced migration [84]. Additional research indicates that CRH and UCN2 induce concentration-dependent apoptosis in cancer cells through upregulation of androgen and vitamin D receptors, as well as activation of heat shock protein 27 (HSP27) [85]. Moreover, CRH inhibits transforming growth factor-β1(TGF-β1)-induced epithelial-mesenchymal transition (EMT), a process often considered the first step in the metastatic cascade, by upregulating E-cadherin expression via both CRF_1 and CRF_2, suggesting a metastasis-suppressive role of CRH in breast cancer [86]. Subsequent studies reveal that UCN inhibits TGF-β1-induced Snail1 and Slug mRNA expression, disrupting TGF-β1-mediated EMT signaling, and attenuates small mothers against decapentaplegic2/3 (Smad2/3)-TGF-β1 signaling through Smad7 upregulation [87]. Snail1 and Slug are considered negative transcriptional regulators of E-cadherin and play a critical role in the EMT transformation of cancer cells through TGF-β1 upregulation. A recent study has linked CRFr signaling with the inhibition of autophagy in malignant tumors. Both CRF_1 and CRF_2 are found to inhibit autophagosome formation by activating the phospholipase C β (PLCβ)-inositol 1,4,5-trisphosphate (IP3)-mammalian target of rapamycin (mTOR) signaling pathway, thereby impeding the conversion of the key marker of autophagy, LC3B-I to LC3B-II. All the data suggest that CRFr activation suppresses autophagy and reduces the migratory potential of malignant MCF-7 cells [88]. These effects may present potential targets for the development of specific CRF_1 or CRF_2 inhibitors.

2.6 Prostate Cancer

Prostate cancer is one of the most common malignancies among men, typically occurring in older males, and is one of the leading causes of cancer-related mortality worldwide [89]. Treatment options include surgery, radiotherapy, chemotherapy, and endocrine therapy. Prostate cancer diagnosed at an early stage generally has a favorable prognosis; however, advanced cases may metastasize, leading to poorer outcomes. Both CRH and UCN1 are expressed in normal epithelial cells, basal cells, stromal smooth muscle, and prostate cancer tissues [90]. CRF_1 and CRF_2 are also expressed in prostate cancer tissues [91, 92]. The loss of CRF_2 expression in prostate cancer and its associated neovasculature has been linked to the initiation, progression, and angiogenesis of prostate tumors [92, 93]. Furthermore, studies have demonstrated that CRH, through CRFr, inhibits the migration of breast cancer cells induced by TGF-β and upregulates $cPLA_2$ expression by increasing IL-1β. In human embryonic kidney 293 (HEK293) cells, CRH/CRF_1 upregulates $cPLA_2$ expression, thereby inducing apoptosis, while UCN2/CRF_2 acts the opposite role. Additionally, both CRH and UCN2 have been shown to induce the migration of prostate cancer RM-1 cells [94]. Similar findings are observed in prostate cancer RM-1 and LNCaP cell lines, where CRH promotes apoptosis, while UCN2 exerts the opposite effect. In addition, it is demonstrated that CRH induces apoptosis by reducing Bcl-2 expression, increasing Bax expression, and hyperpolarizing mitochondrial membrane potential to activate caspase-9, an enzyme that plays a crucial role in the apoptotic process. Conversely, UCN2 increases Bcl-2 expression and decreases Bax expression. The effects of CRH and UCN2 are abolished by selective antagonists of CRF_1 and CRF_2, respectively [91]. In summary, these findings demonstrate the opposing apoptotic roles of CRH/CRF_1 and UCN2/CRF_2 in prostate cancer, suggesting their potential as effective therapeutic targets in future clinical applications.

3 Role of CRFp in Skin Tumors: Melanoma

Melanoma is a malignant tumor originating from melanocytes, commonly found in the skin but also occurring in other areas such as the eyes and ears. It is the most malignant form of skin cancer, characterized by high rates of tumor cell migration and metastasis [95]. Early diagnosis is crucial for treatment. Treatment options include surgical resection, chemotherapy, radiotherapy, targeted therapy, and immunotherapy. The prognosis is generally better in the early stages of melanoma, but the prognosis is poorer in advanced stages due to the high likelihood of metastasis. CRH and UCN1 are expressed in melanocytes, keratinocytes, and fibroblasts in the skin. CRF_1 is expressed in major cell populations in the skin, including the epidermis, dermis, and subcutaneous tissue, while CRF_2 is expressed more limitedly, primarily in follicular keratinocytes and papillary fibroblasts [93, 96].

CRH is a key neuroendocrine regulator traditionally believed to function within the HPA axis by stimulating the production of pro-opiomelanocortin (POMC) through binding to CRFr in the pituitary gland. However, CRH and POMC peptides are not only active in the central nervous system but have also been detected peripherally, particularly in the skin, suggesting that the skin may possess a "local stress response system" [97, 98]. In the skin, the production of CRH and POMC is regulated by inflammatory cells and autocrine mechanisms, like the HPA axis, but with effects confined to the local environment. Under pathological conditions, especially in advanced melanoma, the expression levels of CRH and POMC are significantly increased and are closely associated with tumor progression [99, 100]. This altered expression pattern suggests a potential role for the CRH-POMC axis in skin tumor development. At the molecular level, CRH activates the production of cyclic adenosine monophosphate (cAMP) and IP3 by binding to its receptor CRF_1, thereby regulating cell proliferation through Camp-dependent protein kinase A (PKA) and Ca^{2+}-dependent signaling pathways [101, 102] dependent on cell type and environmental conditions.

In melanocytes, the role of CRH is more complex, exhibiting a dichotomous effect. In serum-containing media, CRH inhibits melanocyte proliferation by blocking the G2 phase, whereas under serum-free conditions, it promotes DNA synthesis [103]. Additionally, CRH induces both early and late apoptotic inhibition in melanocytes, suggesting it may play a significant role in cell survival [103]. These findings highlight the diversity and complexity of CRF_1 in regulating cell viability and proliferation. The expression and function of CRF_1 are also modulated by other signaling pathways, such as the cAMP-dependent pathway and 12-O-tetradecanoylphorbol-13-acetate (TPA), which may affect CRF_1 splicing variants and activity. Furthermore, the function of CRF_1 may be associated with immune cells in the tumor microenvironment. For instance, reduced CRF_1 expression in mast cells can be linked to diminished anti-tumor responses in squamous cell carcinoma and basal cell carcinoma [104]. Moreover, CRFp, such as UCN1, regulate the expression of the tyrosinase-related protein 1 (TRP1) gene, which is involved in pigment production in response to stress, through Nurr-1/Nur77 in human melanoma HMV-II cells [105]. Finally, CRH also participates in the regulation of melanoma cell migration via the ERK1/2 signaling pathway, indicating that CRH plays a crucial role in melanoma cell behavior in the skin, especially under stress conditions [106]. These findings provide new insights into the role of CRH in skin pathophysiology and may offer new therapeutic targets for melanoma treatment.

4 Summary

As pathologic cell proliferation and neoangiogenesis are prerequisite for tumorigenesis and tumor progression, a link between the CRFp/CRFr system and human malignancies has been demonstrated [14, 90, 107]. It is believed that the inhibition of proliferation and the control of angiogenesis are mainly modulated through CRF_2 [32, 108]. These peptide hormones exhibit tissue-specific expression in different tumors and participate in tumor progression by affecting key cellular functions such as proliferation, migration, invasion, and apoptosis. Furthermore, CRFp are involved in the activation and regulation of several important signaling pathways, with abnormal activation of these pathways contributing to tumor progression. Although studies have revealed connections between the CRFp and various systemic cancers, the precise mechanisms through which CRFp influence tumorigenesis and tumor progression still require further elucidation. Future in-depth exploration of the mechanisms by which CRFp operate in tumors holds promise for providing new molecular targets for cancer diagnosis and treatment. It is anticipated that with ongoing research, targeted therapeutic strategies involving CRFp will lead to new breakthroughs in cancer prevention, diagnosis, and treatment, offering patients more hope and more effective treatment options.

References

1. Jehn CF, et al. Association of IL-6, hypothalamus-pituitary-adrenal axis function, and depression in patients with cancer. Integr Cancer Ther. 2010;9(3):270–5.
2. Wu YH, Luo LX. Six transmembrane epithelial antigens of the prostate to illustrate inflammatory response in gastrointestinal cancers. World J Clin Oncol. 2024;15(8):961–4.

3. Bernabe DG, et al. Increased plasma and salivary cortisol levels in patients with oral cancer and their association with clinical stage. J Clin Pathol. 2012;65(10):934–9.
4. Mussi C, et al. Alteration of hypothalamus-pituitary-adrenal glands axis in colorectal cancer patients. Hepato-Gastroenterology. 2003;50(Suppl 2):ccxxviii–ccxxxi.
5. Eagan RT, et al. Lack of value for cisplatin added to mitomycin-doxorubicin combination chemotherapy for carcinoma of unknown primary site. A randomized trial. Am J Clin Oncol. 1987;10(1):82–5.
6. Kaprara A, et al. The corticotropin releasing factor system in cancer: expression and pathophysiological implications. Cell Mol Life Sci. 2010;67(8):1293–306.
7. Ciocca DR, et al. Corticotropin-releasing hormone, luteinizing hormone-releasing hormone, growth hormone-releasing hormone, and somatostatin-like immunoreactivities in biopsies from breast cancer patients. Breast Cancer Res Treat. 1990;15(3):175–84.
8. Faraj Tabrizi P, et al. Cancer-specific loss of Urocortin 3 in human renal cancer. Adv Ther. 2020;37(1):288–99.
9. Dimas A, et al. The expression and possible role of corticotropin-releasing hormone family peptides and their corresponding receptors in gynaecological malignancies and premalignant conditions: a systematic review. Prz Menopauzalny. 2023;22(4):227–35.
10. Balogh B, et al. Urocortin stimulates ERK1/2 phosphorylation and proliferation but reduces ATP production of MCF7 breast cancer cells. Mol Cell Endocrinol. 2022;547:111610.
11. Zhu C, et al. Urocortin affects migration of hepatic cancer cell lines via differential regulation of cPLA2 and iPLA2. Cell Signal. 2014;26(5):1125–34.
12. Jin L, et al. CRH suppressed TGFbeta1-induced epithelial-mesenchymal transition via induction of E-cadherin in breast cancer cells. Cell Signal. 2014;26(4):757–65.
13. Graziani G, et al. Corticotropin-releasing hormone receptor-1 in human endometrial cancer. Oncol Rep. 2006;15(2):375–9.
14. Florio P, et al. Urocortin expression is downregulated in human endometrial carcinoma. J Endocrinol. 2006;190(1):99–105.
15. Kobayashi M, et al. Hypermethylation of corticotropin releasing hormone receptor-2 gene in ulcerative colitis associated colorectal cancer. In Vivo. 2020;34(1):57–63.
16. Dekker E, et al. Colorectal cancer. Lancet. 2019;394(10207):1467–80.
17. Baritaki S, et al. Chronic stress, inflammation, and colon cancer: a CRH system-driven molecular crosstalk. J Clin Med. 2019;8(10)
18. Yamaoka K, Uotsu N, Hoshino E. Relationship between psychosocial stress-induced prefrontal cortex activity and gut microbiota in healthy participants-a functional near-infrared spectroscopy study. Neurobiol Stress. 2022;20:100479.
19. Yi SQ, et al. The role of corticotropin-releasing hormone (CRH) family in tumors. Neoplasma. 2021;68(5):907–16.
20. Herman JP, et al. Regulation of the hypothalamic-pituitary-adrenocortical stress response. Compr Physiol. 2016;6(2):603–21.
21. Dai S, et al. Chronic stress promotes cancer development. Front Oncol. 2020;10:1492.
22. Cui B, et al. Stress-induced epinephrine enhances lactate dehydrogenase a and promotes breast cancer stem-like cells. J Clin Invest. 2019;129(3):1030–46.
23. Grivennikov SI, Greten FR, Karin M. Immunity, inflammation, and cancer. Cell. 2010;140(6):883–99.
24. Labanski A, et al. Stress and the brain-gut axis in functional and chronic-inflammatory gastrointestinal diseases: a transdisciplinary challenge. Psychoneuroendocrinology. 2020;111:104501.
25. Fukudo S, Kanazawa M. Gene, environment, and brain-gut interactions in irritable bowel syndrome. J Gastroenterol Hepatol. 2011;26(Suppl 3):110–5.
26. Rivier J, Spiess J, Vale W. Characterization of rat hypothalamic corticotropin-releasing factor. Proc Natl Acad Sci USA. 1983;80(15):4851–5.
27. Perrin MH, Vale WW. Corticotropin releasing factor receptors and their ligand family. Ann N Y Acad Sci. 1999;885:312–28.

28. Fukudo S. Role of corticotropin-releasing hormone in irritable bowel syndrome and intestinal inflammation. J Gastroenterol. 2007;42(Suppl 17):48–51.
29. Chaniotou Z, et al. Corticotropin-releasing factor regulates TLR4 expression in the colon and protects mice from colitis. Gastroenterology. 2010;139(6):2083–92.
30. Fang X, et al. CRH promotes human colon cancer cell proliferation via IL-6/JAK2/STAT3 signaling pathway and VEGF-induced tumor angiogenesis. Mol Carcinog. 2017;56(11):2434–45.
31. Lee Y, et al. Corticotropin-releasing hormone receptor alters the tumor development and growth in Apcmin/+ mice and in a chemically-induced model of colon cancer. Int J Mol Sci. 2021;22(3)
32. Wang J, et al. Urocortin's inhibition of tumor growth and angiogenesis in hepatocellular carcinoma via corticotrophin-releasing factor receptor 2. Cancer Investig. 2008;26(4):359–68.
33. Guo X, et al. Urocortin-1 promotes colorectal cancer cell migration and proliferation and inhibits apoptosis via inhibition of the p53 signaling pathway. J Cancer Res Clin Oncol. 2024;150(3):163.
34. Lewandowska A, et al. Risk factors for the diagnosis of colorectal cancer. Cancer Control. 2022;29:10732748211056692.
35. Pothoulakis C, et al. CRHR2/Ucn2 signaling is a novel regulator of miR-7/YY1/Fas circuitry contributing to reversal of colorectal cancer cell resistance to Fas-mediated apoptosis. Int J Cancer. 2018;142(2):334–46.
36. Liu Y, et al. The role of corticotropin-releasing hormone receptor 1 in the development of colitis-associated cancer in mouse model. Endocr Relat Cancer. 2014;21(4):639–51.
37. Rodriguez JA, et al. Diminished expression of CRHR2 in human colon cancer promotes tumor growth and EMT via persistent IL-6/Stat3 signaling. Cell Mol Gastroenterol Hepatol. 2015;1(6):610–30.
38. Ducarouge B, et al. CRF2 signaling is a novel regulator of cellular adhesion and migration in colorectal cancer cells. PLoS One. 2013;8(11):e79335.
39. Ramírez-Guerrero AA, et al. Association between genetic variant rs2267716 of CRHR2 gene with colorectal cancer. J Investig Med. 2022;70(4):947–52.
40. Gong SS, et al. Mucosa repair mechanisms of Tong-Xie-Yao-Fang mediated by CRH-R2 in murine, dextran sulfate sodium-induced colitis. World J Gastroenterol. 2018;24(16):1766–78.
41. Hoffman JM, et al. Corticotropin-releasing hormone receptor 2 signaling promotes mucosal repair responses after colitis. Am J Pathol. 2016;186(1):134–44.
42. Panagopoulou M, et al. Methylation status of corticotropin-releasing factor (CRF) receptor genes in colorectal cancer. J Clin Med. 2021;10(12)
43. Im E, et al. Corticotropin-releasing hormone family of peptides regulates intestinal angiogenesis. Gastroenterology. 2010;138(7):2457–67.
44. Llovet JM, et al. Hepatocellular carcinoma. Nat Rev Dis Primers. 2021;7(1):6.
45. Massarweh NN, El-Serag HB. Epidemiology of hepatocellular carcinoma and intrahepatic cholangiocarcinoma. Cancer Control. 2017;24(3):1073274817729245.
46. Charalampopoulos I, et al. Neuropeptide urocortin and its receptors are expressed in rat Kupffer cells. Neuroendocrinology. 2006;84(1):49–57.
47. Zhao Y, et al. CRHR1 mediates p53 transcription induced by high altitude hypoxia through ERK 1/2 signaling in rat hepatic cells. Peptides. 2013;44:8–14.
48. Simopoulos C, et al. Neuropeptide urocortin 1 and its receptors are expressed in the human liver. Neuroendocrinology. 2009;89(3):315–26.
49. Paschos KA, et al. The corticotropin releasing factor system in the liver: expression, actions and possible implications in hepatic physiology and pathology. Hormones (Athens). 2013;12(2):236–45.
50. Behan DP, et al. Cloning and structure of the human corticotrophin releasing factor-binding protein gene (CRHBP). Genomics. 1993;16(1):63–8.
51. Xia HB, et al. Decreased CRHBP expression is predictive of poor prognosis in patients with hepatocellular carcinoma. Oncol Lett. 2018;16(3):3681–9.

52. Wang Z, et al. CRHBP is degraded via autophagy and exerts anti-hepatocellular carcinoma effects by reducing cyclin B2 expression and dissociating cyclin B2-CDK1 complex. Cancer Gene Ther. 2022;29(8–9):1217–27.
53. Smyth EC, et al. Gastric cancer. Lancet. 2020;396(10251):635–48.
54. Yang S, et al. Corticotropin releasing hormone is correlated with tumorigenesis of gastric cancer. Cancer Investig. 2013;31(3):167–71.
55. Chatzaki E, et al. Corticotropin-releasing factor (CRF) receptor type 2 in the human stomach: protective biological role by inhibition of apoptosis. J Cell Physiol. 2006;209(3):905–11.
56. Cheng MF, et al. The association of urocortin expression with clinicopathologic parameters of gastric adenocarcinomas. Appl Immunohistochem Mol Morphol. 2014;22(4):288–94.
57. Weller M, et al. Glioma. Nat Rev Dis Prim. 2024;10(1):33.
58. Feng Y, et al. Human corticotrophin releasing factor inhibits cell proliferation and promotes apoptosis through upregulation of tumor protein p53 in human glioma. Oncol Lett. 2018;15(6):8378–86.
59. Moroz MA, et al. Comparison of corticotropin-releasing factor, dexamethasone, and temozolomide: treatment efficacy and toxicity in U87 and C6 intracranial gliomas. Clin Cancer Res. 2011;17(10):3282–92.
60. Hsieh JJ, et al. Renal cell carcinoma. Nat Rev Dis Prim. 2017;3(1):17009.
61. Czarnecka AM, et al. Hormone signaling pathways as treatment targets in renal cell cancer (review). Int J Oncol. 2016;48(6):2221–35.
62. Tezval H, et al. Urocortin and corticotropin-releasing factor receptor 2 in human renal cell carcinoma: disruption of an endogenous inhibitor of angiogenesis and proliferation. World J Urol. 2009;27(6):825–30.
63. Ma S, et al. A novel gene signature related to oxidative stress predicts the prognosis in clear cell renal cell carcinoma. PeerJ. 2023;11:e14784.
64. Yang K, et al. Integrative analysis reveals CRHBP inhibits renal cell carcinoma progression by regulating inflammation and apoptosis. Cancer Gene Ther. 2020;27(7–8):607–18.
65. Tezval H, et al. Tumor specific epigenetic silencing of corticotropin releasing hormone -binding protein in renal cell carcinoma: Association of Hypermethylation and Metastasis. PLoS One. 2016;11(10):e0163873.
66. Dyrskjøt L, et al. Bladder Cancer Nat Rev Dis Primers. 2023;9(1):58.
67. Hanna-Mitchell AT, et al. Corticotropin-releasing factor family peptide signaling in feline bladder urothelial cells. J Endocrinol. 2014;222(1):113–21.
68. LaBerge J, et al. Expression of corticotropin-releasing factor and CRF receptors in micturition pathways after cyclophosphamide-induced cystitis. Am J Physiol Regul Integr Comp Physiol. 2006;291(3):R692–703.
69. Mavridis C, et al. mRNA expression of CRF family members in urothelial bladder cancer. Oncol Lett. 2024;27(1):13.
70. Mao R, et al. CRH upregulates supervillin through ERK and AKT pathways to promote bladder cancer cell migration. Cell Biol Int. 2024:1–12.
71. Kuroki L, Guntupalli SR. Treatment of epithelial ovarian cancer. BMJ. 2020;371:m3773.
72. Kemppainen J, et al. PET/CT for evaluation of ovarian cancer. Semin Nucl Med. 2019;49(6):484–92.
73. Mastorakos G, et al. Immunoreactive corticotropin-releasing hormone and its binding sites in the rat ovary. J Clin Invest. 1993;92(2):961–8.
74. Morrison AH, Byrne KT, Vonderheide RH. Immunotherapy and prevention of pancreatic cancer. Trends Cancer. 2018;4(6):418–28.
75. Minas V, et al. Intratumoral CRH modulates immuno-escape of ovarian cancer cells through FasL regulation. Br J Cancer. 2007;97(5):637–45.
76. Makker V, et al. Endometrial cancer. Nat Rev Dis Primers. 2021;7(1):88.
77. Makrigiannakis A, et al. Regulation of the promoter of the human corticotropin-releasing hormone gene in transfected human endometrial cells. Neuroendocrinology. 1996;64(2):85–92.

78. Graziani G, et al. CRH inhibits cell growth of human endometrial adenocarcinoma cells via CRH-receptor 1-mediated activation of cAMP-PKA pathway. Endocrinology. 2002;143(3):807–13.
79. Jo YH, et al. Corticotropin-releasing hormone enhances the invasiveness and migration of Ishikawa cells, possibly by increasing matrix metalloproteinase-2 and matrix metalloproteinase-9. J Int Med Res. 2011;39(6):2067–75.
80. Owens GL, et al. Urocortin suppresses endometrial cancer cell migration via CRFR2 and its system components are differentially modulated by estrogen. Cancer Med. 2017;6(2):408–15.
81. Kolak A, et al. Primary and secondary prevention of breast cancer. Ann Agric Environ Med. 2017;24(4):549–53.
82. Kaprara A, et al. Distinct distribution of corticotropin releasing factor receptors in human breast cancer. Neuropeptides. 2010;44(5):355–61.
83. Androulidaki A, et al. Corticotropin releasing factor promotes breast cancer cell motility and invasiveness. Mol Cancer. 2009;8:30.
84. Koureta M, et al. Corticotropin releasing factor receptors in breast cancer: expression and activity in hormone-dependent growth in vitro. Peptides. 2020;129:170316.
85. Jin L, et al. Role of corticotropin-releasing hormone family peptides in androgen receptor and vitamin D receptor expression and translocation in human breast cancer MCF-7 cells. Eur J Pharmacol. 2012;684(1–3):27–35.
86. Jin L, et al. CRH suppressed TGFβ1-induced epithelial-mesenchymal transition via induction of E-cadherin in breast cancer cells. Cell Signal. 2014;26(4):757–65.
87. Jin L, et al. Urocortin attenuates TGFβ1-induced Snail1 and slug expressions: inhibitory role of Smad7 in Smad2/3 signaling in breast cancer cells. J Cell Biochem. 2015;116(11):2494–503.
88. Jin L, et al. Activated CRH receptors inhibit autophagy by repressing conversion of LC3BI to LC3BII. Cell Signal. 2019;58:119–30.
89. Rizzo A, et al. Microbiota and prostate cancer. Semin Cancer Biol. 2022;86(Pt 3):1058–65.
90. Arcuri F, et al. Expression of urocortin mRNA and peptide in the human prostate and in prostatic adenocarcinoma. Prostate. 2002;52(3):167–72.
91. Jin L, et al. Different effects of corticotropin-releasing factor and urocortin 2 on apoptosis of prostate cancer cells in vitro. J Mol Endocrinol. 2011;47(2):219–27.
92. Tezval H, et al. The involvement of altered corticotropin releasing factor receptor 2 expression in prostate cancer due to alteration of anti-angiogenic signaling pathways. Prostate. 2009;69(4):443–8.
93. Slominski A, et al. Differential expression of a cutaneous corticotropin-releasing hormone system. Endocrinology. 2004;145(2):941–50.
94. Jin L, et al. Corticotropin-releasing hormone receptors mediate apoptosis via cytosolic calcium-dependent phospholipase a_2 and migration in prostate cancer cell RM-1. J Mol Endocrinol. 2014;52(3):255–67.
95. Schadendorf D, et al. Melanoma. Nat Rev Dis Prim. 2015;1(1):15003.
96. Pisarchik A, Slominski AT. Alternative splicing of CRH-R1 receptors in human and mouse skin: identification of new variants and their differential expression. FASEB J. 2001;15(14):2754–6.
97. Kono M, et al. In situ expression of corticotropin-releasing hormone (CRH) and proopiomelanocortin (POMC) genes in human skin. FASEB J. 2001;15(12):2297–9.
98. Sato H, et al. The expression of corticotropin-releasing hormone in melanoma. Pigment Cell Res. 2002;15(2):98–103.
99. Funasaka Y, et al. Expression of proopiomelanocortin, corticotropin-releasing hormone (CRH), and CRH receptor in melanoma cells, nevus cells, and normal human melanocytes. J Investig Dermatol Symp Proc. 1999;4(2):105–9.
100. Kim MH, et al. Investigation of the corticotropin-releasing hormone-proopiomelanocortin axis in various skin tumours. Br J Dermatol. 2006;155(5):910–5.
101. Carlson KW, et al. Inhibition of mouse melanoma cell proliferation by corticotropin-releasing hormone and its analogs. Anticancer Res. 2001;21(2a):1173–9.

102. Wiesner B, et al. Intracellular calcium measurements of single human skin cells after stimulation with corticotropin-releasing factor and urocortin using confocal laser scanning microscopy. J Cell Sci. 2003;116(Pt 7):1261–8.
103. Slominski A, et al. CRH functions as a growth factor/cytokine in the skin. J Cell Physiol. 2006;206(3):780–91.
104. Haimakainen S, Harvima IT. Corticotropin-releasing hormone receptor-1 is increased in mast cells in psoriasis and actinic keratosis, but not markedly in keratinocyte skin carcinomas. Exp Dermatol. 2023;32(10):1794–804.
105. Watanuki Y, et al. Involvement of Nurr-1/Nur77 in corticotropin-releasing factor/urocortin1-induced tyrosinase-related protein 1 gene transcription in human melanoma HMV-II cells. Mol Cell Endocrinol. 2013;370(1–2):42–51.
106. Yang Y, et al. Enhancement of cell migration by corticotropin-releasing hormone through ERK1/2 pathway in murine melanoma cell line, B16F10. Exp Dermatol. 2007;16(1):22–7.
107. Wang J, Li S. Corticotropin-releasing factor family and its receptors: tumor therapeutic targets? Biochem Biophys Res Commun. 2007;362(4):785–8.
108. Hao Z, et al. Urocortin2 inhibits tumor growth via effects on vascularization and cell proliferation. Proc Natl Acad Sci USA. 2008;105(10):3939–44.

Chapter 8
CRF Peptides in the Reproductive System

Shengnan Li and Chao Zhu

The evolution of stress response and fertility are considered important aspects driving the fitness of a species [1, 2], which are associated with the central nervous system through the hypothalamic-pituitary-adrenal (HPA) axis and hypothalamic-pituitary-gonadal (HPG) axis, respectively [3, 4]. And a cross talk between HPA and HPG is found [5], stress exerting an influence on fertility, causing fertility reduction and fitness loss threatening species persistence while the end products of HPG helping tune HPA axis-derived stress hormones [2, 5, 6]. Peripherally, many studies demonstrate that reproductive organs/tissues also play an important role in both the fertility and stress via corticotropin-releasing hormone (factor) family system (CRF system), the latter (stress) being precedingly described. In the peripheral reproductive system, CRF peptides (CRFp), including corticotropin-releasing hormone (CRH) and urocortins (UCNs, (UCN1–3)), emerge as critical factors in the process of fertilization and have attracted wide attention [7–10]. CRFp are observed to express similarly to the relevant receptors (CRFr, CRF_1, and CRF_2) in both the female and the male reproductive systems, functioning in an autocrine/paracrine way [11–13]. Moreover, CRF-binding protein (CRF-BP) is found to modulate CRFp levels participating in the process of reproductivity [14, 15]. Understanding the role of the CRF system in the reproductive system is beneficial for exploring therapeutic approaches of CRFp relevance, and indeed, the development of CRH knockout mice has been an important tool for addressing the physiologic and pathologic roles of CRH in fetal development and postnatal life [16]. This chapter will mainly focus on the distribution and role of CRFp in the peripheral reproductive organs.

S. Li · C. Zhu (✉)
Department of Pharmacology, School of Basic Medical Sciences,
Nanjing Medical University, Nanjing, Jiangsu, China
e-mail: czhu@njmu.edu.cn

© The Author(s), under exclusive license to Springer Nature Singapore Pte Ltd. 2025

C. Zhu et al. (eds.), *The Peripheral Existence and Effects of Corticotropin-releasing Factor Family*, https://doi.org/10.1007/978-981-96-5322-5_8

1 CRFp in the Female Reproductive System

Both CRH and UCN1 are reported to exist in the placenta and play a significant role in the pregnancy [17, 18]. Changes in plasma CRH levels during pregnancy are becoming important markers for further exploring the physiological and pathological processes of life birth [19, 20]. It is observed that ovary, endometrium, placenta, and fetal membranes (amnion and chorion) and myometrium are all sources of UCN1, CRFr, and CRF-BP, suggesting that UCN1 function in these tissues in an auto−/paracrine way. In vitro data show that UCN1 plays a critical role in human placenta, stimulating the secretion of corticotrophin (ACTH), prostaglandins, and activin A from cultured human placental cells and regulating placental vessel resistance. UCN1 is also found to stimulate uterine contractility when incubated with myometrial strips [18]. These results suggest that UCN1 plays important roles in the physiology of pregnancy and parturition.

1.1 CRFp in the Placenta

CRFp are found to be highly related to pregnancy due to their role in the placenta. CRH, the selective CRF_1 ligand, is detected in the extracts of human placentas obtained at full term from spontaneous deliveries [17]. Plasma CRH levels are low in nonpregnant women and those in the first trimester of pregnancy [21, 22], even not detectable in some cases [22]. However, in the second trimester of pregnancy, plasma CRH levels become exponentially higher, rising steadily until about 35 weeks and then increasing more rapidly until term from placenta origin [17, 20, 23]. The placental CRH release is bidirectional, into maternal and fetal compartments associated with regulating delivery timing, remodeling the fetal nervous system, and influencing developmental trajectories [17, 24]. Fetal exposure to placental CRH during early and late gestation is linked to unique patterns of cortical thinning in school-age children. Placental CRH is elevated in response to stress, likely being an integrative marker of early adversity [17, 24, 25]. In primary trophoblast cell cultures, it is observed CRH functions in its typical cAMP pathway, stimulating ACTH secretion via cAMP accumulation. In addition, placental CRH secreted into the fetal circulation stimulates fetal pituitary ACTH and adrenal gland dehydroepiandrosterone release in vitro [17]. Plasma CRH level varies in the delivery process, and vaginal delivery is a condition associated with the highest values of maternal CRH levels [26]. It is also reported that both maternal plasma CRH and UCN1 levels are higher in labor than those during pregnancy, almost maintained during the different stages of spontaneous labor [27]. And both term and preterm labor are associated with increased expression of placental CRH [28]. Interestingly, it is observed that CRH in fetal plasma is much lower than in maternal circulation, while the umbilical cord venous plasma has a high CRH level in preterm infants with chronic fetal distress. Moreover, increased cortisol levels in cord plasma are associated with spontaneous vaginal delivery, but not with chronic fetal distress [29]. These findings suggest that the fetal plasma CRH of placental origin may be enhanced in pregnancy complications with chronic fetal distress, while there may not exist any relationship between placental CRH and fetal adrenal function.

On the other hand, increased maternal plasma CRH levels may characterize some gestational diseases. For instance, women with chronic hypertension and pre-eclampsia have high CRH levels [30, 31]. In women delivering preterm, the midgestational plasma CRH levels are higher, and hence, CRH level may be a preterm birth predictor [32, 33], although it is also observed that CRH levels do not significantly change in women delivering preterm [34]. Moreover, in the various pathologic states, maternal plasma and cord CRF-BP levels undergo opposite changes, decreasing to very low levels [17, 35]. The reported results together suggest that the autocrine/paracrine CRH/CRF-BP interaction may play a crucial role in the mechanism of human parturition.

UCN1 is expressed by human placenta, trophoblast, and fetal membranes, which has the same biologic effects as CRH [36, 37], but the expression is observed lower than CRH [7]. UCN1 stimulates myometrial contractility and ACTH and prostaglandin release from cultured human placental cells [18]. Research results reveal that both maternal plasma UCN1 (and CRH) levels are increased in labor, without significant change during the different stages of labor [27]. Leitch and colleagues report that UCN1 exerts potent vasodilatory effects on the human fetal placental circulation in vitro. The vasoactive properties of UCN1 are observed in the human fetal placental vasculature in vitro with single placental lobules bilaterally perfused, showing that the $PGF_{2\alpha}$-induced vasoconstriction is antagonized by arterial infusion of UCN1 causing concentration-dependent vasodilatation, which is significantly attenuated by the CRFr antagonist, α-helical-CRH(9–41) [38]. The vasodilatory effects lead to a hypothesis that UCN1 is produced locally in the placenta to regulate uteroplacental vascular tone during pregnancy, which is confirmed by Clifton and colleagues [39], who report the distribution features of UCN1 in the human placenta, fetal membranes, and uterine tissue at term in both the presence and absence of labor. UCN1 is observed in the vascular smooth muscle of the myometrium, decidual stromal cells, syncytiotrophoblast, and amnion epithelium. Staining intensity for immunoradioactive UCN1 is the greatest in the decidua suggesting decidua being a site of UCN1 production during pregnancy, which is supported by the in vitro experimental data that positive staining for UCN1 is observed in choriodecidual cells with many of them being able to secrete UCN1 under basal conditions. Moreover, UCN1 is detectable also in maternal plasma [39]. These results well address the hypothesis that UCN1 is secreted locally by the placenta (decidua) and may act to regulate uteroplacental blood flow in an auto−/paracrine way. However, there are also reports that UCN1 is not detectable in the placenta and maternal human plasma [40–42]. Only a low concentration of UCN1 in the amniotic fluid at mid-term is detected, which is considered a sign of predisposition to preterm birth [41]. On the other hand, no statistical significant differences are found between amniotic fluid UCN1 concentrations in women with potential preterm labor and those with term delivery, suggesting that UCN1 in the amniotic fluid may not be predictive of preterm labor [42].

The gestational tissues express UCN2 and UCN3 mRNA in cytotrophoblast and syncytiotrophoblast cells, with UCN2 only found in the maternal and fetal vessels and amniotic cells [41]. Despite the expression of UCN2 and UCN3, they do not stimulate placental ACTH secretion as CRH and UCN1. Consistently by location, UCN2 and UCN3 are literally localized in cytotrophoblast and syncytiotrophoblast cells except UCN2 (but not UCN3) being present in maternal and fetal vessels and in amniotic cells [43]. Furthermore, UCN2 and UCN3 are found to affect uterine quiescence by modulating the estradiol secretion from the adjacent placenta. Pepels and colleagues examine UCN2 and UCN3 peptide characterization in third trimester plasma pools, demonstrating that UCN2 stimulates the placental estradiol secretion, which is inhibited by anti-sauvagine-30 (aSvg30), a selective CRF_2 antagonist [44]. Collectively, these reports indicate that placentas of healthy pregnant women do not secrete UCN2 and UCN3 into the plasma, and UCNs can regulate the estradiol secretion from placental tissues via the CRF_2, functioning as auto–/paracrine messengers other than as systemic endocrine messengers.

1.2 CRFp in the Ovary and Endometrium

The ovary and endometrium are the most important female reproductive organ/tissues. The ovarian steroid hormones exert significant influences on endometrial cells, producing and interacting with a variety of growth factors and peptide hormones participating in physiological growth and differentiation during the endometrial cycle, decidualization, and pathological growth and differentiation in endometriosis and cancer [45–49]. CRFp are recognized to be among the significant peptide hormones playing a role in ovary–endometrium functions [18, 50].

The presence of CRH in rat and human ovary is reported [51, 52], and CRH is demonstrated to have an inhibitory effect on fertilized oocytes and suppress ovarian steroidogenesis in vitro [53]. Moreover, CRH is observed to suppress estrogen production by rat and human granulosa cells in vitro [54], whereas granulosa cells are devoid of CRH and CRF_1 mRNAs and proteins [14]. Consistently, CRH and its mRNA are found localized in thecal cells of small antral and mature follicles, with a low abundance in stromal cells, and with CRF_1 mRNA exclusively in thecal cells, higher in mature follicles than in small antral follicles. CRF-BP, but not its gene transcript, is detected in thecal cells and capillary vessels of the thecal/stromal compartment of mature follicles, suggesting its origin out of the ovarian. It is also observed that the increases in intensity of CRH, CRF_1, and 17α-hydroxylase are parallel with follicular maturation [14]. However, a contrary effect of CRH on luteinizing hormone (LH)-stimulated 17α-hydroxylase gene expression and androgen production by isolated thecal cells from human ovarian follicles is presented, i.e., a potent inhibitory effect of CRH on LH-stimulated dehydroepiandrosterone and androstenedione production that appears to be mediated through the reduction of 17α-hydroxylase gene expression [55]. Taken together, these results may suggest that the intraovarian CRF system plays a balancing role in modulating androgen and estrogen biosynthesis, conditioned by the presence of circulating CRF-BP [54, 55]. In the epithelial and stromal cells of the human endometrium, CRH is also expressed in increasing pattern from the endometrial proliferative to the secretory phase. An enhanced expression of CRH in the pregnant endometrium is also observed from early in the pregnancy until term. In addition, progesterone induces CRH gene expression and release from decidualized cells and decidualizing cultured stromal endometrial cells [50]. On the contrary, in women with endometriosis, the endometrial CRH expression and function are abated [56].

In normal cycling human ovaries, UCN1 is detected in luteinized thecal cells of regressing corpora lutea, in which only luteinized thecal cells have the capacity for steroidogenesis [57]. UCN1 is also observed in luteinized granulosa and thecal cells of functioning corpora lutea, in which both cell components are capable of producing steroids. And levels of UCN1 (and CRH, CRF_1, and $CRF_{2\alpha}$) appear significantly higher in the regressing corpus luteum than in the functioning corpus luteum [57]. These findings suggest that UCN1 is locally synthesized in steroidogenic luteal cells and acts on them as an autocrine/paracrine regulator of ovarian steroidogenesis, especially during luteal regression. Moreover, UCN1 gene expression and synthesis are reported in epithelial and stromal cells of the human endometrium [50, 58]. In human endometrium secretory cells (HESCs) isolated from human endometrium collected from healthy volunteers with normal menstrual cycle, it is showed that UCN1 expression is highest in the secretory phase of the menstrual cycle (higher in the late than the early secretory phase). After decidualization of HESCs with cAMP, UCN1 levels rise in parallel with prolactin concentrations. The addition of UCN1 to HESCs induces the release of prolactin [59]. Collectively, these results suggest a possible role of UCN1 in the ovarian-endometrial physiology.

Moreover, UCN1 is found by Petraglia and colleagues to be significantly reduced in endometrial adenocarcinoma compared to healthy controls. Immunohistochemistry assay reveals that immunoreactive UCN1 is expressed in luminal and glandular epithelial cells in healthy, but not in neoplastic, samples [60]. However, a study by the same group report that plasma UCN1 levels are twice as high in endometrioma patients as in the control group (patients with benign ovarian cyst), the peptide being immunolocalized in endometrioma glands and stromal capillary vessels. Moreover, the elevated plasma UCN1 levels detect 88% of the cases of endometrioma, whereas the standard marker, CA125, detects only 65% of the cases [61]. These data suggest that plasma UCN1 may be a useful marker for screening endometrioma and distinguishing endometriomas from other benign ovarian cysts. Furthermore, in vitro experiments reveal that UCN1 suppresses migration of endometrial cancer cells, which is completely eliminated by selective antagonism of CRF_2 but not CRF_1. Activation of estrogen receptor A (ERA) reduces UCN1 expression but only has a small effect on the expression of CRF_1. However, expression of CRF_2 is more notably reduced by activation of ERB. UCN1 in turn reduces both ERA and ERB expression [62]. These findings demonstrate that UCN1 suppresses the migration of endometrial cancer cells via CRF_2 associated with ERs and that loss of UCN1 in endometrial cancer may promote invasion and metastatic spread. In addition, in patients with endometriosis, the serum and peritoneal fluid levels of UCN1 are significantly upregulated, corresponding with more advanced stages of the disease [63]. The predictive value of UCN1 in detecting endometriosis in symptomatic women is carried out by Maia and colleagues. Enrolling prospectively 97 women submitted to endometriosis symptoms, they analyze the sample UCN1 levels. It is observed that patients with endometriosis have higher plasma UCN1 levels, parallel with the increase in chronic pelvic pain, infertility, or both symptoms of endometriosis [64]. The findings suggest that high plasma UCN1 levels may become a marker for endometriosis diagnosis. However, opposite data are also reported, i.e., UCN1 expression and function, as with CRH, are impaired in women with endometriosis [56].

UCN2 and UCN3, the selective CRF_2 ligands, are also found in human ovary–endometrium [65, 66]. Both peptides are immunolocalized in epithelial, stromal, and endothelial cells. And it is observed that UCN2 mRNA is significantly higher in the early proliferative phase of the menstrual cycle than in other phases and maternal decidua (MD) and UCN3 mRNA the highest in MD [66]. Moreover, it is found that UCN3 and CRF_2 mRNAs and proteins are expressed in granulosa lutein cells. And UCN3 is detected in culture media of granulosa lutein cells and follicular fluid. Treatment of cultured granulosa lutein cells with UCN3 decreases progesterone secretion, which is counteracted by the CRF_2 antagonist aSvg30 [9]. These results suggest that UCN2,3/CRF_2 are present in human ovaries inhibiting progesterone production from granulosa lutein cells through interaction with CRF_2. Interestingly, patients with endometriosis show lower endometrial UCN2 and UCN3 mRNA expression, and the expression levels display no endometrial cycle-related changes, suggesting a possible involvement of UCN2 and UCN3 in endometriosis [65].

The expression of CRFr has mostly been described together with the action peptides in the above content. Most recently, CRF_1 and CRF_2 are reported to be associated with polycystic ovarian syndrome. It is observed that CRF_1 and CRF_2 may function as risk factors promoting negative chromatin activation of their related genes in the ovaries, potentially affecting the female cycle and ovulation [67].

1.3 CRFp in the Uterus and Myometrium

Although CRH acting on the myometrium is often considered to be derived from the placenta [68–70], CRH is also found expressed in the myometrium [68, 71]. Most importantly, both CRF_1 and CRF_2 exist in human myometrium, on which CRFp act participating in labor [68, 70, 72], supported by the reports that CRH potently regulates human myometrial contractility [73, 74]. Moreover, expression of CRF-BP, CRF_1, and CRF_2 in uterine tissues is downregulated during pregnancy, with the most pronounced inhibition of CRH-BP and CRF_2 in laboring cervix. The detection of substantial expression of the CRH and the receptor proteins in the cervix suggests that the cervix may be a target site for CRH action [75]. CRF_1 and CRF_2 are found to be predominantly localized at myometrial smooth muscle cells in upper and lower segment myometrium. Interestingly, there exists a modulation variety between the receptors in the upper part and those in the lower part of the myometrium. The level of CRF_1 in the upper segment is significantly downregulated in pregnancy, with a further decrease at the onset of labor, with no change of CRF_1 expression in the lower segment during pregnancy and labor. In contrast, CRF_2 expression remains unchanged in both segments; moreover, $CRF_{2\alpha}$ is identified in pregnant myometrium, while $CRF_{2\beta}$ is observed in nonpregnant myometrium [76]. Furthermore, it is discovered that CRH stimulates production of a number of chemokines and cytokines including IL-1β, IL-6, and TNF-α in cultured uterine smooth muscle cells (USMCs), inducing chemotaxis of monocytes via CRF_1. And cocultures of CRH-treated USMCs with monocytes greatly enhance the levels of these cytokines and chemokines as well as prostaglandins and increase the expression of uterine activation proteins [77], suggesting CRH's participation in uterus inflammation and parturition.

UCN1 is found to be expressed in the myometrium, as well as endometrial epithelial and stromal cells, in the nonpregnant uterus, with no differences between proliferative and secretory phase being observed by immunohistochemistry assay, which are confirmed by reverse PCR analysis of isolated myometrial, endometrial epithelial, and stromal cell specimens [58]. In cultured human pregnant myometrial cells, UCN1 but not CRH is able to induce mitogen-activated protein kinases (MAPK) phosphorylation and activation, suggesting that in the human myometrium UCN1 has distinct action mechanisms and biological roles, which is supported by the observation that CRF_1 and $CRF_{2\beta}$ mediate UCN1-induced MAPK activation via Gq-IP3-protein kinase C (PKC) pathway [78]. On the other hand, in human gestational myometrium, mRNA expression of UCN1 is low but with high expression of CRF_1 and CRF_2 [7], suggesting that the reported UCN1 participating in the myometrial contractility and labor may come from placenta or fetal secretion [8, 79].

Expression of UCN2/CRF_2 in human/mouse myometrium and inflammatory mediators in myometrial cell lines is also reported [11, 80, 81]. UCN2 but not CRF_2 is observed to be upregulated in human tissues in labor. In myometrium cell lines, UCN2 is upregulated by TNF-α via NF-κB through CRF_2 [11]. Consistently, both UCN2 and CRF_2 mRNAs are found expressed in human nonpregnant and pregnant myometrium [80]. Treatment of primary human myometrial cells with UCN2 results in a dose-dependent increase of myosin light chain (MLC) phosphorylation contributing to the contractility enhancement, involving the activation of PKC and extracellular signal-regulated kinase (ERK1/2). Inhibitors of MAPK kinase 1 (U0126) and PKC (bisindolylmaleimide) blunt the UCN2-induced phosphorylation of MLC [80]. In cultured human uterine smooth muscle cells from pregnant women at term, UCN1 and UCN3 treatment promote PGE_2 and $PGF_{2\alpha}$ secretion in a dose-dependent manner. In contrast, UCN2 inhibits PGE_2 and $PGF_{2\alpha}$ secretion. Furthermore, UCN1 and UCN3 suppress cAMP production and lead to Gi activation, while UCN2 stimulates cAMP production and activates Gs signaling [81].

1.4 CRFp in the Breast

Data about CRFp in the breast are relatively few, of which most are focused on their possible relation with breast tumors.

CRH stimulates cell motility and invasiveness of breast carcinoma cell line, MCF-7 cells [82]. In human breast tumors, CRF_1 transcripts are found in 20^+ percent of benign and malignant biopsies while CRF_{2a} in 22.2% of benign and 36.0% of malignant biopsies [83]. Similarly to breast cancer biopsies, the predominant receptor type expressed in the MCF-7 cell line is $CRF_{2\alpha}$. The transcription of CRF_1 and CRF_2 is up- and downregulated, respectively, by exposure to estradiol, and CRF_1 methylation is found to be positively associated with the presence of steroid hormone receptors. And specific activation of CRF_2 increases the cells' migration and potentiates an estrogen-inducing effect [84]. In the estrogen receptor-positive (ER+) malignant mammary epithelial cell line MCF-7, CRH activates numerous kinases and downstream effectors via CRF_1 and increases the transcription of genes encoding factors associated with estrogen signaling [85]. Interestingly, CRH is observed to inhibit the migration of human breast cancer cells through downregulation of the hallmark of epithelial-mesenchymal transition (EMT), Snail1, and Twist1 [86]. Moreover, CRH significantly inhibits cell growth induced by estradiol, which is not associated with the induction of apoptosis. CRH inhibition of cell proliferation is counteracted by the nonselective CRFr antagonist, astressin, as well as by a CRF_1 selective receptor antagonist, antalarmin [87].

1.5 CRF-BP Modulation of CRFp Effects

As already mentioned above, a local CRF-BP is found in placenta and intrauterine tissues to modulate the paracrine effects of CRH and UCN1, participating in the processes of pregnancy and labor [8, 15, 35]. In nonpregnant women, plasma CRH levels are low. During the first and second trimesters of pregnancy, CRH levels become higher, and a clear increase is obvious at term, while CRF-BP levels decrease. Moreover, women with preterm labor show high CRH and low CRF-BP levels. These results support an involvement of CRF-BP modulating CRFp levels in pregnancy and parturition [8].The human ovaries may not be an origin of CRF-BP since its transcript is not detected [14].

2 CRFp in the Male Reproductive System

Central CRH exerts an inhibitory action on male reproductive process, supported by the facts that in the male rats, intraventricular injection of synthetic oCRH causes a significant decrease in plasma LH and testosterone levels [88] and that CRH-induced activation of cells in the brain decreases the ability of gonadotropin to release testosterone independently of the pituitary [89]. The distribution and direct roles of CRFp (CRH and UCNs) in reproductive organs (mainly testis and prostate) have also attracted much attention, which is summarized as follows.

2.1 *CRFp in the Testis*

Analysis performed on extracts of adult rat testes reveals a high concentration of CRH, while the peripheral blood level of CRH is extremely low [90], suggesting that the detected CRH originates from the local sites (also consistent with the fact that central CRH is bound to CRF-BP [91] and has a short half-life in plasma [92]). Immunocytochemical studies show strong CRH-specific staining in the Leydig cells, germ cells, and epididymal spermatozoa in normal adult rat testis. And neither hemicastration nor unilateral cryptorchidism influences the CRH levels in the contralateral testis, further confirming a local production of CRH influencing Leydig cell function and sperm maturation [90]. Moreover, cultured rat Leydig cells secret considerable amounts of CRH. And in the testis, CRH is found to act as an anti-reproductive hormone and a major local inhibitory regulator of Leydig cell function. In contrast, the Leydig cell-derived CRH is mainly stimulated by the trophic hormone LH/human chorionic gonadotropin (hCG) [93]. Ulisse and colleagues find that in cultured fetal and adult Leydig cells, CRH inhibits hCG-induced androgen production, with no effect on basal testosterone secretion. And a marked reduction of steroid precursors of the androgen by CRH is observed during hCG stimulation, which is fully reversed by 8-bromo-cAMP but is not affected by pertussis toxin. Interestingly, CRH causes no changes in hCG binding to Leydig cells, and in contrast to other target tissues, CRH does not stimulate cAMP production, which can be interpreted by that the CRH/CRFr are not coupled to Gs in Leydig cells [94], suggesting a novel mechanism of CRH's anti-reproductive effect at the testicular level. Subsequently, participation of PKC in these CRH actions in the Leydig cells is observed [95], which is in line with the CRH action mechanism of elevating intracellular Ca^{2+} via PKC in the rat pheochromocytoma cell line [96]. It is observed that CRH causes a rapid translocation of PKC in Leydig cells, which is prevented by PKC inhibitors or 12-O-tetradecanoylphorbol-13-acetate (TPA)-induced depletion of PKC. And binding of ^{125}I-oCRH to Leydig cell membranes is reduced by GTP and guanyl-5′-yl imidodiphosphate (Gpp(NH)p). Moreover, CRH causes a time-dependent inhibition of hCG-induced cAMP generation and steroidogenesis, which is reversed by 8-bromo-cAMP. Also, CRH and TPA are able to inhibit the stimulation of cAMP and testosterone production by forskolin. In CRH-treated cells, adenylate cyclase stimulation by Gpp(NH)p is also markedly inhibited [95]. Taken together, these results suggest that CRFr interact with a pertussis toxin-insensitive G protein in the Leydig cell and that the inhibitory action of CRH is exerted mainly on the catalytic subunit of adenylate cyclase through a direct or indirect action of PKC. In addition, in hamster Leydig cells, CRH is shown to activate tyrosine phosphatases and subsequently reduce the phosphorylation levels of kinases ERK and JNK, inhibiting the production of testosterone [97].

Interestingly, the secretion of CRH by the Leydig cell is stimulated by LH, acting via release of serotonin (5-HT) and autocrine activation of 5-HT2 receptors [10, 98], and in turn, 5-HT stimulates CRH secretion, being even more effective than hCG, which is inhibited by the 5-HT2A inhibitor, ketanserin. Moreover, 5-HT-stimulated CRH inhibits basal and hCG-induced cAMP generation and steroidogenesis. Furthermore, 5-HT mediates the stimulatory action of LH/hCG on CRH secretion from Leydig cells [99]. And ketanserin inhibits testosterone secretion by rat Leydig cells in vitro [100]. Immunohistochemical studies reveal specific staining of 5-HT in interstitial cells of the adult rat testis, and adult Leydig cells are found to be able to secret considerable quantities of 5-HT, acutely stimulated by hCG and forskolin, while TPA is much less effective, indicating a major role for cAMP in hCG-induced 5-HT release. Similar increases of 5-HT release by hCG are observed in the absence of extracellular Ca^{2+}. However, ionomycin is a potent stimulus of 5-HT release, indicating that elevation of cytoplasmic Ca^{2+} could also induce the secretion. [98]. Moreover, as described above, 5-HT stimulates CRH secretion but inhibits basal and hCG-stimulated cAMP generation and testosterone production, the latter inhibitory action of 5-HT being prevented by a CRH antibody and α-helical CRH(9–41). In accordance, the selective 5-HT2 receptor agonist 1-[2,5-dimethoxy-4-iodophyryl]2-amino propane hydrochloride (DOI) mimics 5-HT stimulating CRH secretion and inhibiting hCG-stimulated cAMP generation and testosterone production, while agonists of other types of 5-HT receptors are less effective. Moreover, the selective 5-HT2 receptor antagonist ketanserin prevents the effects of CRH and DOI. Also, ketanserin increases sensitivity to hCG and raises maximal cAMP and testosterone production [99].

On the contrary, CRH is also reported to directly stimulate testosterone production in mouse Leydig cells [13, 101–104], although it does not influence the maximum hCG-induced testosterone production. The effect is antagonized by the CRFr antagonist α-helical CRH(9–41) and accompanied by intracellular cAMP elevation. Furthermore, the positive response of mouse Leydig cells to oCRH corresponds to that measured in COS cells expressing CRF_1 instead of $CRF_{2\alpha}$ or $CRF_{2\beta}$ [104]. These results demonstrate that mouse Leydig cells express CRF_1, mediating elevation of testosterone production, which is inconsistent with the most reported negative regulating effects described above. The difference may be attributed to different species, supported by the findings that CRFp have no influence on the basal testosterone and that both CRFr agonists and antagonist do not change the hCG-stimulated testosterone production in rat Leydig cells [104].

Interestingly, CRH regulation of testosterone varies by age, which is supported by the results that mouse fetal Leydig cells and adult Leydig cells differ in CRFr expression and testosterone synthesis mechanism [105]. In neonatal rats, the promoting role of CRH in the regulation of testicular functions is found, CRH being a local stimulator of steroidogenesis. Using anti-CRH-antiserum injected intratesticularly to newborn rats with two testes and to hemicastrates, it is observed that the anti-CRH serum has an obvious effect on the hemicastration, resulting in a decrease in serum testosterone concentration and basal testosterone secretion in vitro. Unilateral testicular injection of the anti-CRH serum in rats with two testes also results in a significant drop in serum testosterone level with no change in basal testosterone production [106]. Similar stimulatory effects of CRH are reported in fetal testes. A comparative analysis of rodent fetal testis microarray datasets reveals 54 candidate fetal Leydig cell-specific genes, of which CRF_1 expression in fetal mouse testis is verified by in situ hybridization, which is tested for a steroidogenic function using ex vivo fetal testes through the selective agonist, CRH. The results show that CRH increases expression of the steroidogenic genes in mouse and rat testes and testosterone production is increased, which is blunted by CRF_1 antagonist. Similarly, CRH exposure of MA-10 Leydig cells increases steroidogenic pathway mRNA and progesterone levels, showing CRH can enhance steroidogenesis by directly targeting Leydig cells [13]. In addition, in vivo investigations show that CRH exerts similar dual effects on β-endorphin (β-EP) secretion in the rat testis. In the pubertal rat, intratesticular infusion of CRH results in a three-fold stimulation of β-EP levels in testicular interstitial fluid, which is reversed by the antagonist CRH(12–41); however, in adult animals, CRH is found without effect, suggesting a developmental regulation of CRH action on β-EP secretion in the rat testis [107]. Inconsistently, CRH is also observed to stimulate β-EP secretion from adult rat Leydig cells in vitro. A reverse hemolytic plaque assay and immunocytochemistry with Leydig cell-specific antibodies indicate that in normal rat primary Leydig cell cultures, increasing concentrations of CRH result in a drastic increase in both the percentage of plaque-forming cells and the mean plaque size, which is abolished by the CRH antagonist, CRH(9–41), demonstrating that Leydig cells have functional CRFr and that their β-EP secretion is stimulated by CRH [108].

Besides CRH, strong signals for UCN1 in the rat testis are observed, with weaker levels of UCN2 and UCN3. UCN1 gene expression is corroborated by immunohistochemical detection, which is restricted to Leydig cells. Moreover, in rats exposed to alcohol, significant increase in testicular UCN1 is observed, but not UCN2, UCN3, CRH, CRF_1, or CRF_2 mRNA levels [109], implying a relationship among alcohol, UCN1, and male reproduction. In human adult testes, UCN1 mRNA is present, and the peptide is expressed in elongating spermatids, mature spermatozoa, and peritubular myoid cells, but to a lesser extent in Leydig cells. But the two distinct CRFr are located differently, with CRF_1 mainly in spermatogonia, spermatocytes, and Leydig cells, and CRF_2 mostly in spermatogonia [110]. The separate location of UCN1 and CRFr may indicate a complicated action of UCN1 in the course of spermatogenesis. UCN1 and the CRF_1-selective peptide Stressin1, but not UCN2 or UCN3, significantly inhibit the rat testosterone response to hCG. Moreover, the effects of exogenous UCN1 systemically or directly used into the testes are reversed by the unselective CRFr antagonist astressin, but not interfered by blockade of GnRH receptors, eliminating the pituitary LH's involvement in this rat model [111]. It is noteworthy that CRFr antagonists are unable to reverse the inhibitory effect exerted by alcohol on hCG-induced testosterone release, which is hard to interpret since alcohol upregulates gonadal UCN1 gene expression as mentioned above [111]. In mouse testis, both UCN1 mRNA and peptide are obviously expressed in mature spermatozoa, whereas CRF_1 and CRF_2 are expressed in spermatocytes and spermatogonia, respectively. Double-immunostaining results show that UCN1 expression decreases with acrosome reaction proceeding with UCN1 significantly inhibiting acrosome reaction initiated by progesterone and decreasing spermatozoa motility, which is also un-interpretably not affected by astressin, an unselective CRFr antagonist. In addition, UCN1 decreases intracellular Ca^{2+} in spermatozoa [112].

Adding to the above contents, CRH is also isolated and sequenced from ovine testes [113]. And rare reports about CRH and UCNs' roles in ovine testicular functions are available.

2.2 CRFp in the Prostate

In the human prostates and some prostate-related cells, the expression of CRFp and CRFr is reported and referred as being associated with prostate cancer [18, 114, 115]. It shows that UCN1 mRNA and peptide are demonstrated in the human gland. In nonneoplastic prostate tissues, UCN1 is localized in the secretory luminal epithelial and basal layer cells, in the smooth muscle component of the stroma, and in lymphoid infiltrates. And in prostate adenocarcinoma cells, UCN1 expression is also observed, suggesting a potential involvement of UCN1 in prostate physiopathology [115]. Moreover, both CRF_1 and CRF_2 are expressed in the mouse prostate cancer cell line RM-1. CRH promotes apoptosis, while UCN2 exerts the opposite effect, CRH reducing Bcl-2 but inducing Bax expression, which is abolished by CRF_1 selective antagonist, antalarmin, while UCN2 increasing Bcl-2 but decreasing Bax expression, which is reversed by CRF_2 selective antagonist, aSvg30 [116]. Furthermore, cytosolic calcium-dependent phospholipase A_2 ($cPLA_2$) is found to bridge CRFr activations-Bcl-2/Bax ratio and cell migration. Silencing of $cPLA_2$ attenuates CRH-induced apoptosis and the decrease in Bcl-2/Bax ratio whereas aggravates UCN2-inhibited apoptosis and the increase in Bcl-2/Bax ratio, demonstrating $cPLA_2$'s participation in CRF_1-induced apoptosis and CRF_2-inhibited apoptosis [117].

As reported, activation of CRF_2 inhibits tumor growth by regulation of proliferation and apoptosis as well as suppression of vascularization [118–121]. It is observed that human normal prostate lysates exhibit specific signals for CRF_2 mRNA while lysates of prostate cancer exhibit no signal for CRF_2 mRNA. Moreover, the smooth muscle components of the stroma and endothelial cells of blood vessels highly express CRF_2 [114, 122], whereas the tumoral neovascular system and stroma exhibit no indication for CRF_2. These results demonstrate that human benign prostate tissue and prostate cancer specimen differentially express CRF_2 and the loss of CRF_2 in prostate cancer and its neovascularization may contribute to prostate tumorigenesis, progression, and neoangiogenesis [122]. Moreover, besides the abundancy of mRNA of CRF_2 in human prostate lysates, CRF_2 is expressed in the cytoplasm of basal and luminal epithelial cells as well as in cystic glands. Smooth muscle components of the stroma and vascular endothelial cells show extensive expression of CRF_2 [114].

On the other hand, the relationship of CRF_1 with human prostate cancer is rarely reported. In accordance, in a case report of a man with a large pituitary tumor and a prostatic cancer, the histological examinations reveal that anti-CRH antibodies do not show any binding in the prostatic cancer [123], suggesting the CRF_1-selective ligand, CRH, is absent in the prostatic cancer tissue.

3 Summary

The major content of this chapter is as summarized in Fig. 8.1. Besides CRH's central inhibitory effect on reproduction, CRFp have been found to play a direct role in the peripheral reproductive system. Both CRH and UCNs and the two distinct

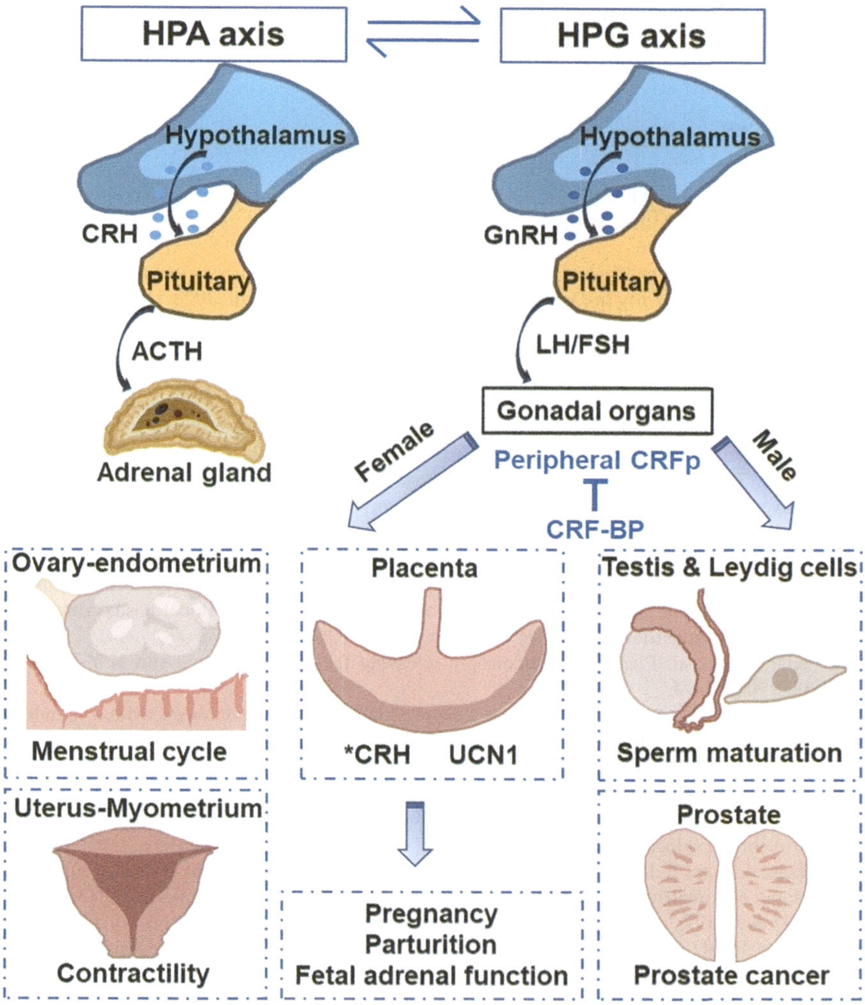

Fig. 8.1 The distribution and role of CRFp in the reproductive system. *Plasma CRH level also increases during pregnancy originating from the placenta

receptors, CRF_1 and CRF_2, are locally expressed in the reproductive system. Up-to-date, more data about CRFp are obtained with the female reproductive functions. CRH and UCNs are observed to have a significant association with human pregnancy and may function actively during the labor. Moreover, CRFp levels' change may be associated with some diseases, both maternal and fetal. In the male reproductive system, CRH and UCN1 are found in the testis Leydig cells, influencing the production of testosterone. And in human prostate, CRFp, especially UCN1, is found to be related to prostate cancer via CRF_2 regulating neovascularization. Attention worth being paid to is that locally produced CRF-BP in placenta and intrauterine tissues is reported to be related to CRH and UCN1 levels during pregnancy and labor. Taken together, given their significant influence, the local CRF system may become a useful target for disorders of reproductive relevance.

References

1. Lovejoy DA, Barsyte-Lovejoy D. Systems approaches to genomic and epigenetic inter-regulation of peptide hormones in stress and reproduction. Prog Biophys Mol Biol. 2013;113(3):375–86.
2. Canal Domenech B, Fricke C. Developmental heat stress interrupts spermatogenesis inducing early male sterility in *Drosophila melanogaster*. J Therm Biol. 2023;114:103589.
3. Smith SM, Vale WW. The role of the hypothalamic-pituitary-adrenal axis in neuroendocrine responses to stress. Dialogues Clin Neurosci. 2006;8(4):383–95.
4. Spaziani M, et al. Hypothalamo-pituitary axis and puberty. Mol Cell Endocrinol. 2021;520:111094.
5. Oyola MG, Handa RJ. Hypothalamic-pituitary-adrenal and hypothalamic-pituitary-gonadal axes: sex differences in regulation of stress responsivity. Stress. 2017;20(5):476–94.
6. Kozicz T, et al. Chronic psychosocial stress affects corticotropin-releasing factor in the paraventricular nucleus and central extended amygdala as well as urocortin 1 in the non-preganglionic Edinger-Westphal nucleus of the tree shrew. Psychoneuroendocrinology. 2008;33(6):741–54.
7. Sehringer B, et al. mRNA expression profiles for corticotrophin-releasing hormone, urocortin, CRH-binding protein and CRH receptors in human term gestational tissues determined by real-time quantitative RT-PCR. J Mol Endocrinol. 2004;32(2):339–48.
8. Fadalti M, et al. Placental corticotropin-releasing factor. An update. Ann N Y Acad Sci. 2000;900:89–94.
9. Yata A, et al. Suppression of progesterone production by stresscopin/urocortin 3 in cultured human granulosa-lutein cells. Hum Reprod. 2009;24(7):1748–53.
10. Dufau ML, Tinajero JC, Fabbri A. Corticotropin-releasing factor: an antireproductive hormone of the testis. FASEB J. 1993;7(2):299–307.
11. Voltolini C, et al. Urocortin 2 role in placental and myometrial inflammatory mechanisms at parturition. Endocrinology. 2015;156(2):670–9.
12. Vergetaki A, et al. Differential expression of CRH, UCN, CRHR1 and CRHR2 in eutopic and ectopic endometrium of women with endometriosis. PLoS One. 2013;8(4):e62313.
13. McDowell EN, et al. A transcriptome-wide screen for mRNAs enriched in fetal Leydig cells: CRHR1 agonism stimulates rat and mouse fetal testis steroidogenesis. PLoS One. 2012;7(10):e47359.
14. Asakura H, Zwain IH, Yen SS. Expression of genes encoding corticotropin-releasing factor (CRF), type 1 CRF receptor, and CRF-binding protein and localization of the gene products in the human ovary. J Clin Endocrinol Metab. 1997;82(8):2720–5.

15. Petraglia F, et al. Corticotropin-releasing factor-binding protein is produced by human placenta and intrauterine tissues. J Clin Endocrinol Metab. 1993;77(4):919–24.
16. Vuppaladhadiam L, et al. Corticotropin-releasing factor family: a stress hormone-receptor system's emerging role in mediating sex-specific signaling. Cells. 2020;9(4)
17. Reis FM, et al. Putative role of placental corticotropin-releasing factor in the mechanisms of human parturition. J Soc Gynecol Investig. 1999;6(3):109–19.
18. Florio P, Vale W, Petraglia F. Urocortins in human reproduction. Peptides. 2004;25(10):1751–7.
19. Kalantaridou SN, et al. Roles of reproductive corticotropin-releasing hormone. Ann N Y Acad Sci. 2003;997:129–35.
20. Mastorakos G, Ilias I. Maternal hypothalamic-pituitary-adrenal axis in pregnancy and the postpartum period. Postpartum-related disorders. Ann N Y Acad Sci. 2000;900:95–106.
21. Liapi CA, et al. Corticotropin-releasing-hormone levels in pregnancy-induced hypertension. Eur J Obstet Gynecol Reprod Biol. 1996;68(1–2):109–14.
22. Goland RS, et al. High levels of corticotropin-releasing hormone immunoactivity in maternal and fetal plasma during pregnancy. J Clin Endocrinol Metab. 1986;63(5):1199–203.
23. Sandman CA. Prenatal CRH: an integrating signal of fetal distress. Dev Psychopathol. 2018;30(3):941–52.
24. Mastorakos G, Ilias I. Maternal and fetal hypothalamic-pituitary-adrenal axes during pregnancy and postpartum. Ann N Y Acad Sci. 2003;997:136–49.
25. Weinstock M. The potential influence of maternal stress hormones on development and mental health of the offspring. Brain Behav Immun. 2005;19(4):296–308.
26. Okamoto E, et al. Immunoreactive corticotropin-releasing hormone, adrenocorticotropin and cortisol in human plasma during pregnancy and delivery and postpartum. Horm Metab Res. 1989;21(10):566–72.
27. Florio P, et al. Levels of maternal plasma corticotropin-releasing factor and urocortin during labor. J Soc Gynecol Investig. 2002;9(4):233–7.
28. Torricelli M, et al. Labor (term and preterm) is associated with changes in the placental mRNA expression of corticotrophin-releasing factor. Reprod Sci. 2007;14(3):241–5.
29. Ruth V, Hallman M, Laatikainen T. Corticotropin-releasing hormone and cortisol in cord plasma in relation to gestational age, labor, and fetal distress. Am J Perinatol. 1993;10(2):115–8.
30. Campbell EA, et al. Plasma corticotropin-releasing hormone concentrations during pregnancy and parturition. J Clin Endocrinol Metab. 1987;64(5):1054–9.
31. Laatikainen T, et al. Corticotropin-releasing hormone in maternal and cord plasma in preeclampsia. Eur J Obstet Gynecol Reprod Biol. 1991;39(1):19–24.
32. Herrera CL, et al. Revisiting the placental clock: early corticotrophin-releasing hormone rise in recurrent preterm birth. PLoS One. 2021;16(9):e0257422.
33. Ruiz RJ, et al. CRH as a predictor of preterm birth in minority women. Biol Res Nurs. 2016;18(3):316–21.
34. Torricelli M, et al. Amniotic fluid urocortin, CRF, oestriol, dehydroepiandrosterone sulfate and cortisol concentrations at mid-trimester: putative relationship with preterm delivery. Eur J Obstet Gynecol Reprod Biol. 2009;146(2):169–73.
35. Petraglia F, et al. Cord plasma corticotropin-releasing factor-binding protein (CRF-BP) in term and preterm labour. Placenta. 1997;18(2–3):115–9.
36. Petraglia F, et al. Human placenta and fetal membranes express human urocortin mRNA and peptide. J Clin Endocrinol Metab. 1996;81(10):3807–10.
37. Li W, Challis JR. Corticotropin-releasing hormone and urocortin induce secretion of matrix metalloproteinase-9 (MMP-9) without change in tissue inhibitors of MMP-1 by cultured cells from human placenta and fetal membranes. J Clin Endocrinol Metab. 2005;90(12):6569–74.
38. Leitch IM, et al. Vasodilator actions of urocortin and related peptides in the human perfused placenta in vitro. J Clin Endocrinol Metab. 1998;83(12):4510–3.
39. Clifton VL, et al. Localization and characterization of urocortin during human pregnancy. Placenta. 2000;21(8):782–8.

40. Glynn BP, et al. Urocortin in pregnancy. Am J Obstet Gynecol. 1998;179(2):533–9.
41. Vitale SG, et al. Role of urocortin in pregnancy: an update and future perspectives. World J Clin Cases. 2016;4(7):165–71.
42. Iavazzo C, et al. Urocortin in second trimester amniotic fluid: its role as predictor of preterm labor. Mediat Inflamm. 2009;2009:947981.
43. Imperatore A, et al. Urocortin 2 and urocortin 3 are expressed by the human placenta, deciduas, and fetal membranes. Am J Obstet Gynecol. 2006;195(1):288–95.
44. Pepels PP, et al. Placental urocortin-2 and -3: endocrine or paracrine functioning during healthy pregnancy? Placenta. 2010;31(6):475–81.
45. Jeon SY, Hwang KA, Choi KC. Effect of steroid hormones, estrogen and progesterone, on epithelial mesenchymal transition in ovarian cancer development. J Steroid Biochem Mol Biol. 2016;158:1–8.
46. Gellersen B, Brosens J. Cyclic AMP and progesterone receptor cross-talk in human endometrium: a decidualizing affair. J Endocrinol. 2003;178(3):357–72.
47. Bishop CV, et al. Evaluation of antral follicle growth in the macaque ovary during the menstrual cycle and controlled ovarian stimulation by high-resolution ultrasonography. Am J Primatol. 2009;71(5):384–92.
48. Chou CH, Chen MJ. The effect of steroid hormones on ovarian follicle development. Vitam Horm. 2018;107:155–75.
49. Liu YX, et al. Regulation of follicular development and differentiation by intra-ovarian factors and endocrine hormones. Front Biosci (Landmark Ed). 2019;24(5):983–93.
50. Florio P, et al. Paracrine regulation of endometrial function: interaction between progesterone and corticotropin-releasing factor (CRF) and activin a. Steroids. 2003;68(10–13):801–7.
51. Mastorakos G, et al. Immunoreactive corticotropin-releasing hormone and its binding sites in the rat ovary. J Clin Invest. 1993;92(2):961–8.
52. Mastorakos G, et al. Presence of immunoreactive corticotropin-releasing hormone in normal and polycystic human ovaries. J Clin Endocrinol Metab. 1994;79(4):1191–7.
53. Dinopoulou V, et al. The effect of CRH and its inhibitor, antalarmin, on in vitro growth of preantral mouse follicles, early embryo development, and steroidogenesis. Endocrinology. 2013;154(1):222–31.
54. Ghizzoni L, et al. Corticotropin-releasing hormone (CRH) inhibits steroid biosynthesis by cultured human granulosa-lutein cells in a CRH and interleukin-1 receptor-mediated fashion. Endocrinology. 1997;138(11):4806–11.
55. Erden HF, et al. Corticotropin-releasing factor inhibits luteinizing hormone-stimulated P450c17 gene expression and androgen production by isolated thecal cells of human ovarian follicles. J Clin Endocrinol Metab. 1998;83(2):448–52.
56. Novembri R, et al. Impaired CRH and urocortin expression and function in eutopic endometrium of women with endometriosis. J Clin Endocrinol Metab. 2011;96(4):1145–50.
57. Muramatsu Y, et al. Urocortin and corticotropin-releasing factor receptor expression in normal cycling human ovaries. J Clin Endocrinol Metab. 2001;86(3):1362–9.
58. Florio P, et al. Identification of urocortin mRNA and peptide in the human endometrium. J Endocrinol. 2002;173(2):R9–14.
59. Torricelli M, et al. Secretory endometrium highly expresses urocortin messenger RNA and peptide: possible role in the decidualization process. Hum Reprod. 2007;22(1):92–6.
60. Florio P, et al. Urocortin expression is downregulated in human endometrial carcinoma. J Endocrinol. 2006;190(1):99–105.
61. Florio P, et al. Plasma urocortin levels in the diagnosis of ovarian endometriosis. Obstet Gynecol. 2007;110(3):594–600.
62. Owens GL, et al. Urocortin suppresses endometrial cancer cell migration via CRFR2 and its system components are differentially modulated by estrogen. Cancer Med. 2017;6(2):408–15.
63. Abramiuk M, et al. Possible correlation between Urocortin 1 (Ucn1) and immune parameters in patients with endometriosis. Int J Mol Sci. 2023;24(9)

64. Maia LM, et al. Plasma urocortin-1 as a preoperative marker of endometriosis in symptomatic women. Gynecol Endocrinol. 2018;34(3):202–5.
65. Novembri R, et al. Urocortin 2 and urocortin 3 in endometriosis: evidence for a possible role in inflammatory response. Mol Hum Reprod. 2011;17(9):587–93.
66. Florio P, et al. Human endometrium expresses urocortin II and III messenger RNA and peptides. Fertil Steril. 2006;86(6):1766–70.
67. Amin M, et al. Novel corticotropin-releasing hormone receptor genes (CRHR1 and CRHR2) linkage to and association with polycystic ovary syndrome. J Ovarian Res. 2023;16(1):155.
68. Grammatopoulos DK, Hillhouse EW. Role of corticotropin-releasing hormone in onset of labour. Lancet. 1999;354(9189):1546–9.
69. Grammatopoulos DK, Hillhouse EW. Basal and interleukin-1beta-stimulated prostaglandin production from cultured human myometrial cells: differential regulation by corticotropin-releasing hormone. J Clin Endocrinol Metab. 1999;84(6):2204–11.
70. Grammatopoulos DK. Placental corticotrophin-releasing hormone and its receptors in human pregnancy and labour: still a scientific enigma. J Neuroendocrinol. 2008;20(4):432–8.
71. Karteris E, et al. Expression and signalling characteristics of the corticotrophin-releasing hormone receptors during the implantation phase in the human endometrium. J Mol Endocrinol. 2004;32(1):21–32.
72. Rodriguez-Linares B, Linton EA, Phaneuf S. Expression of corticotrophin-releasing hormone receptor mRNA and protein in the human myometrium. J Endocrinol. 1998;156(1):15–21.
73. Grammatopoulos DK. The role of CRH receptors and their agonists in myometrial contractility and quiescence during pregnancy and labour. Front Biosci. 2007;12:561–71.
74. Tyson EK, Smith R, Read M. Evidence that corticotropin-releasing hormone modulates myometrial contractility during human pregnancy. Endocrinology. 2009;150(12):5617–25.
75. Klimaviciute A, et al. Corticotropin-releasing hormone, its binding protein and receptors in human cervical tissue at preterm and term labor in comparison to non-pregnant state. Reprod Biol Endocrinol. 2006;4:29.
76. Cong B, et al. Reduced expression of CRH receptor type 1 in upper segment human myometrium during labour. Reprod Biol Endocrinol. 2009;7:43.
77. You X, et al. Corticotropin-releasing hormone (CRH) promotes inflammation in human pregnant myometrium: the evidence of CRH initiating parturition? J Clin Endocrinol Metab. 2014;99(2):E199–208.
78. Grammatopoulos DK, et al. Urocortin, but not corticotropin-releasing hormone (CRH), activates the mitogen-activated protein kinase signal transduction pathway in human pregnant myometrium: an effect mediated via R1alpha and R2beta CRH receptor subtypes and stimulation of Gq-proteins. Mol Endocrinol. 2000;14(12):2076–91.
79. Florio P, et al. High fetal urocortin levels at term and preterm labor. J Clin Endocrinol Metab. 2005;90(9):5361–5.
80. Karteris E, Hillhouse EW, Grammatopoulos D. Urocortin II is expressed in human pregnant myometrial cells and regulates myosin light chain phosphorylation: potential role of the type-2 corticotropin-releasing hormone receptor in the control of myometrial contractility. Endocrinology. 2004;145(2):890–900.
81. You X, et al. Urocortins exhibit differential effects on PGE2 and PGF2alpha output via CRHR2 in human myometrium. Reproduction. 2021;162(1):11–20.
82. Androulidaki A, et al. Corticotropin releasing factor promotes breast cancer cell motility and invasiveness. Mol Cancer. 2009;8:30.
83. Kaprara A, et al. Distinct distribution of corticotropin releasing factor receptors in human breast cancer. Neuropeptides. 2010;44(5):355–61.
84. Koureta M, et al. Corticotropin releasing factor receptors in breast cancer: expression and activity in hormone-dependent growth in vitro. Peptides. 2020;129:170316.
85. Lal S, et al. Estrogen alters the splicing of type 1 corticotropin-releasing hormone receptor in breast cancer cells. Sci Signal. 2013;6(282):ra53.

86. Jin L, et al. CRH suppressed TGFbeta1-induced epithelial-mesenchymal transition via induction of E-cadherin in breast cancer cells. Cell Signal. 2014;26(4):757–65.
87. Graziani G, et al. Evidence that corticotropin-releasing hormone inhibits cell growth of human breast cancer cells via the activation of CRH-R1 receptor subtype. Mol Cell Endocrinol. 2007;264(1–2):44–9.
88. Miskowiak B, et al. Reproductive functions in the adult male rats after prolonged intraventricular administration of corticotropin-releasing factor (CRF). Exp Clin Endocrinol. 1986;88(1):25–30.
89. Selvage DJ, Rivier C. Importance of the paraventricular nucleus of the hypothalamus as a component of a neural pathway between the brain and the testes that modulates testosterone secretion independently of the pituitary. Endocrinology. 2003;144(2):594–8.
90. Yoon DJ, Sklar C, David R. Presence of immunoreactive corticotropin-releasing factor in rat testis. Endocrinology. 1988;122(2):759–61.
91. Petraglia F, et al. Corticotropin-releasing factor-binding protein: origins and possible functions. Horm Res. 1996;45(3–5):187–91.
92. Nieman LK, Loriaux DL. Corticotropin-releasing hormone: clinical applications. Annu Rev Med. 1989;40:331–9.
93. Fabbri A, Tinajero JC, Dufau ML. Corticotropin-releasing factor is produced by rat Leydig cells and has a major local antireproductive role in the testis. Endocrinology. 1990;127(3):1541–3.
94. Ulisse S, Fabbri A, Dufau ML. Corticotropin-releasing factor receptors and actions in rat Leydig cells. J Biol Chem. 1989;264(4):2156–63.
95. Ulisse S, et al. A novel mechanism of action of corticotropin releasing factor in rat Leydig cells. J Biol Chem. 1990;265(4):1964–71.
96. Dermitzaki I, et al. Roles of protein kinase a (PKA) and PKC on corticotropin-releasing hormone (CRH)-induced elevation of cytosolic calcium from extra-and intra-cellular sources. Hormones (Athens). 2004;3(4):252–8.
97. Rossi SP, et al. New insights into melatonin/CRH signaling in hamster Leydig cells. Gen Comp Endocrinol. 2012;178(1):153–63.
98. Tinajero JC, et al. Serotonin secretion from rat Leydig cells. Endocrinology. 1993;133(6):3026–9.
99. Tinajero JC, Fabbri A, Dufau ML. Regulation of corticotropin-releasing factor secretion from Leydig cells by serotonin. Endocrinology. 1992;130(4):1780–8.
100. Piescikowska I, et al. Ketanserin, an antagonist of 5-HT2A receptor of serotonin, inhibits testosterone secretion by rat Leydig cells in vitro. Folia Histochem Cytobiol. 1999;37(3):223–4.
101. Huang BM, Stocco DM, Norman RL. The cellular mechanisms of corticotropin-releasing hormone (CRH)-stimulated steroidogenesis in mouse Leydig cells are similar to those for LH. J Androl. 1997;18(5):528–34.
102. Huang BM, et al. Corticotropin-releasing hormone stimulates steroidogenesis in mouse Leydig cells. Biol Reprod. 1995;53(3):620–6.
103. Huang BM, et al. Corticotropin-releasing hormone stimulates the expression of the steroidogenic acute regulatory protein in MA-10 mouse cells. Biol Reprod. 1997;57(3):547–51.
104. Heinrich N, et al. Corticotropin-releasing factor (CRF) agonists stimulate testosterone production in mouse leydig cells through CRF receptor-1. Endocrinology. 1998;139(2):651–8.
105. Sararols P, et al. Specific transcriptomic signatures and dual regulation of steroidogenesis between fetal and adult mouse Leydig cells. Front Cell Dev Biol. 2021;9:695546.
106. Gerendai I, Nemeskeri A, Csernus V. Effect of intratesticular administration of anti-corticotropin-releasing factor antiserum (a-CRF) on testicular function in neonatal rats. Andrologia. 1993;25(4):211–5.
107. Eskeland NL, Molineaux CJ, Schachter BS. Regulation of beta-endorphin secretion by corticotropin-releasing factor in the intact rat testis. Endocrinology. 1992;130(3):1173–9.
108. Eskeland NL, et al. Stimulation of beta-endorphin secretion by corticotropin-releasing factor in primary rat Leydig cell cultures. Endocrinology. 1989;124(6):2914–9.

109. Lee S, et al. Urocortins are present in the rat testis. Neuropeptides. 2011;45(2):131–7.
110. Tezval H, et al. Differential expression of urocortin in human testicular germ cells in course of spermatogenesis: role for urocortin in male fertility? Urology. 2009;73(4):901–5.
111. Rivier CL. Urocortin 1 inhibits rat leydig cell function. Endocrinology. 2008;149(12):6425–32.
112. Tao J, et al. Separate locations of urocortin and its receptors in mouse testis: function in male reproduction and the relevant mechanisms. Cell Physiol Biochem. 2007;19(5–6):303–12.
113. Audhya T, et al. Structural characterization and localization of corticotropin-releasing factor in testis. Biochim Biophys Acta. 1989;995(1):10–6.
114. Tezval H, et al. Expression of corticotropin releasing factor receptor 2 (CRFR2) in the human prostate. A new potential target for medical therapy of benign prostatic hyperplasia. Urologe A. 2008;47(9):1079–80.
115. Arcuri F, et al. Expression of urocortin mRNA and peptide in the human prostate and in prostatic adenocarcinoma. Prostate. 2002;52(3):167–72.
116. Jin L, et al. Different effects of corticotropin-releasing factor and urocortin 2 on apoptosis of prostate cancer cells in vitro. J Mol Endocrinol. 2011;47(2):219–27.
117. Jin L, et al. Corticotropin-releasing hormone receptors mediate apoptosis via cytosolic calcium-dependent phospholipase A(2) and migration in prostate cancer cell RM-1. J Mol Endocrinol. 2014;52(3):255–67.
118. Hao Z, et al. Urocortin2 inhibits tumor growth via effects on vascularization and cell proliferation. Proc Natl Acad Sci USA. 2008;105(10):3939–44.
119. Wang J, et al. Urocortin's inhibition of tumor growth and angiogenesis in hepatocellular carcinoma via corticotrophin-releasing factor receptor 2. Cancer Investig. 2008;26(4):359–68.
120. Tezval H, et al. Urocortin and corticotropin-releasing factor receptor 2 in human renal cell carcinoma: disruption of an endogenous inhibitor of angiogenesis and proliferation. World J Urol. 2009;27(6):825–30.
121. Bale TL, Giordano FJ, Vale WW. A new role for corticotropin-releasing factor receptor-2: suppression of vascularization. Trends Cardiovasc Med. 2003;13(2):68–71.
122. Tezval H, et al. The involvement of altered corticotropin releasing factor receptor 2 expression in prostate cancer due to alteration of anti-angiogenic signaling pathways. Prostate. 2009;69(4):443–8.
123. Yamada Y, et al. Cushing's syndrome with a large pituitary adenoma producing both corticotropin-releasing hormone (CRH) and adrenocorticotropin (ACTH). Intern Med. 2002;41(7):549–54.

Chapter 9
CRF Peptides in Non-mammals

Shengnan Li and Chao Zhu

As described in the previous chapters, mammals have four mature corticotropin-releasing hormone (factor) family peptides (CRF peptides, CRFp), namely, corticotropin-releasing hormone (CRH), urocortin (UCN1), UCN2, and UCN3, which are the evolutionary results from an ancestral peptide precursor early in metazoan ancestry [1, 2]. These neuropeptides may induce intricating physiological responses by exerting their actions on two distinct types of CRF receptors (CRFr), CRF_1 and CRF_2, which belong to the class B1 family of G-protein-coupled receptors (GPCRs) (Chap. 3) [3]. Among non-mammals, CRFp are relatively more investigated in fish and insects, representing vertebrates and invertebrates, respectively. Vertebrates' CRFp consist of four distinct paralogous lineages found on separate chromosomes, which are CRH, urotensin-I (UTI)/UCN1/sauvagine (Svg), UCN2, and UCN3, the former two representing a gene duplication from one lineage, while the latter two being results from the other similar lineage [1, 4]. Invertebrates' CRFp are relatively characterized well in insects, which evolve in ancestral species before the Precambrian times. And diuretic hormones (DHs) in insects are found to be highly similar to CRFp [4–6]. Collectively, non-mammal CRFp originate from a gene duplication of a single ancestral CRH-like peptide conserved from a horizontal gene transfer event, having some difference from mammal CRFp [1]. This chapter will focus on the distribution and main function of non-mammal CRFp.

S. Li · C. Zhu (✉)
Department of Pharmacology, School of Basic Medical Sciences, Nanjing Medical University, Nanjing, Jiangsu, China
e-mail: czhu@njmu.edu.cn

© The Author(s), under exclusive license to Springer Nature Singapore Pte Ltd. 2025

C. Zhu et al. (eds.), *The Peripheral Existence and Effects of Corticotropin-releasing Factor Family*, https://doi.org/10.1007/978-981-96-5322-5_9

1 CRFp in Non-mammal Vertebrates

Peptide signaling systems, such as CRFp signal pathways, are critical mediators for stress and reproduction [7, 8], the evolution of which is among the most important aspects driving the fitness of a species [9]. Correspondingly, changes of CRFp and gonadotropin-releasing hormone (GnRH) are often used as approaches to illustrate the importance in understanding neuropeptides [10].

The CRFp, CRH, UTI, UCN1, and Svg are found throughout chordate taxa [2, 11–13]. As mentioned above, in vertebrates, it is suggested that CRH and UTI/UCN1/Svg and UCN2/UCN3 form different paralogous lineages. Moreover, UCN1 and Svg represent tetrapod orthologs of fish UTI, while on the other hand, Svg's unique structure may be distinctly derived characterizing the evolutionary history of amphibia [2]. As in mammals, these peptides function via CRF_1 and CRF_2 and are also modulated by CRF-binding protein (CRF-BP). The different paralogous neuropeptides may follow distinct pathways in the vertebrates, leading to their functional differences [2]. Teleost fishes, the most diverse type of vertebrates, have species of more than 6000 comprising 1/10 of total vertebrate biodiversity [14] and hence are frequently studied on about their CRFp.

1.1 CRH in Non-mammal Vertebrates

As in mammals, CRH is active both centrally and peripherally in non-mammal vertebrates. And central CRH functions through the hypothalamic-pituitary-interrenal (head kidney) (HPI)/the hypothalamic-pituitary-adrenal (HPA) axis [15].

In the central nervous system (CNS) of different vertebrate classes, immunocytochemical staining with an antiserum to ovine CRH(oCRH)shows multiple locations of CRH perikaryal and CRH containing fibers and terminals. CRH fibers end at the median eminence against the hypophysial portal vessels in vertebrates as in birds [16] (also see Chap. 1 for the portal system in mammals [17]); however, in fish, CRH fibers terminate in the peripheral area near corticotrophs [18]. For fish, HPI axis (equivalent to other vertebrate and mammal HPA axis) is responsible for stress response, corresponding hormones being CRH-adrenocorticotrophic hormone (ACTH)-cortisol [19, 20]. Also, melanocyte-stimulating hormone (MSH) is considered to be a mild corticotrope in chronic stress responses in fish functioning via MSH receptor 2 and 5 (MCR2 and MCR5) in the head kidney, which seems to have a positive feedback effect on CRH release [21]. Inconsistently, however, in carp, it is reported that MSH does not have corticotropic effects, which is in accordance with the absence of MCR5 in carp's head kidney. Interestingly, CRH can activate ACTH cells only when these cells undergo blockade of dopaminergic action, and hypothalamic endorphin is observed to reverse the stimulatory CRH action of β-endorphin releasing on MSH cells in vitro with MSH release unaffected [22]. Similarly in amphibians, CRH/CRH-like peptides are found throughout the brain and regulate ACTH-cortisol level through HPA/HPI axis in stress response [23, 24].

By reversed-phase HPLC combined with a radioimmunoassay for oCRH, a peptide with CRH-like immunoreactivity (IR) is isolated from an extract of the caudal spinal cord region of the spotted dogfish, *Scyliorhinus canicula*. The primary structure of the peptide is established as Pro-Ala-Glu-Thr-Pro-Asn-Ser-Leu-Asp-Leu-Thr-Phe-His-Leu-Leu-Arg-Glu-Met-Ile-Glu-Ile-Ala-Lys-His-Glu-Asn-Gln-Gln-Met-Gln-Ala-Asp-Ser-Asn-Arg-Arg-Ile-Met-Asp-Thr-Ile-NH2. This amino acid (AA) sequence shows moderate structural similarity to human CRH (hCRH) (56%) and to *Catostomus* UTI (51%) [25] (Table 9.1).

CRH is found to be the main vertebrate ACTH-releasing peptide, while UTI/Svg are often observed to be associated with a variety of peripheral activities [26]. An additional *crh* gene, *crh2*, paralog of *crh* (*crh1*) is identified in fishes and lizards, such as the spotted gar, a holocephalan chondrichthyan, sauropsids, and a non-teleost actinopterygian holostean [27, 28]. It is recognized that *crh2* is recurrently lost in some vertebrate groups including teleosts [27], consistent with the report that some species have *crh1*, *crh2*, and *ucn1* and some get *ucn2* and *ucn3* in the slowly evolving genomes while *crh2* gene gets lost independently in placental mammals and in teleost fish, but is present in birds [29]. However, a recent work by Maugars et al. on the fate of *crh1* and *crh2* in vertebrates shows different results. They report the presence of *crh1a* and *crh1b* in most teleosts with *crh1a* lost independently in some species but *crh2* gene being identified in additional vertebrate groups. For instance, the presence of *crh2* in teleosts is revealed, while it is shown lost in Euteleostei. Importantly, all the *crh1a*-, *crh1b*-, and *crh2*-derived peptides conserve

Table 9.1 The sequence comparison among UTI, CRH, and Svg

Peptides	Amino acid sequences
UTI[a]	H-Asn-Asp-Asp-Pro-Pro-Ile-Ser-Ile-Asp-Leu-Thr-Phe-His-Leu-Leu-Arg-Asn-Met-Ile-Glu-Met-Ala-Arg-Ile-Glu-Asn-Glu-Arg-Glu-Gln-Ala-Gly-Leu-Asn-Arg-Lys-Tyr-Leu-Asp-Glu-Val
UCN1	Asp-Asn-Pro-Ser-Leu-Ser-Ile-Asp-Leu-Thr-Phe-His-Leu-Leu-Arg-Thr-Leu-Leu-Glu-Leu-Ala-Arg-Thr-Gln-Ser-Gln-Arg-Glu-Arg-Ala-Glu-Gln-Asn-Arg-Ile-Ile-Phe-Asp-Ser-Val
oCRH	Ser-Gln-Glu-Pro-Pro-Ile-Ser-Leu-Asp-Leu-Thr-Phe-His-Leu-Leu-Arg-Glu-Val-Leu-Glu-Met-Thr-Arg-Ala-Glu-Gln-Leu-Ala-Gln-Gln-Ala-His-Ser-Asn-Arg-Lys-Leu-Met-Asp-Ile-Ala
hCRH	Ser-Glu-Glu-Pro-Pro-Ile-Ser-Leu-Asp-Leu-Thr-Phe-His-Leu-Leu-Arg-Glu-Val-Leu-Glu-Met-Ala-Arg-Ala-Glu-Gln-Leu-Ala-Gln-Gln-Ala-His-Ser-Asn-Arg-Lys-Leu-Met-Glu-Ile-Ile
Fish CRH	Pro-Ala-Glu-Thr-Pro-Asn-Ser-Leu-Asp-Leu-Thr-Phe-His-Leu-Leu-Arg-Glu-Met-Ile-Glu-Ile-Ala-Lys-His-Glu-Asn-Gln-Gln-Met-Gln-Ala-Asp-Ser-Asn-Arg-Arg-Ile-Met-Asp-Thr-Ile
Svg	Pyr-Gly-Pro-Pro-Ile-Ser-Ile-Asp-Leu-Ser-Leu-Glu-Leu-Leu-Arg-Lys-Met-Ile-Glu-Ile-Glu-Lys-Gln-Glu-Lys-Glu-Lys-Gln-Gln-Ala-Ala-Asn-Asn-Arg-Leu-Leu-Leu-Asp-Thr-Ile

[a]56% identity with hCRH

the structural characteristics of human CRH, with *crh1b* mainly expressed in the brain, supporting *crh1b* paralogs' central role in controlling HPI axis and *crh1a* paralogs' peripheral one in tissues such as muscle and heart in teleosts [28].

Findings suggest that HPI axis exists in the earliest vertebrates, which is maintained by natural selection owing to the critical adaptation to the environment. Similar to HPA axis (see Chap. 1), HPI axis is controlled centrally by peptides of the CRFp, responding to stressors [30]. Importantly as in mammals, central CRH is the major hypophysiotropin for adrenocorticotropin via HPI axis [22]. The hypothalamic CRH stimulates the pituitary ACTH resulting in cortisol production by the interrenal cells in fish head kidney, in a well-established feedback loop way [31–33]. Moreover, CRH also functions as the major thyrotropin (TSH)-releasing factor in the vertebrates [34, 35]. Direct evidence is presented, i.e., homologous CRH enhances the release of TSH from the bullfrog (*Rana catesbeiana*) pituitary. And the in vitro study on the anterior pituitary cells of adult bullfrogs demonstrates that synthetic frog CRH (fCRH) causes the TSH release concentration-dependently, equivalently to the mammalian oCRH. Interestingly, similar TSH releasing results are also observed with human UCN3, a CRF_2 specific agonist, indicating the involvement of CRF_2 in this CRH-induced TSH release in the bullfrogs [35]. Moreover, it is well established that the combined effects of the hypothalamus-produced CRH in stimulating the synthesis and secretion of both thyroid and corticosteroid hormones are associated with the tadpole metamorphosis [34]. Furthermore, in social animals, it is observed that hierarchical rank governs the rights and rank order changing depends on dynamic behaviors and emotions [36, 37], adding evidence to the combined effects of CRH in stress and reproduction. And there is also report that subordinate rats show suppressed vasopressin (AVP)-ACTH-cortisol responses to interaction with dominant males, likely exerting a positive feedback effect on CRH neurons [38]. By analyzing the CRF system during social encounters, it is observed that among African cichlid fish (*Astatotilapia burtoni*), the social status regulates reproduction, ascending fish having lower plasma cortisol levels than subordinate conspecifics, but similar levels compared to dominant animals. In the preoptic area (location of GnRH cells) and pituitary gland (location of ACTH cells), CRH and CRF_1 levels, respectively, are rapidly down-regulated in ascending males. Correspondingly, in a forebrain region (location of CRH cells), levels of mRNA coding for both CRF_1 and CRF_2 are reduced in ascending fish [37]. Because of the typical inhibitory effects of CRH on the neuroendocrine reproductive axis in vertebrates (both mammal and non-mammal) [39–41], inhibition of CRH activity may quickly activate the axis and facilitate the transition to dominance [37]. Finally, in rainbow trout, it is observed that most fish receiving CRH or UTI treatment show a series of behaviors including opercula flaring, mouth opening, and violent head shaking. Furthermore, fish receiving exogenous CRH become subordinate. In addition, isolated fish receiving the CRH antagonist, α-helical-CRH, has got lower concentrations of 5-hydroxyindoleacetic acid, serotonin, 3,4-dihydroxyphenylacetic acid, and dopamine in the brain stem [42]. Collectively, these results indicate that CRH is likely to attenuate competitive ability, and both CRH and UTI may take an important part in social behavior.

In the periphery, CRH roles have attracted much attention, too. Widespread expression of CRH together with UCNs, CRFr and CRF-BP genes, is shown in the frog, *Xenopus laevis*. In the tadpole tail, CRH is present and found to be cytoprotective, which is blocked by CRF-BP hastening the death of tail muscle cell. At metamorphic climax, CRF-BP expression is strongly upregulated in the tadpole tail where it neutralizes CRH bioactivity, thus promoting tail resorption [43]. Moreover, a vasorelaxant effect of CRH is reported in fish (*Catostomus commersonii*) [44]. In the gills and skin of common carp *Cyprinus carpio*, CRH, CRF-BP, and CRF_1 are expressed in macrophage-like cells, which are involved in stress and infection. After both infection and restraint, the expression of CRH-BP and CRF_1 genes is downregulated [45]. In zebrafish heart, the cardiac CRF system plays an important role. All genes of the CRF system, including CRH, UTI, UCN3, CRF_1 and CRF_2, and CRF-BP, are expressed in the heart of zebrafish. Both in vivo and in vitro, CRH or UCN3 are found cardioprotective. The nonselective CRFr antagonist α-helical-CRH(9–41) prevents the cytoprotective effects [46]. In addition, CRH has been detected in the endocrine pancreas in many species of vertebrates such as fishes, amphibians, reptiles, and birds [47, 48], although not many reports about its role associated with the pancreas functions are presented.

1.2 UTI/UCN1/Svg in Non-mammal Vertebrates

1.2.1 UTI/UCN1

The discovery of UTI in Lederis laboratory, along with the discovery of urotensin II (UTII) in Bern laboratory, and CRH in Vale laboratory (also see Chap. 2) [11], has made a great difference in the research area of CRFp relevance. Fish UTI and amphibian Svg are considered to be homologs of CRH until UCN1 is identified in these same vertebrate classes. UCN1 is with 63% sequence identity to UTI and 45% sequence identity to CRH [49]. Identified first in mammalians, UCN1 (and other UCNs) is then observed in bony fish, amphibians, and birds, having unique phylogenies, pharmacology, and tissue distributions [50]. By increasing α-helix-forming potential through AA substitutions from carp and sucker UTI, as from other native known sequences (rat/human/ovine CRH, Svg), more potent peptides can be synthesized in vitro. Moreover, certain N-terminally shortened fragments, such as α-helical CRH/CRH(8–41), CRH(9–41), and CRH(10–41), are obtained, being competitive inhibitors [51].

UTI is a 41-residue peptide purified from extracts of the urophysis of a teleost fish (*Catostomus commersonii*), having a potent hypotensive effect and ACTH-releasing activity. The primary structure of UTI is determined to be H-Asn-Asp-Asp-Pro-Pro-Ile-Ser-Ile-Asp-Leu-Thr-Phe-His-Leu-Leu-Arg-Asn-Met-Ile-Glu-Met-Ala-Arg-Ile-Glu-Asn-Glu-Arg-Glu-Gln-Ala-Gly-Leu-Asn-Arg-Lys-Tyr-Leu-Asp-Glu-Val-NH2, which exhibits a high sequence homology with oCRH and frog Svg, as listed in Table 9.1.

Also, UTI, oCRH, and Svg exhibit similar activities in biological test systems [52]. Moreover, extraction of urophyses cleaves an N-terminal tripeptide yielding a fully active UTI(4–41). Functionally, UTI peptides are equipotent with CRH and Svg in releasing mammalian pituitary ACTH, but UTI is much more potent than the mammalian CRH in releasing fish pituitary ACTH [53].

Fish endocrinology study is helpful and fundamental for basic understanding and agricultural practice [54, 55], leading to applications in many areas, from aquaculture to conservation biology and ecology/evolution [56]. The activity changes of fish are highly associated with stress increasing plasma cortisol levels, due to changed HPI axis leading to a changed CRFp expression [57]. It is well recognized that the caudal neurosecretory system (CNSS) is unique to fish [58], important for keeping homeostasis in osmoregulation and reproduction [59]. Anatomically, the neurosecretory cells (Dahlgren cells) in the spinal cord project to the urophysis, which neuropeptides are released from. For instance, in the euryhaline flounder *Platichthys flesus*, Dahlgren cells synthesize neuropeptides, including UTI, UTII, and CRH [59, 60]. UTII is observed to have a role in adaptation to hyperosmotic conditions, and its distribution in the zebrafish spinal cord is different from that of UTI [61]. Moreover, based on the observations about the responses to stress, a shared role for CRH and UTI released from the CNSS is plausible [62]. Collectively, these results suggest the presence of homologs of UTI in vertebrates playing different roles. Furthermore, an in vitro investigation in salmon pituitary cell culture is carried out to examine regulation of TSH secretion by oCRH, carpUTI, and frog Svg. The results demonstrate that UTI, oCRH, and Svg cause a significant increase in TSH secretion, which is suppressed by the CRFr antagonist, α-helical-CRH(9–41) [63].

Peripherally, UTI has significant function in cardiovascular system. In zebrafish heart, UTI is expressed and upregulated by hypoxia, being cytoprotective. Moreover, other CRF system components including CRH, UCN3, CRF_1 and CRF_2, and CRF-BP are also found in the heart of zebrafish. In vivo exposure to ischemia/reperfusion injury results in four- to five-fold increases in *crh1b* and *ucn3* mRNA levels (whole heart) but does not affect the gene expression of UTI and other CRF system components, consistent with the in vitro pretreatment of excised whole hearts with CRH or UCN3 stopping the increase in apoptosis, which is prevented by the nonselective CRFr antagonist, α-helical-CRH(9–41) [46]. Moreover, trout UTI exerts a relaxation of preconstricted isolated trout arterial rings, suggesting its vasodilatory effect via relaxing vascular smooth muscles [64]. Consistently, UTI is found to exert a long-lasting hypotensive action in mammals, and the mechanism is unique, i.e., selectively dilating the vessels in the superior (anterior) mesenteric vascular bed, with higher potency than the mammalian CRH [53]. These results support a role of UTI in changing hemodynamic patterns in species from fishes to mammals. For elucidation of the difference between UTI and the mammalian CRH, a comparative analysis of the CRH paralog sequences suggests that CRH is the most derived peptide among CRFp and may have lost many of its ancestral characteristics after becoming associated with the HPA/I axis. And in vertebrates, UTI group of orthologs (including Svg and UCNs) possess shared characteristics indicative of the ancestral peptide, while others are distantly related to the present CRFp [65].

1.2.2 Svg in Non-mammal Vertebrates

The primary structure of Svg, a polypeptide extracted from the skin of *Phyllomedusa sauvagii* (PS-Svg), a frog of Central and South America, is determined by combined procedures, specific remove of the N-terminal pyrrolidonecarboxylic acid, cleavages at the single methionine and the two arginine residues, and then automated liquid-phase procedure. The AA sequence is Pyr-Gly-Pro-Pro-Ile-Ser-Ile-Asp-Leu-Ser-Leu-Glu-Leu-Leu-Arg-Lys-Met-Ile-Glu-Ile -Glu-Lys-Gln-Glu-Lys-Glu-Lys-Gln-Gln-Ala-Ala-Asn-Asn-Arg-Leu-Leu-Leu-Asp-Thr-Ile-NH2 (Table 9.1). In vitro studies show that Svg, like UTI, is unable to stimulate ACTH release in amphibian anterior pituitary cells while CRH and vasopressin have releasing effects [66], contrary to mammalian CRH inducing a potent response from amphibian pituitaries [67], suggesting that the main function of Svg is not associated with ACTH regulation, and therefore, there must exist an additional CRH-like peptide in amphibia influencing ACTH release, which is supported by the successful isolation of frog CRH, sharing more than 93% homology with mammalian CRH, yet only 50% homology with Svg [68]. Moreover, an Svg-like peptide is isolated from a different frog species, *Pachymedusa dacnicolor* (PD-Svg). PD-Svg is a high-affinity CRFr agonist, and its radioiodinated analog, [^{125}I-Tyr0-Glu1, Nle17]-PD-Svg, shows improved biochemical properties, compared to the earlier iodinated agonist, ^{125}I-Tyr0-Svg [69, 70]. This PD-Svg radioligand binds both CRF_1 and CRF_2 with high affinity and detects much more sites on the two receptors. PD-Svg is also very potent at stimulating cAMP production in cells expressing the native receptors. Furthermore, PD-Svg shows robust specific binding to both rodent brain and peripheral tissues expressing CRFr [71]. These results suggest that analogs of PD-Svg may become useful tools for investigations on CRFr.

Svg has a significant peripheral role, possessing important pharmacological actions on diuresis and the cardiovascular system, being considered the prototype of a new family of amphibian peptides [72]. As UTI, Svg is also found to have a long-lasting hypotensive action in mammals (rats), further leading to the intense antidiuresis effect [73, 74]. Specifically, Svg is observed to dilate mesenteric vessels in mammals (dogs), reducing intestinal vascular resistance but having no influence on systemic arterial blood pressure [75]. By investigations on the endothelium-denuded rings of rat thoracic aorta (RTA) and the isolated perfused superior mesenteric arterial vasculature (SMA), it is revealed that Svg is a much more potent vasodilator than CRH on RTA and SMA. And the vasodilatory molecular mechanisms are related to nitric oxide [76].

1.2.3 UCN2/3 in Non-mammal Vertebrates

UCN3, discovered in 2001, has a variety of central and peripheral biological functions in mammals [77–79]. Then, in fish Siberian sturgeon (*Acipenser baerii* Brandt), UCN3 cDNAs sequence is also cloned, and UCN3 mRNA levels is investigated. The Siberian sturgeon UCN3 cDNA sequence encodes 148 AA with a mature peptide of 40 AA. Moreover, UCN3 is widely distributed with highest expression in brain. Functional studies show that the UCN3 mRNA expression in brain is significantly enhanced after feeding, decreased after fasting, and increased back after re-feeding. In accordance, exogenous UCN3 can reduce food intake [80]. These results indicate that Siberian sturgeon UCN3 acts as a satiety factor inhibiting food intake. It is noteworthy that human and mouse UCN3 share 90% identity in the 38 AA peptide while in the peptide coding region, both human and mouse UCN3 are 76% identical to pufferfish UCN-related peptide [78]. In the elephant shark, UCN3 (also UTI) is found in the genome. Interestingly, the UCN2 peptide seems to be lost and is identified as a pseudogene in *Callorhinchus milii* [81]. In a rainbow trout, a clone, the 40 residue teneurin-3, is identified, which possesses a primary structure similarity to UCNs. The peptide is potent at increasing cAMP level and stimulating neuronal cell proliferation [82]. Moreover, similar to CRH, exogenous UCN3 is found to induce TSH release in the bullfrogs [35].

In mammals as well as in fish, UCN2/3 are selective CRF_2 agonists, whose effects are prevented by the selective CRF_2 antagonist, anti-Svg-30 (aSvg30), which is supported by the finding that ^{125}I-aSvg30 exclusively binds to both $hCRF_2$ and xenopus CRF_2 with high affinity [83].

2 CRFp in Invertebrates

In the invertebrates, the stress responses are relatively simple, mainly involving CRH and CRH-related peptides, the diuretic hormones (DHs) [84–86]. DH family found in insects share about 20% AA sequence homology to other CRFp [87]. In addition, CRF-BP, as in vertebrates, participates in modulating CRFp levels and hence the CRFp actions. Invertebrates also possess a responding ability to stressors. Honey bees, for example, have a stress response pathway analogous to the mammalian HPA (or fish HPI) axis, involving the brain and the neurohemal organ corpus cardiacum and peripheral targets such as fat body and crop, although there lacks an equivalent HPA/HPI axis [87, 88].

Similar antigenic determinants of CRH in vertebrates and insects are observed, bespeaking the long evolutionary history. It has been decades since the reports on the presence of CRH in the CNS of mammals, non-mammal vertebrates, and insects [89, 90]. In cockroach, CRH is observed in the brain as well as the corpus cardiacum and corpus allatum [90]. The sequence of a cDNA encoding CRH precursor is identified by screening *lambda gt11* libraries, which are constructed from the hypothalamic RNA of the white sucker brain using oligonucleotide probes deduced from rat CRH. And the AA sequence of this sucker CRH is found strikingly conserved from rat CRH, differing in only two positions at the C-terminus [91]. Moreover, using an antibody against rat UCN1 and CRH for determining and comparing the distribution of UCN1- and CRH-like IR in the earthworm nervous system, it is found that they are distributed differently, the majority of UCN1-like IR cells being in the ventral ganglia, whereas CRH-like IR cells being mainly in the cerebral ganglion. No co-localization of UCN1 and CRH is observed [92]. Moreover, a CRH-type neuropeptide, ArCRH, is verified in the starfish *Asterias rubens* (phylum Echinodermata), which is a 40 AA peptide with N-terminus pyroglutamylated and C-terminus amidated, being abundant in the peripheral organs including papulae, the apical muscle, and the digestive system [93].

In insects, DHs are vital neuropeptides in maintaining the life [94, 95]. As we know, keeping internal osmolarity balance is essential for insects' survival, due to their susceptibility to osmotic stress because of the high surface-to-volume ratio. And the functions of CRFp are associated with osmoregulation and diuresis, in which the CRH-similar peptides, DHs, play the most significant role [96]. For example, in the largest group of insects, beetles, it is demonstrated that the brain responds to internal osmolarity alterations by releasing DH37 and DH47 homologs of vertebrate CRFp, which are capable of controlling systemic water balance. The effects are supported by the finding that knockdown of DHs gene reduces Malpighian tubule secretion and restricts organismal fluid loss, which can be reversed by injection of DH37 or DH47 [97]. DHs related to the vertebrate CRH (CRH/DH) and calcitonin are identified in diverse insect species [6, 98]. In the migratory locust, a DH is found to mimic the effect of vasopressin, causing diuretic effect via cAMP [99, 100]. Moreover, the diuretic effect of DHs is proved to be associated with feeding, i.e., the post-feeding diuresis [101, 102]. In the lepidopteran *Hyles lineata*, two DHs, DH41 and DH30, are identified from extracts of whole heads, very similar to those from the tobacco hornworm *Manduca sexta*, another type of sphingid moths [103]. Manduca sexta DH (Mas-DH) stimulates fluid secretion by adult Malpighian tubules and cAMP production by both larval and adult tubules. Moreover, Mas-DH- and CRFp-related DHs cause similar increases in the production of cAMP by the Malpighian tubules of both larval and adult *Manduca sexta*. It is worth noticing that insect CRH-related DHs exhibit varying degrees of potency among different species, while Svg, bovine-CRH, and hCRH have a much lower effect on cAMP production [5]. Interestingly, the hemipteran insect *Rhodnius prolixus* is observed to undergo rapid post-feeding diuresis. During this kind of post-feeding diuresis, CRH/DH and serotonin are found to work synergistically, increasing fluid secretion rate from Malpighian tubules [104, 105]. In *Rhodnius prolixus*'s hemolymph, the presence of CRH/DH is also identified. Correspondingly, the CRH/DH receptor transcript is isolated and characterized from this insect, which as CRFr belongs to the family of B1 GPCRs [96].

CRH/DH also exert an important role in the modulation of feeding and reproduction [102, 106]. In the migratory locust, CRH/DH, whose release varies on age and feeding status [107], are found to be localized in the same neurosecretory cells as the ovary maturating parsin (OMP), stimulating oocyte growth and vitellogenesis and influencing hemolymph ecdysteroid levels in adult females [108]. Furthermore, in the desert locust, two similar CRH/DH precursor cDNAs are identified, both encoding OMP isoforms. The precursor transcripts mainly occur in CNS, being highest expressed in the brain, influencing food intake and reproduction. Moreover, exogenous locust CRH/DH causes a remarkably lower food intake, while RNAi knockdown of CRH/DH has an opposite effect. Furthermore, in adult females, exogenous CRH/DH is observed to retard oocyte growth and reduce ecdysteroid titers in hemolymph and ovaries, opposite to the results with RNAi knockdown [109]. Moreover, as described above, CRH/DH plays a key role in feeding (and feeding-related diuresis) in a blood-gorging insect, *Rhodnius prolixus* [102], which may also relate to CRH/DH effects on reproduction. In adult female *Rhodnius prolixus*, immunohistochemistry assay reveals the co-localization of CRH and the glycoprotein hormone subunit in the neurosecretory cells, suggesting a working-together among these peptides regulating physiological processes. Further analysis indicates presence of the transcript for CRH/DH receptor 2 (Rhopr-CRH/DH-R2) in reproductive tissues and fat body in adult female *Rhodnius prolixus*, the expression of which increases post blood meal, an influencer of diuresis, growth, and reproduction [106, 110]. Furthermore, downregulation of CRH/DH-R2 results in accelerated oogenesis, increased number of eggs produced, and reduced hatching rate, due to the increased expression of the crucial reproductive factor, yolk protein (vitellogenin), in the fat body and ovaries [111]. The gonad inhibitory effect is supported by the ex vivo observation that CRH/DH inhibits the transcript expression of ecdysteroid biosynthetic enzymes and reduces ecdysteroid titer in isolated ovaries [106].

3 The Distribution and Functions of CRFr in Non-mammals

As precedingly described, similar to the CRFr in mammals belonging to B1 GPCRs (see *Chap. 3*), non-mammal receptors for CRFp also exist as two distinct forms, CRF_1 and CRF_2 [112].

In vertebrates such as fish and frog, CRF_1 and CRF_2 are isolated and characterized [112–114]. The complete structure of CRF_1 is partially characterized by using the compact genome of the Japanese pufferfish, *Fugu rubripes*, as a model. The Fugu CRF_1 gene, with 14 exons, is about 27 kb in length. The receptor exists mainly in the liver, gonads, heart, and brain, also detectable in the kidney, gut, and gills [113]. The fish-derived CRFp, UCNs, are potent CRF_2 agonists causing vasodilation, and central injections of UTI induce dose-dependent reductions in fish food intake, both of which can be reversed by pretreatment with a CRFr antagonist [115, 116]. In anuran amphibians, CRFr activation by CRH leads to a potent stimulation of TSH release and modulation of food intake, while intracerebroventricular administration of CRH induces a significant decrease of food intake, which is blocked by the unselective CRF_1/CRF_2 antagonist, α-helical-CRH(9–41) [117].

Molecular cloning of cDNAs encoding CRFr in the bullfrog, *Rana catesbeiana*, is reported. Specific cDNAs are amplified using reverse-transcribed PCR of a total RNA isolated from frog hypothalamus. Two types of full-length CRFr cDNAs (CRF_1 2275 bp, CRF_2 1600 bp) are obtained from a hypothalamic cDNA library. The deduced AA sequences of CRF_1 and CRF_2 show 79–94% and 81–92% identity with other vertebrates' CRF_1 and CRF_2, respectively. Furthermore, CRF_1 mRNA is detected mainly in the brain and pituitary, whereas CRF_2 is found in the peripheral tissues as well as in CNS [118]. The isolation and functional expression of two cDNAs encoding orthologs of the mammalian and amphibian CRF_1 and CRF_2 from salmon are also reported. Radioligand competition binding experiments reveal that the two salmon receptors, CRF_1 and CRF_2, bind UTI with approximately eight-fold higher affinity than rat/human CRH, potently stimulating cAMP production [119]. Also, as described above, CRH/DH receptor is isolated and characterized from insect, belonging to B1 GPCR, too [96]. Moreover, as precedingly mentioned, TSH releasing effects are observed with frog CRH and human UCN3, a CRF_2 specific ligand, indicating CRF_2 involvement in the CRH-induced TSH release in the bullfrogs [35].

In beetles, a CRFr-like receptor for CRH/DH, urinate receptor (Urn8R), is found to exist exclusively in functionally unique secondary cells in the tubules, functioning in osmolarity modulation [97]. In *Drosophila*, two CRFr-related GPCRs, DH44-R1 and DH44-R2, are identified. DH44-R2 is less sensitive than DH44-R1 to the ligand, DH44. And specific RNAi knockdown of DH44-R2 leads to enhanced sensitivity to osmotic challenges [120]. Moreover, an orphan GPCR of DH is observed to be related to the calcitonin receptor-like receptor (CLR) family, which may require accessory protein (ligand), DH31, for proper functioning. In both larval and adult brain, most DH31 receptor-expressing neurons also express the CRFr-related receptor for DH44 [121]. Moreover, SEB-3, a CRFr-like GPCR in *Caenorhabditis elegans*, is reported. SEB-3 is observed to participate in the regulation of stress responses, causing an enhanced active state of locomotion, behavioral arousal, and tremor, which is associated with CRF_1 [122], belonging to B1 GPCRs, which are identified in the invertebrate genomes of some species [123].

Interestingly, infection of an enveloped RNA virus, the Chikungunya virus (CHIKV), which is considered a growing threat to public health, is found to be efficiently suppressed by several compounds related to CRFr blockade. It is observed that CP-154,526, a non-peptide antagonist of the CRF_1, shows a strong anti-CHIKV activity, inhibiting CHIKV infection in Huh-7 cells [124]. Moreover, in both vertebrates and invertebrates, CRH is observed to be an important factor in neuroimmune and autoimmunoregulatory processes, and the specific inhibitor of CRH, α-helical-CRH, antagonizes CRH-induced cellular immunosuppression, via specific CRFr in immunocytes [125–127].

4 The Distribution and Functions of CRF-BP in Non-mammals

In non-mammals, as in mammals, CRF system also includes an evolutionarily conserved CRF-BP, which is a secreted glycoprotein binding CRFp and hence modulating their levels. CRF-BP has a higher affinity to CRFp than the receptors (CRFr) [88, 128]. CRF-BP exists in both the CNS and periphery of vertebrates and invertebrates, influencing central or tissue-local CRFp activities [88, 129, 130].

CRF-BP's functional properties are reported in a teleost fish. In vitro experiments show that carp CRF-BP inhibits CRH- and UTI-mediated CRFr activation, with its potency varying between the receptor and peptide ligand [131]. Together with CRH/CRF_1, CRF-BP is found in the tadpole brain and tail, participating in the tadpole metamorphosis via both centrally and locally modulating CRFp levels. This role of CRF-BP is supported by that CRF-BP is remarkably upregulated in the relevant brain area and tail of tadpoles during metamorphosis [43]. It is observed that CRH activating CRF_1 slows spontaneous tail regression, while overexpression of CRF-BP in vivo accelerates the loss of tail during spontaneous metamorphosis [132]. Moreover, upon metamorphosis, tadpoles losing their tails are associated with programmed cell death by thyroid hormone (T3) influenced by CRFp [133]. On the other hand, it is interesting that the silver nanoparticles (AgNPs), which are often used in medical and consumer products, do not influence HPI axis in zebrafish, although the transcript levels of CRH, CRF-BP, and CRF_2 are significantly decreased by Ag(+), which need more investigations for interpretation [134].

In rainbow trout, the mRNA levels of CRF-BP are observed to be closely associated with those of CRH and UTI. The hypoxia challenge suppresses the mRNA levels of CRH and CRF-BP, with no effect on the expression of UTI [130]. Moreover, the intensity and duration of stress are found to be related to CRH and CRF-BP mRNA. Pituitary CRF-BP is also observed to participate in the modulation of the stress axis activity, by reducing CRFp access to CRF_1 in the corticotropes [129]. In common carp, it is shown that CRH and CRF-BP are mostly expressed in the head kidney, being localized in chromaffin cells, suggesting that a mutual interaction between the two components of CRF system is present in the fish head kidney [135].

5 Summary

This chapter briefly summarizes the distribution and role of CRFp and CRFp-similar peptides, diuretic hormones, in non-mammals including non-mammal vertebrates and invertebrates, represented mainly by fish and insects, respectively (Fig. 9.1). The goal is to share a basic knowledge of their varieties, existence, and functions in non-mammals, presenting an overall comparison of CRFp among the different species and mammals described in all the other chapters. Knowing of these non-mammal CRFp may also be helpful for widening our knowledge of the CRF system, including their evolution.

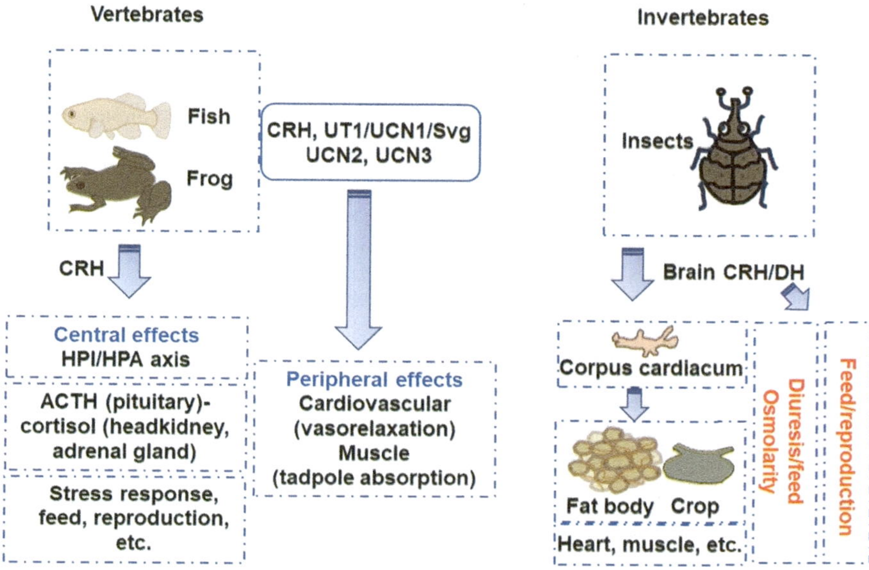

Fig. 9.1 The CRF system in non-mammal vertebrates and invertebrates. In vertebrates, HPI/HPA axis is the main stress response pathway. And in invertebrates, a similar pathway, brain-neural organ (corpus cardiacum)-peripheral organs, functions in response to stress, and DHs play important roles in feed/diuresis and feed/reproduction

References

1. Lovejoy DA, de Lannoy L. Evolution and phylogeny of the corticotropin-releasing factor (CRF) family of peptides: expansion and specialization in the vertebrates. J Chem Neuroanat. 2013;54:50–6.
2. Lovejoy DA, Balment RJ. Evolution and physiology of the corticotropin-releasing factor (CRF) family of neuropeptides in vertebrates. Gen Comp Endocrinol. 1999;115(1):1–22.
3. Grammatopoulos DK. Insights into mechanisms of corticotropin-releasing hormone receptor signal transduction. Br J Pharmacol. 2012;166(1):85–97.
4. Lovejoy DA, Jahan S. Phylogeny of the corticotropin-releasing factor family of peptides in the metazoa. Gen Comp Endocrinol. 2006;146(1):1–8.
5. Audsley N, et al. Cross reactivity studies of CRF-related peptides on insect Malpighian tubules. Comp Biochem Physiol A Physiol. 1995;110(1):87–93.
6. Lee G, Jang H, Oh Y. The role of diuretic hormones (DHs) and their receptors in *Drosophila*. BMB Rep. 2023;56(4):209–15.
7. Phumsatitpong C, Moenter SM. Estradiol-dependent stimulation and suppression of gonadotropin-releasing hormone neuron firing activity by corticotropin-releasing hormone in female mice. Endocrinology. 2018;159(1):414–25.
8. Vermeulen A. Environment, human reproduction, menopause, and andropause. Environ Health Perspect. 1993;101(Suppl 2):91–100.
9. Lovejoy DA, Barsyte-Lovejoy D. Systems approaches to genomic and epigenetic inter-regulation of peptide hormones in stress and reproduction. Prog Biophys Mol Biol. 2013;113(3):375–86.

10. Sherwood NM, Parker DB. Neuropeptide families: an evolutionary perspective. J Exp Zool Suppl. 1990;4:63–71.
11. Pittman QJ, Hollenberg MD. Urotensin I-CRF-Urocortins: a mermaid's tail. Gen Comp Endocrinol. 2009;164(1):7–14.
12. Suda T, et al. Physiological roles of urocortins, human homologues of fish urotensin I, and their receptors. Peptides. 2004;25(10):1689–701.
13. Lovejoy DA, Rotzinger S, Barsyte-Lovejoy D. Evolution of complementary peptide systems: teneurin C-terminal-associated peptides and corticotropin-releasing factor superfamilies. Ann N Y Acad Sci. 2009;1163:215–20.
14. Brandl SJ, et al. The hidden half: ecology and evolution of cryptobenthic fishes on coral reefs. Biol Rev Camb Philos Soc. 2018;93(4):1846–73.
15. Paul B, et al. Thyroid and corticosteroid signaling in amphibian metamorphosis. Cells. 2022;11(10)
16. Singh KB, Dominic CJ. Anterior and posterior groups of portal vessels in the avian pituitary: incidence in forty nine species. Arch Anat Microsc Morphol Exp. 1975;64(4):359–74.
17. Fink G. 60 years of neuroendocrinology: memoir: Harris' neuroendocrine revolution: of portal vessels and self-priming. J Endocrinol. 2015;226(2):T13–24.
18. Fellmann D, et al. The CRF neuron: immunocytochemical study. Peptides. 1984;5(Suppl 1):19–33.
19. Ganesh CB. The stress - Reproductive axis in fish: The involvement of functional neuroanatomical systems in the brain. J Chem Neuroanat. 2021;112:101904.
20. Harris BN, Carr JA. The role of the hypothalamus-pituitary-adrenal/interrenal axis in mediating predator-avoidance trade-offs. Gen Comp Endocrinol. 2016;230-231:110–42.
21. Metz JR, et al. ACTH, alpha-MSH, and control of cortisol release: cloning, sequencing, and functional expression of the melanocortin-2 and melanocortin-5 receptor in *Cyprinus carpio*. Am J Physiol Regul Integr Comp Physiol. 2005;289(3):R814–26.
22. Flik G, et al. CRF and stress in fish. Gen Comp Endocrinol. 2006;146(1):36–44.
23. Boorse GC, Denver RJ. Expression and hypophysiotropic actions of corticotropin-releasing factor in *Xenopus laevis*. Gen Comp Endocrinol. 2004;137(3):272–82.
24. Hernandez SE, Sernia C, Bradley AJ. Adrenocortical function in cane toads from different environments. Comp Biochem Physiol A Mol Integr Physiol. 2016;195:65–72.
25. Waugh D, et al. A peptide from the caudal neurosecretory system of the dogfish *Scyliorhinus canicula* that is structurally related to urotensin I. Gen Comp Endocrinol. 1995;99(3):333–9.
26. Lovejoy DA. Peptide hormone evolution: functional heterogeneity within GnRH and CRF families. Biochem Cell Biol. 1996;74(1):1–7.
27. Grone BP, Maruska KP. A second corticotropin-releasing hormone gene (CRH2) is conserved across vertebrate classes and expressed in the hindbrain of a basal neopterygian fish, the spotted gar (*Lepisosteus oculatus*). J Comp Neurol. 2015;523(7):1125–43.
28. Maugars G, et al. New insights into the evolution of corticotropin-releasing hormone family with a special focus on teleosts. Front Endocrinol (Lausanne). 2022;13:937218.
29. Cardoso JC, et al. Corticotropin-releasing hormone family evolution: five ancestral genes remain in some lineages. J Mol Endocrinol. 2016;57(1):73–86.
30. Denver RJ. Structural and functional evolution of vertebrate neuroendocrine stress systems. Ann N Y Acad Sci. 2009;1163:1–16.
31. Jeffrey JD, et al. Modulation of hypothalamic-pituitary-interrenal axis function by social status in rainbow trout. Gen Comp Endocrinol. 2012;176(2):201–10.
32. Pham V, et al. Nesfatin-1 stimulates the hypothalamus-pituitary-interrenal axis hormones in goldfish. Am J Physiol Regul Integr Comp Physiol. 2021;321(4):R603–13.
33. Alderman SL, et al. Central and peripheral glucocorticoid receptors are involved in the plasma cortisol response to an acute stressor in rainbow trout. Gen Comp Endocrinol. 2012;176(1):79–85.
34. Crespi EJ, Denver RJ. Ancient origins of human developmental plasticity. Am J Hum Biol. 2005;17(1):44–54.

35. Ito Y, et al. Molecular cloning of bullfrog corticotropin-releasing factor (CRF): effect of homologous CRF on the release of TSH from pituitary cells in vitro. Gen Comp Endocrinol. 2004;138(3):218–27.
36. Komori T, Makinodan M, Kishimoto T. Social status and modern-type depression: a review. Brain Behav. 2019;9(12):e01464.
37. Carpenter RE, et al. Social opportunity rapidly regulates expression of CRF and CRF receptors in the brain during social ascent of a teleost fish, *Astatotilapia burtoni*. PLoS One. 2014;9(5):e96632.
38. De Goeij DC, Dijkstra H, Tilders FJ. Chronic psychosocial stress enhances vasopressin, but not corticotropin-releasing factor, in the external zone of the median eminence of male rats: relationship to subordinate status. Endocrinology. 1992;131(2):847–53.
39. Rivier C, Rivest S. Effect of stress on the activity of the hypothalamic-pituitary-gonadal axis: peripheral and central mechanisms. Biol Reprod. 1991;45(4):523–32.
40. Zhou H, Chen A, Lu W. Corticotropin-releasing hormone reduces basal estradiol production in zebrafish follicular cells. Mol Cell Endocrinol. 2021;527:111222.
41. Yang L, Zha J, Wang Z. Pentachlorophenol affected both reproductive and interrenal systems: In silico and in vivo evidence. Chemosphere. 2017;166:174–83.
42. Backstrom T, et al. CRF and urotensin I effects on aggression and anxiety-like behavior in rainbow trout. J Exp Biol. 2011;214(Pt 6):907–14.
43. Boorse GC, Denver RJ. Widespread tissue distribution and diverse functions of corticotropin-releasing factor and related peptides. Gen Comp Endocrinol. 2006;146(1):9–18.
44. Okawara Y, Lederis K. Vasorelaxant effects of fish (*Catostomus commersoni*) corticotropin releasing factor. Proc West Pharmacol Soc. 1990;33:163–5.
45. Mazon AF, et al. Corticotropin-releasing hormone-receptor 1 (CRH-R1) and CRH-binding protein (CRH-BP) are expressed in the gills and skin of common carp *Cyprinus carpio* L. and respond to acute stress and infection. J Exp Biol. 2006;209(Pt 3):510–7.
46. Williams TA, et al. CRF and urocortin 3 protect the heart from hypoxia/reoxygenation-induced apoptosis in zebrafish. Am J Physiol Regul Integr Comp Physiol. 2017;313(2):R91–R100.
47. Petrusz P, et al. Corticotropin-releasing factor (CRF)-like immunoreactivity in the gastro-entero-pancreatic endocrine system. Peptides. 1984;5(Suppl 1):71–8.
48. Petrusz P, et al. Corticotropin-releasing factor (CRF)-like immunoreactivity in the vertebrate endocrine pancreas. Proc Natl Acad Sci USA. 1983;80(6):1721–5.
49. Vaughan J, et al. Urocortin, a mammalian neuropeptide related to fish urotensin I and to corticotropin-releasing factor. Nature. 1995;378(6554):287–92.
50. Fekete EM, Zorrilla EP. Physiology, pharmacology, and therapeutic relevance of urocortins in mammals: ancient CRF paralogs. Front Neuroendocrinol. 2007;28(1):1–27.
51. Rivier J, Rivier C, Vale W. Synthetic competitive antagonists of corticotropin-releasing factor: effect on ACTH secretion in the rat. Science. 1984;224(4651):889–91.
52. Lederis K, et al. Complete amino acid sequence of urotensin I, a hypotensive and corticotropin-releasing neuropeptide from *Catostomus*. Science. 1982;218(4568):162–5.
53. Lederis K, et al. Isolation, analysis of structure, synthesis, and biological actions of urotensin I neuropeptides. Can J Biochem Cell Biol. 1983;61(7):602–14.
54. Bieniarz K, Epler P. Advances in reproductive endocrinology of fish. J Physiol Pharmacol. 1992;43(4 Suppl 1):215–22.
55. Takei Y, et al. Contribution of comparative fish studies to general endocrinology: structure and function of some osmoregulatory hormones. J Exp Zool A Comp Exp Biol. 2006;305(9):787–98.
56. Tache Y, et al. Brain and gut CRF Signaling: Biological Actions And Role In The Gastrointestinal Tract. Curr Mol Pharmacol. 2018;11(1):51–71.
57. Saiz N, et al. Assessing chronodisruption distress in goldfish: the importance of multimodal approaches. Animals (Basel). 2023;13(15)
58. Rousseau K, et al. The caudal neurosecretory system: a still enigmatic second neuroendocrine complex in fish. Neuroendocrinology. 2024;115:1.

59. Lu W, et al. Seasonal changes in peptide, receptor and ion channel mRNA expression in the caudal neurosecretory system of the European flounder (*Platichthys flesus*). Gen Comp Endocrinol. 2007;153(1–3):262–72.
60. Onstott D, Elde R. Coexistence of urotensin I/corticotropin-releasing factor and urotensin II immunoreactivities in cells of the caudal neurosecretory system of a teleost and an elasmobranch fish. Gen Comp Endocrinol. 1986;63(2):295–300.
61. Parmentier C, et al. Comparative distribution of the mRNAs encoding urotensin I and urotensin II in zebrafish. Peptides. 2008;29(5):820–9.
62. McCrohan CR, et al. Fish caudal neurosecretory system: a model for the study of neuroendocrine secretion. Gen Comp Endocrinol. 2007;153(1–3):243–50.
63. Larsen DA, et al. In vitro thyrotropin-releasing activity of corticotropin-releasing hormone-family peptides in coho salmon, *Oncorhynchus kisutch*. Gen Comp Endocrinol. 1998;109(2):276–85.
64. Mimassi N, et al. Cardiovascular actions of centrally and peripherally administered trout urotensin-I in the trout. Am J Physiol Regul Integr Comp Physiol. 2000;279(2):R484–91.
65. Lovejoy DA. Structural evolution of urotensin-I: reflections of life before corticotropin releasing factor. Gen Comp Endocrinol. 2009;164(1):15–9.
66. Tonon MC, et al. Comparative effects of corticotropin-releasing factor, arginine vasopressin, and related neuropeptides on the secretion of ACTH and alpha-MSH by frog anterior pituitary cells and neurointermediate lobes in vitro. Gen Comp Endocrinol. 1986;61(3):438–45.
67. Malagon MM, et al. Effects of ovine CRF on amphibian pituitary ACTH and TSH cells in vivo: a quantitative ultrastructural study. Gen Comp Endocrinol. 1991;83(3):487–97.
68. Stenzel-Poore MP, et al. Characterization of the genomic corticotropin-releasing factor (CRF) gene from *Xenopus laevis*: two members of the CRF family exist in amphibians. Mol Endocrinol. 1992;6(10):1716–24.
69. Rominger DH, et al. Characterization of [125I]sauvagine binding to CRH2 receptors: membrane homogenate and autoradiographic studies. J Pharmacol Exp Ther. 1998;286(1):459–68.
70. Grigoriadis DE, et al. 125I-Tyro-sauvagine: a novel high affinity radioligand for the pharmacological and biochemical study of human corticotropin-releasing factor 2 alpha receptors. Mol Pharmacol. 1996;50(3):679–86.
71. Perrin MH, et al. Characterization of a *Pachymedusa dacnicolor*-Sauvagine analog as a new high-affinity radioligand for corticotropin-releasing factor receptor studies. J Pharmacol Exp Ther. 2015;353(2):307–17.
72. Montecucchi PC, Henschen A. Amino acid composition and sequence analysis of sauvagine, a new active peptide from the skin of *Phyllomedusa sauvagei*. Int J Pept Protein Res. 1981;18(2):113–20.
73. Erspamer V, et al. Sauvagine, a new polypeptide from *Phyllomedusa sauvagei* skin. Occurrence in various *Phyllomedusa* species and pharmacological actions on rat blood pressure and diuresis. Naunyn Schmiedeberg's Arch Pharmacol. 1980;312(3):265–70.
74. Improta G. The mechanism of the antidiuretic effect of sauvagine in rats. Pharmacol Res Commun. 1980;12(3):185–93.
75. MacCannell KL, et al. Use of selective mesenteric vasodilator peptides in experimental nonocclusive mesenteric ischemia in the dog. Gastroenterology. 1986;90(3):669–76.
76. Barker DM, Corder R. Studies of the role of endothelium-dependent nitric oxide release in the sustained vasodilator effects of corticotrophin releasing factor and sauvagine. Br J Pharmacol. 1999;126(1):317–25.
77. Venihaki M, et al. Urocortin III, a brain neuropeptide of the corticotropin-releasing hormone family: modulation by stress and attenuation of some anxiety-like behaviours. J Neuroendocrinol. 2004;16(5):411–22.
78. Lewis K, et al. Identification of urocortin III, an additional member of the corticotropin-releasing factor (CRF) family with high affinity for the CRF2 receptor. Proc Natl Acad Sci USA. 2001;98(13):7570–5.

79. Saruta M, et al. Urocortin 3/stresscopin in human colon: possible modulators of gastrointestinal function during stressful conditions. Peptides. 2005;26(7):1196–206.
80. Zhang X, et al. Intraperitoneal injection urocortin-3 reduces the food intake of Siberian sturgeon (*Acipenser baerii*). Peptides. 2016;85:80–8.
81. Nock TG, Chand D, Lovejoy DA. Identification of members of the gonadotropin-releasing hormone (GnRH), corticotropin-releasing factor (CRF) families in the genome of the holocephalan, *Callorhinchus milii* (elephant shark). Gen Comp Endocrinol. 2011;171(2):237–44.
82. Qian X, et al. Cloning and characterization of teneurin C-terminus associated peptide (TCAP)-3 from the hypothalamus of an adult rainbow trout (*Oncorhynchus mykiss*). Gen Comp Endocrinol. 2004;137(2):205–16.
83. Higelin J, et al. 125I-Antisauvagine-30: a novel and specific high-affinity radioligand for the characterization of corticotropin-releasing factor type 2 receptors. Neuropharmacology. 2001;40(1):114–22.
84. Blackburn MB, et al. Isolation and identification of a new diuretic peptide from the tobacco hornworm, *Manduca sexta*. Biochem Biophys Res Commun. 1991;181(3):927–32.
85. Coast GM. Diuresis in the housefly (*Musca domestica*) and its control by neuropeptides. Peptides. 2001;22(2):153–60.
86. Te Brugge VA, et al. The distribution of a kinin-like peptide and its co-localization with a CRF-like peptide in the blood-feeding bug, *Rhodnius prolixus*. Peptides. 2001;22(2):161–73.
87. Even N, Devaud JM, Barron AB. General stress responses in the honey bee. Insects. 2012;3(4):1271–98.
88. Ketchesin KD, Stinnett GS, Seasholtz AF. Corticotropin-releasing hormone-binding protein and stress: from invertebrates to humans. Stress. 2017;20(5):449–64.
89. Vale W, et al. Characterization of a 41-residue ovine hypothalamic peptide that stimulates secretion of corticotropin and beta-endorphin. Science. 1981;213(4514):1394–7.
90. Verhaert P, et al. Localization of CRF immunoreactivity in the central nervous system of three vertebrate and one insect species. Cell Tissue Res. 1984;238(1):49–53.
91. Okawara Y, et al. Cloning and sequence analysis of cDNA for corticotropin-releasing factor precursor from the teleost fish *Catostomus commersoni*. Proc Natl Acad Sci USA. 1988;85(22):8439–43.
92. Lubics A, et al. Comparative distribution of urocortin- and CRF-like immunoreactivities in the nervous system of the earthworm *Lumbricus terrestris*. Peptides. 2003;24(2):205–13.
93. Cai W, et al. Molecular identification and cellular localization of a corticotropin-releasing hormone-type neuropeptide in an echinoderm. Neuroendocrinology. 2023;113(2):231–50.
94. Lovejoy DA, Barsyte-Lovejoy D. Characterization of a corticotropin-releasing factor (CRF)/diuretic hormone-like peptide from tunicates: insight into the origins of the vertebrate CRF family. Gen Comp Endocrinol. 2010;165(2):330–6.
95. Koyama T, Rana DW, Halberg KV. Managing fuels and fluids: network integration of osmoregulatory and metabolic hormonal circuits in the polymodal control of homeostasis in insects. BioEssays. 2023;45(9):e2300011.
96. Lee HR, et al. Isolation and characterization of the corticotropin-releasing factor-related diuretic hormone receptor in *Rhodnius prolixus*. Cell Signal. 2016;28(9):1152–62.
97. Koyama T, et al. A unique Malpighian tubule architecture in *Tribolium castaneum* informs the evolutionary origins of systemic osmoregulation in beetles. Proc Natl Acad Sci USA. 2021;118(14)
98. Furuya K, et al. Cockroach diuretic hormones: characterization of a calcitonin-like peptide in insects. Proc Natl Acad Sci USA. 2000;97(12):6469–74.
99. Proux JP, Herault JP. Cyclic AMP: a second messenger of the newly characterized AVP-like insect diuretic hormone, the migratory locust diuretic hormone. Neuropeptides. 1988;12(1):7–12.
100. Picquot M, Proux J. Biosynthesis and degradation of the arginine-vasopressin-like insect diuretic hormone, a neurohormone in the migratory locust. Regul Pept. 1990;31(3):139–56.

101. Te Brugge VA, Schooley DA, Orchard I. The biological activity of diuretic factors in *Rhodnius prolixus*. Peptides. 2002;23(4):671–81.
102. Mollayeva S, Orchard I, Lange AB. The involvement of Rhopr-CRF/DH in feeding and reproduction in the blood-gorging insect *Rhodnius prolixus*. Gen Comp Endocrinol. 2018;258:79–90.
103. Furuya K, et al. Isolation and characterization of CRF-related diuretic hormones from the whitelined sphinx moth *Hyles lineata*. Insect Biochem Mol Biol. 2000;30(2):127–33.
104. Zandawala M, Orchard I. Post-feeding physiology in *Rhodnius prolixus*: the possible role of FGLamide-related allatostatins. Gen Comp Endocrinol. 2013;194:311–7.
105. Te Brugge V, Ianowski JP, Orchard I. Biological activity of diuretic factors on the anterior midgut of the blood-feeding bug, *Rhodnius prolixus*. Gen Comp Endocrinol. 2009;162(1):105–12.
106. Al-Dailami AN, Orchard I, Lange AB. Corticotropin-releasing factor-like diuretic hormone acts as a gonad-inhibiting hormone in adult female, *Rhodnius prolixus*. Front Endocrinol (Lausanne). 2023;14:1279929.
107. Audsley N, Goldsworthy GJ, Coast GM. Quantification of Locusta diuretic hormone in the central nervous system and corpora cardiaca: influence of age and feeding status, and mechanism of release. Regul Pept. 1997;69(1):25–32.
108. Tamarelle M, Coast GM, Veenstra JA. Ovary maturing parsin and diuretic hormone are produced by the same neuroendocrine cells in the migratory locust, *Locusta migratoria*. Peptides. 2000;21(5):737–9.
109. Van Wielendaele P, et al. CRF-like diuretic hormone negatively affects both feeding and reproduction in the desert locust, *Schistocerca gregaria*. PLoS One. 2012;7(2):e31425.
110. Orchard I, et al. Malpighian tubules of *Rhodnius prolixus*: more than post-prandial diuresis. Front Insect Sci. 2023;3:1167889.
111. Husain M, et al. RNAi-mediated silencing of vitellogenin gene curtails oogenesis in the almond moth *Cadra cautella*. PLoS One. 2021;16(2):e0245928.
112. Qi J, et al. The suppression effects of feeding and mechanisms in CRF system of animals. Gene. 2020;733:144363.
113. Cardoso JC, et al. Isolation and characterisation of the corticotropin releasing factor receptor 1 (CRFR1) gene in a teleost fish, *Fugu rubripes*. DNA Seq. 2003;14(3):215–8.
114. Boorse GC, et al. Urocortins of the South African clawed frog, *Xenopus laevis*: conservation of structure and function in tetrapod evolution. Endocrinology. 2005;146(11):4851–60.
115. Bernier NJ. The corticotropin-releasing factor system as a mediator of the appetite-suppressing effects of stress in fish. Gen Comp Endocrinol. 2006;146(1):45–55.
116. Takahashi K. Translational medicine in fish-derived peptides: from fish endocrinology to human physiology and diseases. Endocr J. 2004;51(1):1–17.
117. Morimoto N, et al. Inhibitory effect of corticotropin-releasing factor on food intake in the bullfrog, *Aquarana catesbeiana*. Peptides. 2011;32(9):1872–5.
118. Ito Y, et al. Cloning and distribution of the bullfrog type 1 and type 2 corticotropin-releasing factor receptors. Gen Comp Endocrinol. 2006;146(3):291–5.
119. Pohl S, et al. Cloning and functional pharmacology of two corticotropin-releasing factor receptors from a teleost fish. Eur J Pharmacol. 2001;430(2–3):193–202.
120. Hector CE, et al. Functional differences between two CRF-related diuretic hormone receptors in *Drosophila*. J Exp Biol. 2009;212(19):3142–7.
121. Johnson EC, et al. A novel diuretic hormone receptor in *Drosophila*: evidence for conservation of CGRP signaling. J Exp Biol. 2005;208(Pt 7):1239–46.
122. Jee C, et al. SEB-3, a CRF receptor-like GPCR, regulates locomotor activity states, stress responses and ethanol tolerance in *Caenorhabditis elegans*. Genes Brain Behav. 2013;12(2):250–62.
123. Cardoso JC, et al. Evolution of secretin family GPCR members in the metazoa. BMC Evol Biol. 2006;6:108.

124. Watanabe Y, et al. Identification of the corticotropin-releasing factor receptor 1 antagonists as inhibitors of Chikungunya virus replication using a Gaussia luciferase-expressing subgenomic replicon. Biochem Biophys Res Commun. 2022;637:181–8.
125. Smith EM, et al. Corticotropin-releasing factor-induced immunosuppression in human and invertebrate immunocytes. Cell Mol Neurobiol. 1992;12(5):473–81.
126. Karalis K, et al. CRH and the immune system. J Neuroimmunol. 1997;72(2):131–6.
127. Bamberger CM, Bamberger AM. The peripheral CRH/urocortin system. Ann N Y Acad Sci. 2000;917:290–6.
128. Seasholtz AF, Valverde RA, Denver RJ. Corticotropin-releasing hormone-binding protein: biochemistry and function from fishes to mammals. J Endocrinol. 2002;175(1):89–97.
129. Doyon C, Trudeau VL, Moon TW. Stress elevates corticotropin-releasing factor (CRF) and CRF-binding protein mRNA levels in rainbow trout (*Oncorhynchus mykiss*). J Endocrinol. 2005;186(1):123–30.
130. Fuzzen ML, et al. Ontogeny of the corticotropin-releasing factor system in rainbow trout and differential effects of hypoxia on the endocrine and cellular stress responses during development. Gen Comp Endocrinol. 2011;170(3):604–12.
131. Manuel R, et al. Corticotropin-releasing factor-binding protein (CRF-BP) inhibits CRF- and urotensin-I-mediated activation of CRF receptor-1 and -2 in common carp. Gen Comp Endocrinol. 2014;202:69–75.
132. Boorse GC, et al. Corticotropin-releasing factor is cytoprotective in Xenopus tadpole tail: coordination of ligand, receptor, and binding protein in tail muscle cell survival. Endocrinology. 2006;147(3):1498–507.
133. Manzon RG, Denver RJ. Regulation of pituitary thyrotropin gene expression during Xenopus metamorphosis: negative feedback is functional throughout metamorphosis. J Endocrinol. 2004;182(2):273–85.
134. Massarsky A, et al. Acute embryonic exposure to nanosilver or silver ion does not disrupt the stress response in zebrafish (*Danio rerio*) larvae and adults. Sci Total Environ. 2014;478:133–40.
135. Huising MO, et al. Corticotropin-releasing factor (CRF) and CRF-binding protein expression in and release from the head kidney of common carp: evolutionary conservation of the adrenal CRF system. J Endocrinol. 2007;193(3):349–57.

Index

© The Editor(s) (if applicable) and The Author(s), under exclusive license to Springer Nature Singapore Pte Ltd. 2025
C. Zhu et al. (eds.), *The Peripheral Existence and Effects of Corticotropin-releasing Factor Family*, https://doi.org/10.1007/978-981-96-5322-5

D

E

F

G

The manufacturer's authorised representative in the EU is Springer Nature Customer Service Centre GmbH, Europaplatz 3, 69115 Heidelberg, Germany. If you have any concerns regarding our products, please contact ProductSafety@springernature.com

Printed and bound by CPI Group (UK) Ltd, Croydon, CR0 4YY
30/09/2026
02225297-0005